Tai Ji Quan

(fundamentally)

by

Billy Lee Harman

<u>Tai Ji Quan</u>
(fundamentally)

HI
www.hitrt.com
391 South Jefferson Street
Coldwater, MI 49036

Publisher
KDP

ISBN
979-8-512-02111-8

For the All

Returning, one is *dào*'s motion.
Yielding, one is *dào*'s use.
Sky's below's ten thousand things live from having.
Having lives from not having.

Dào Dé Jīng, 40

Contents

Tai Ji Quan

(fundamentally)
Introduction

Primarily, *Tàijíquán* is a kind of *hatha yoga*. Secondarily, it's a method of what modern medical professionals call biofeedback. Tertiarily, it's an alternative to martial arts.

Many *Tàijíquán* practitioners may disagree with that. But *Webster's New World College Dictionary* says intellect is the ability to understand relationships and differences. So let's consider some relevant circumstances that ordinarily may seem disjunct.

The phrase "*tài jí quán*" literally means "extreme polarity fist". And fingers resemble poles, and spreading them apart literally effects the disparity the word "polarize" has come to denote, while folding them into a fist unites them. And *Tàijíquán* practitioners call the traditional circular representation of *yīn* and *yáng* the *tàijí* symbol while originally it symbolized harmony and unity, and fists are somewhat spherical, martial or not.

The words "*yīn*" and "*yáng*", in their use in reference to that diagram, originally referred to the shady and sunny sides of a mountain. And, while sunlight and shade shift across a mountain as the day progresses, the mountain remains one mountain. So that diagram is a depiction of that flow from above the mountain.

And the basic premise of Hinduism is that all differences are illusion. And "*yoga*" is the origin of the English word "yoke" and is a Sanskrit word meaning "union" that Hindus use to refer to realizing the unity of the all, by various means. And "*hatha*" is a Sanskrit word meaning "force", and *hatha yoga* is a Hindu discipline in which the *yogin* forces his or her self to pay attention to her or his breathing and posturing to recognize that the air and space inside one's body is the same as the air and space outside one's body, and the third chapter of the *Maitri Upanishad* plainly specifies the problem of extreme polarity, of one's delusions tossing one about on the horns of various dilemma, dichotomies.

So does other Hindu scripture, but that "*maitri*" is Sanskrit for "benevolence" or "friendship" makes the *Maitri Upanishad* especially pertinent here, and Hinduism has a historical connection with *Tàijíquán*, through both Buddhism and Daoism, both generally and specifically, in many ways.

Daoism is essentially a Chinese approach to *yoga*, not by way of *hatha yoga* in particular, but by *yoga* in general. And, originally, Buddhism was Hinduism with none of the metaphorical rituals and personifications that have claimants to the three Abrahamic dualistic religions calling the monism of Hinduism polytheistic idol worship. And "*buddha*", in both Vedic Sanskrit and the Pali dialect of Sanskrit the Buddha spoke, means "consciousness".

And "*sutta*" is a Pali word for "thread" that Buddhists use to refer to their linguistic expressions of monism. And "*satipatthana*" is Pali for "mindfulness foundation", and the *Satipatthana Sutta* is a Buddhist scripture directing being mindful of the body and mind, to be conscious of how all relates to all. And the historical connection of those circumstances to *Tàijíquán* is through a Buddhist monk.

In the sixth century, about a millennium after the life of the Buddha, Bodhidharma trekked from India across the Himalayas and west to Persia, and then east along the Silk Road to Dunhuang and on across China to the Shaolin Monastery, a Buddhist monastery in China's eastern mountains.

And there, probably having learned of Daoism and Chinese martial arts along the way, he synthesized Daoism and Buddhism into what we now call Zen and into a method of establishing harmony between opponents, not to defeat enemies but to eliminate enmity, essentially uniting the personalities, replacing opposition with unity. And, through the mindfulness of body the *Satipatthana Sutta* purveys, he also incorporated that into a method of biofeedback. So he formulated each of the three principal functions of *Tàijíquán*.

Most *Tàijíquán* practitioners say the Daoist monk Zhang Sanfeng originated *Tàijíquán* at the Daoist monastery on Wudang Mountain. But another question we might consider is why, though an Indian monk originated Zen in China, it has a Japanese name. And part of the answer to that question is that its name originated neither in Japan nor in China.

"Zen" is a Japanese pronunciation of "chan", and "chan" is a Chinese pronunciation of "*dhyana*", which is Sanskrit for "meditation". And the popularity of Zen in Japan began in the twelfth century, the century *Tàijíquán* practitioners say was the century of the life of Zhang Sanfeng, six centuries after the life of Bodhidharma. So the relationship between those circumstances may be that events in that century turned the Shaolin Monastery away from the teachings of Bodhidharma.

Those events may or may not have been shifts in leadership. But, whatever occurred, we also know Buddhist monks emigrated from China to Japan during that century. So a reasonable hypothesis is that Zhang Sanfeng was a Buddhist monk who trekked from the Shaolin Monastery to Wudang Mountain for the same reason those other monks sailed to Japan.

And Wudang Mountain is fewer than three hundred miles from the Shaolin Monastery, and the Daoist monks on Wudang Mountain may have welcomed Zhang Sanfeng for the same reason Bodhidharma assimilated Daoism into Buddhism, and Zhang

Sanfeng may have responded to that welcome by teaching them what we've come to call *Tàijíquán*.

And every book I've read about *Tàijíquán* disagrees with every other in various ways. And, in addition to denials of both the literal and the metaphorical meaning of its current name, factors in that disagreement are both who originated the discipline and when. So I'm presenting in this introduction to this book a synthesis of those books with the history and premises of the two religions to which those books most frequently refer.

And, while many *Tàijíquán* practitioners have said both Bodhidharma and Zhang Sanfeng bear some relevance to the development of their discipline, many now argue against that. So, in this book, I've tried to avoid the extrapolation necessary for formulating a history of the development of *Tàijíquán* during the centuries prior to what people have said of it since the nineteenth century. Instead I've tried to interpolate the flow of all those centuries into terms we use for *Tàijíquán* in this century.

That is, to understand the flow of that development through all of those centuries, I've tried to consider the past in terms of the present.

Tàijíquán practitioners say Zhang Sanfeng composed the *Tàijíquán Jīng*. And *"jīng"*, in that context, literally means "abiding" and idiomatically means "abiding writing", while English-speaking *Tàijíquán* practitioners translate it to mean "classic". And *Tàijíquán* practitioners, also using the term *"Tàijíquán jīng"* to refer to other abiding writings of *Tàijíquán*, also call them the *Tàijíquán* classics.

They disagree about which writings belong in that group, but generally they agree that the *Tàijíquán Jīng* belongs in it and that so does the *Tàijíquán Lùn*, a writing they say Zhang Sanfeng's disciple Wang Zongyue composed. *"Lùn"* in that title means "treatise", and the *Tàijíquán Lùn* begins with a relatively concise statement of the concern Hindus and Buddhists and Daoists share, the dilemma of disparity. It says that *tàijí* and one's *wújí*, while being life and *yīn* and *yáng*, are their mother also.

So, with "*wújí*" meaning "having no polarity" in that context, it effectually defines the primary purpose of *Tàijíquán* and makes "*wújí*" effectually synonymous with the *quán* in *Tàijíquán*. And the 28th segment of the *Dào Dé Jīng* says that knowing the white of below the sky while keeping its black actuates the standard of below the sky. And it says that, actuating its standard, *dé* continually doesn't deviate from returning and reverting to *wújí*. And its 40th segment, the epigraph to this book, effectually says that of *dào*.

And the *Dào Dé Jīng*'s 42nd segment explicitly describes the process of *tàijí*. It says that *dào* engendered one and that one engendered two and that the three engendered the ten thousand things. The ten thousand things are Daoist synecdoche for all the different entities.

And "*dào*" in the title *Dào Dé Jīng* means "way" or "path". And "*dé*" in that title means "virtue" or "power" as in the English phrase "by virtue of". And the *jīng* in that title is the *jīng* in the title *Tàijíquán Jīng*.

And a direct semantic relationship between all of that and *Tàijíquán* is that *Tàijíquán* practitioners call the beginning and ending position of their practice sequence the *wújí* stance. And the 42nd segment of the *Dào Dé Jīng* also says the ten thousand things, to carry *yīn* while embracing *yáng*, absorb *qì* by enacting fusion. And a direct physical relationship between that and *Tàijíquán* is *Tàijíquán* practitioners' use of the word "*qì*".

"*Qì*", in that context, means "breath". And *Tàijíquán* practitioners, using it as though it means "energy", direct using *yì* to direct its flow throughout the body. And "*yì*", in that context, means "intention", making that also an explicitly direct relationship between *Tàijíquán* and both *hatha yoga* and biofeedback.

And all of that's also explicit in Buddhist *sutta*s and *sutra*s. "*Sutra*" is Vedic Sanskrit for "*sutta*", and "*nibbana*" in Pali and "*nirvana*" in Vedic Sanskrit literally mean "*blowing out*" and are the Buddhist equivalent of the Hindu term "*yoga*", and Vedic Sanskrit was the language of the region of India where the Buddha did all of his teaching. So the purpose of the threads that are Buddhist scripture is to help one sew one's recognition into realization of the consciousness that extinguishes the illusion of differences and returns Buddhists from *tàijí* to the *yoga* of *wújí*.

And the *Tàijíquán Lùn* directs stringing and connecting wherein is *xū líng dǐng jìn*, sinking the *qì* to the *dāntián*, and not leaning or inclining. "*Dāntián*" literally means "elixir field" and in *Tàijíquán* refers to the center of the pelvic region. And "*xū líng dǐng jìn*" literally means "empty alert head-top strength".

And the first foundation of mindfulness the *Satipatthana Sutta* designates is mindfulness of the body. And, in that *sutta*, immediately after saying the aspirant keeps his or her body straight and her or his mindfulness alert, the Buddha directs mindfulness of breathing, while experiencing the whole body. And the *Diamond Sutra* is an effort to explain how all relationships are ultimately the same and metaphysical.

But, because "*Tàijíquán*" didn't become the general designation for the discipline until the twentieth century, Zhang Sanfeng probably didn't call anything he wrote the *Tàijíquán Jīng*. And, because humility is also a tenet of both Daoism and Buddhism, also improbable is that either a Daoist monk or a Buddhist monk would call any writing of his or hers a *jīng*. And, of the five main *Tàijíquán* abiding writings, only Wang Zongyue's *lùn* contains either the term "*tàijí*" or the term "*wújí*".

So many *Tàijíquán* practitioners ignore the relevance of Buddhism and Daoism and deny that the discipline they call *Tàijíquán* existed before anyone called it what they call it. Yet, perhaps by way of Chinese respect for tradition or perhaps because returning to *wújí* is as inevitable as the *Dào Dé Jīng* says it is, the *Tàijíquán* abiding writings and various persons have perpetuated its fundamentals through the centuries since the lives of Zhang Sanfeng and Wang Zongyue. And current practitioners at least ostensibly honor some of those persons.

But, in most histories of *Tàijíquán*, the next prominent person is Chen Changxing. And he was no kind of monk, and his life was about six centuries after the lives of Zhang Sanfeng and Wang Zongyue, but his family's village was between Wudang Mountain and the Shaolin Monastery. And his family treated *Tàijíquán* as a family legacy and traced it to Zhang Sanfeng.

But, perhaps partly explaining how Chen Changxing became the next person prominent in the history of *Tàijíquán*, his family also treated that legacy as a family secret. So the next person prominent in *Tàijíquán* history wasn't a Chen. He was a Yang.

He was Yang Luchan. And his association with the Chens was by indenturing himself to them. And his further association with *Tàijíquán* is through several interrelating circumstances.

One is that, through his indenture, he earned enough credence from Chen Changxing for that Chen to teach him that family secret. And another is that, about a generation after he indentured himself to those Chens, when their family member to whom he'd indentured himself died, he left the family's village and went to Beijing, where he taught publicly. That is, he shared with the public what Chen Changxing had taught him, what many *Tàijíquán* practitioners now call Yang style *Tàijíquán*.

And, in the twentieth century, his grandson Yang Chengfu extended that promulgation into publishing two books describing what he learned from his grandfather through one or more of his uncles.

And those two books are the earliest books calling the discipline *Tàijíquán*. And they're also the earliest books both describing and picturing any *Tàijíquán* practice sequence. And they also list the *Tàijíquán* succession of disciples from Zhang Sanfeng, through Chen Changxing, to Yang Chengfu.

And, perhaps more important than the probability that those books are at least the main reason for the fame of Chen Changxing, they contain the five short writings *Tàijíquán* practitioners most often call the *Tàijíquán* abiding writings.

But that publicity also may have led to fragmentation of the legacy. Now *Tàijíquán* practitioners designate what they call various styles of *Tàijíquán*. But the designations for the three most prominent ones also indicate the fallacy of that.

Their designations, in addition to Yang style, are Chen style and Wu style. But, while the Yang style is Yang Chengfu's purveyance of his grandfather Yang Luchan's purveyance of Chen Changxing's style, Chen Changxing is the Chen of the Chen style. And the Wu style is the style of Yang Luchan's student Wu Yuxiang.

So, if Wu Yuxiang didn't deviate from what Yang Luchan conveyed, the Wu style is the Yang style. So, if neither did Yang Luchan or Yang Chengfu deviate from what Chen Changxing taught Yang Luchan, all three styles are the Chen style. So, if neither did Chen Changxing deviate from his family legacy, all three styles ostensibly are the discipline Zhang Sanfeng passed on ultimately from Bodhidharma. And Yang Chengfu's books plainly assert that they pass on what Zhang Sanfeng passed on. But those books also make that questionable.

One factor is that, though Wang Zongyue's life was about six centuries earlier than Chen Changxing's, the list of the succession of disciples at the beginning of Yang Chengfu's 1931 book lists Chen Changxing immediately after Wang Zongyue. And another factor is that, though Yang Luchan died eleven years before Yang Chengfu's birth, Yang Chengfu says in his preface to his 1934 book that he watched Yang Luchan teaching the art. And he also recounts a conversation of his with Yang Luchan.

And another factor is that a factor possibly explaining those and other apparent discrepancies in Yang Chengfu's books makes the books perhaps more questionable.

That explanation would be that Yang Chengfu wasn't the only author of either or both of the books he published. And one indication of that is that, while his 1931 book lists Chen Changxing immediately after Wang Zongyue in the succession of disciples, the conversation with Yang Luchan in his 1934 book lists three disciples between Wang Zongyue and Chen Changxing. But a Chinese tradition may explain much of that.

The Chinese language is basically a language of nouns. Every Chinese word is a one-syllable name for a picture, what English-speaking linguists call pictographs, what Chinese people call *zì*. So, at least partly because grammatical inflection generally requires adding syllables to words, the Chinese language has no grammatical inflection. So it's nearly entirely synthetic.

Because grammatical inflection signifies such as tense and number and gender and parts of speech, the meaning of sentences in synthetic languages depends on context and accordingly on the order of the words in sentences, what linguists call syntax and inflect to call such languages synthetic.

But most literally significant in all that is that, with a result of it being flexibility of interpretation of how Chinese words relate to one another, the resulting ambiguity limits the precision of expressing abstract notions.

So, somewhat offsetting that limitation, the Chinese people have developed and broadly apply a tradition of telling stories to express abstract ideas. And Yang Chengfu's 1931 book tells fabulous stories of Zhang Sanfeng, of Yang Chengfu's uncle the story of the conversation with Yang Chengfu's grandfather says directed Yang Chengfu to learn *Tàijíquán* from him, and of others.

And, more directly suggesting that the story of Yang Luchan's conversing with Yang Chengfu may be an example of that tradition of story telling, Yang Chengfu's 1931 book contains some more plainly fabulous stories of Yang Luchan.

And, though, in the narrative of that conversation, Yang Luchan says the martial arts reputation of the Chen family drew him to them, he mainly informs Yang Chengfu of the health and spiritual functions of *Tàijíquán*.

Yang Chengfu begins the narrative by saying his uncle Yang Banhou directed him to study with him his grandfather's discipline, that Yang Chengfu preferred to learn how to defeat ten thousand opponents, and that he told Yang Banhou that. Next in it he says his father entered the conversation and told him his grandfather had passed the art down as their family's legacy and that he was abandoning his calling. And next he says his grandfather Yang Luchan interrupted the conversation to tell his father one couldn't force the art on a child.

And next in Yang Chengfu's narrative, after soothing him with a hand and asking him to listen, Yang Luchan tells him the purpose of the art isn't to accost enemies but to protect one's body.

Also, in the narrative, Yang Luchan tells Yang Chengfu the art isn't to save the world but to help the nation. But, though that may seem to be a sort of militant nationalism, next in it he says it's because China needs more help than do other nations. He says that, while Chinese people then were saying the troubles of their nation came from poverty, they didn't understand that the nation's sickness lay in its weakness. He says that, while disease was riddling the country, he hadn't heard of a plan for rousing the failing or raising the weak. And he says the first step toward strengthening other nations has been to strengthen their people.

Some may also interpret those references to weakness and strength to be martial. But he also says the basis of their family's art is what's natural and that, while the motion is in the body, it reaches the spiritual. So, basically, that story says Yang Luchan conveyed to Yang Chengfu what the first paragraph of this introduction says are the three principal functions of *Tàijíquán*.

And Yang Chengfu also says in that preface that he accepted what his grandfather told him and that he doesn't dare to forget it. And, introducing instruction in using *Tàijíquán* to deploy spears, his 1931 book also contains an anecdote of Zhang Sanfeng that more overtly exemplifies the Chinese tradition of presenting fables as though they're fact. So here's Paul Brennan's translation of that anecdote:

"Zhang Sanfeng was training in Daoism in the Wudang Mountains. During his quietude, he sat in meditation, training his spirit to return to its primordial state. During his activity, he wandered in the mountains. Each morning Zhang went to a quiet place at the mountain summit to gather in the essential energy of the universe and manipulate it through his breathing. One day Zhang suddenly saw a light to the west where clouds were being parted by mountain peaks. It dazzled and danced. He went toward it but lost sight of it, then found it was coming from a cave by a brook. When he got to the cave opening, he suddenly perceived that inside there were two golden snakes with flashing eyes coming at him. Zhang waved his duster and, with the sunlight better able to penetrate through the clearer air, he saw that they were actually two spears about seven and a half feet in length. What they were made of was not quite rattan and not quite wood, for they were resilient against the cutting of blades, and they could seem either soft or hard. In the cave something else gleamed. He went in to get a better look and what he found was a book in a single volume called Taiji Sticking Spear. It was meant to be shared with everyone, so he delved into its theory and contemplated its subtleties. The text of the book was all poetry and its ingenuities would be obscure to most of us, but Zhang studied every word until it made sense to him, and he turned it into a routine of postures so that everyone can train it by way of his exercises."

Anyone familiar with the *Dào Dé Jīng*, and the *Satipatthana Sutta* and the *Diamond Sutra*, will recognize direct accordance of that anecdote with them and quite literally with the *Dào Dé Jīng*. And its saying that, while the book was for sharing with everyone, it would be obscure to most of us is an especially direct reference to language frequent in the *Dào Dé Jīng*. So easy inference is that the book in that anecdote is the *Dào Dé Jīng* and that the spears are *yīn* and *yáng*.

So, while many *Tàijíquán* practitioners say the fabulous stories of Zhang Sanfeng make his existence questionable and that Yang Chengfu's deviation from literal fact makes anything he says questionable, that may only indicate that those *Tàijíquán* practitioners haven't learned to use the spears to penetrate the obscurity.

And, while Yang Chengfu's books' describing the forms and interpreting the two oldest of the abiding writings in martial arts terms may suggest that neither had he, the validity of that suggestion may depend on how much the others who contributed to his books influenced him and how much of either of those two books they wrote, as the answer to the question of why the list of succession in his 1931 book lacks three of the names his 1934 book says his grandfather listed may be that he didn't write one or the other of those books, or that he wrote neither. And prominent possibilities of who may have written much of either are Yang Chengfu's students Zheng Manqing and Chen Weiming. But factors argue for and against both.

Yang Chengfu says in his 1934 book that a reason he wrote his books is that, though Chen Weiming wrote a book about *Tàijíquán* he asked him to write, it only tells how to teach the practice sequence. And indications that Zheng Manqing may have written all of Yang Chengfu's 1934 book are that it begins with

Zheng Manqing's forward to it and that another of Yang Chengfu's students said Zheng Manquing wrote it. But, in that foreword, Zheng Manqing says he met Yang Chengfu in 1932 and advised him to write a book. So further complicating the question is the question of why he'd advise him in 1932 to do what he'd done in 1931. And Zheng Manqing undercuts his own credibility in other ways also.

That foreword also misrepresents both the *Tàijíquán* abiding writings and the *Dào Dé Jīng*. Effectually denying the *Dào Dé Jīng*'s assertion that nothing's stronger than the pliancy of water, he treats the Chinese word "*lì*" meaning "force" as though it's a synonym for the Chinese word "*jìn*" meaning "strength", and he refers to the reference in the Expositions of Insights into the Practice of the Thirteen Postures to the strength of a hundred chains of steel as though it's referring to the rigidity of steel. That is, while ostensibly touting the *Dào Dé Jīng*, Zheng Manqing effectually says the rigidity of steel is strength while the pliancy of water and chains is weakness.

And the reference to the strength of a hundred chains of steel to which he refers immediately follows an assertion that *qì* everywhere in a person's body is called transporting *jìn*. And, referring to that abiding writing's also saying one has no *lì* when one has *qì* and that one's purely hard when one has no *qì*, Zheng Manqing says it means one should have no *qì*. And under his own name, by writing books elaborating on and aggrandizing the *Yì Jīng*'s notion of the polarity of *yīn* and *yáng*, he established a reputation for scholarship beyond martial arts.

But Yang Chengfu's 1931 book, also aggrandizing the extreme polarity of the *Yì Jīng*, says the *Yì Jīng*'s *bāguà* are the basis for *Tàijíquán*. So many *Tàijíquán* practitioners do the same now. And that further complicates the question.

The *bāguà*, the eight augury trigrams, are the eight possible combinations of three *yīn*s or *yáng*s that are the first step in extending that abstract polarization of *yīn* and *yáng* into the 64 *guà* and interpretations of them that constitute the *Yì Jīng*. And, beyond much other elaboration on the *bāguà* in Yang Chengfu's books, the presentations of the *Tàijíquán Jīng* in his books says the first four components of the segment of the practice sequence immediately following the initial segment beginning with the *wújí* stance reach the first four of the *bāguà* and are also the four main compass directions. But Zheng Manqing, in his foreword to Yang Chengfu's 1934 book, also misrepresents the *Yì Jīng*.

And, suggesting that neither did Zheng Manqing write all of either book, each book contradicts itself fundamentally. That is, while both refer to the primal unity that's the principal subject of the *Dào Dé Jīng*, both also contradict that primacy by referring to *tàijí* as though it's the purpose and justification of *wújí*. And much of both books argues extensively, with no reference of any kind to *wújí*, that the *bāguà* define *Tàijíquán*.

And the 1931 book also lists many examples of apparent polarity and idealizes their polarity while calling that idealizing the *dào*. So much in both books refers to the cycle as though *tàijí* is superior to *wújí* and as though thus the departure into *tàijí* is more important than return to *wújí*. And, to do that, whoever wrote those parts of them misrepresents the *Dào Dé Jīng* beyond the misrepresentations in Zheng Manqing's foreword.

And another indication that Yang Chengfu wasn't the only author of his books is that some sections of the 1931 book refer to him from the third person point of view. And other internal evidence suggests that Yang Chengfu intended from the beginning that his books be compilations of his and others' writings. And that may answer the whole question.

But a factor plainly indicating that the movements the books describe are Yang Chengfu's motion is that both books illustrate the practice sequence they describe with photographs of Yang Chengfu demonstrating it. And, while the 1931 book also has photographs and explanations of him demonstrating the *tàijí* spear form, the anecdote of Zhang Sanfeng finding the spears suggests that the spear form may be metaphorical. So all of the motion the books describe also may be metaphorical.

But, be any of that as it may, whether or not Yang Chengfu understood what anyone says Yang Luchan told him, and whether or not he understood either what he said or what others may or may not have said for him, the perversion of the original meaning of *yīn* and *yáng* into aggrandizing *tàijí* while ignoring *wújí* preceded Bodhidharma. It's at least as old as the *Yì Jīng*, and the *Yì Jīng* originated during the Zhōu Dynasty, which ended more than seven centuries before any probable dates of the life of Bodhidharma. So Bodhidharma may have been trying to counteract its influence.

Originally, what we now call the *Yì Jīng* was a record of Zhōu Dynasty monarchs' extrapolating from a method of augury to use the *bāguà* to determine their efforts to control all of China by military force, and that extrapolation includes calling *yīn* bad and weak and female while calling *yáng* good and strong and male. So it uses *yīn* and *yáng* to extend extreme polarity not only into militance but also into other social and ethical polarity, but most pertinent here is that a result of that is that perverting the original symbolism of *yīn* and *yáng* into symbolizing polarity has become ordinary in Chinese and other epistemology. And now presentations of the *Yì Jīng* include commentary Chinese tradition attributes to Confucius.

And general consensus among historians says Lao Zi and Confucius lived during the Zhōu Dynasty and may have been contemporaries of both one another and the Buddha. And Chinese tradition also says both that Lao Zi wrote the *Dào Dé Jīng* and that Confucius once met him and said he'd never met anyone wiser. But, considering what the *Dào Dé Jīng* says of *wújí* and words, that suggests polar disparity between history and tradition.

So, if the history of *Tàijíquán* after Yang Chengfu, for reasons of either intentional or unintentional ignorance or either intentional or unintentional misrepresentation or for religious or epistemological or commercial reasons, deviates further from both Bodhidharma and the *Tàijíquán* abiding writings than does Yang Chengfu, that shouldn't surprise us.

And a 21st century indicative example of that deviant trend is what Dr. Yang Jwingming does through his organization he calls Yang's Martial Arts Academy.

That the Dr. Yang of that endeavor is from Taiwan suggests that, whatever he intends his name to suggest for marketing or any other purpose, he has no direct genetic relationship to the family of Yang Luchan and Yang Chengfu.

And that's but one indication of his purpose or lack of purpose. Another is that he left Taiwan to earn his doctoral degree in mechanical engineering from Purdue University in Indiana. And another is that he left the mechanical engineering profession to found that "academy" in California.

And he uses that organization not only to teach what he calls classical Yang style Tai Chi Chuan while publishing books and demonstration DVD's but also to market other merchandise. And an indicative example of the merchandise he sells is six-inch wooden balls he calls Tai Chi balls. And he sells them on his website for about the price of an automobile tire.

That example may allude to the traditional circular representation of *yīn* and *yáng*. And, in several of Yang Chengfu's descriptions of forms in his books, he says a component of the motion involving the palms facing one another resembles holding a sphere or ball. But, in Dr. Yang's DVD's, in his nearest approximations to those forms, he hangs one of his hands between his legs in that part of the motion, and that's but one of many ways the sequence he describes varies from Yang Chengfu's.

And another indication of his commercial motive is his misrepresentation of the Grasp Sparrow Tail form on a DVD and in his 2010 edition of his book *Tai Chi Chuan: Classical Yang Style, the Complete Long Form and Qigong.*

In his version, in the second of the four components of that form, he turns his left hand in a small circle. And, in his description of that, he says that "this movement does not have a practical application; instead, it is the signature of Yang Style Taijiquan." So a perhaps definitive element of the discordance of that with Yang Chengfu's books is that, excepting in a section of Yang Chengfu's 1931 book referring to him from the third person point of view, neither of Yang Chengfu's books says the Yang family's style is in any way different from *Tàijíquán* in general.

And Yang Chengfu's 1931 book says the Yang style is the authentic transmission. So one reasonably may suspect that assertion of Dr. Yang's to be an effort to establish a trademark for his commercial efforts he calls classical Yang style Tai Chi Chuan. And his deviations extend far beyond his commercialism.

He also says in that 2010 book that he regrets that *Tàijíquán* is straying from its martial arts origin. And one of many ways he asserts that notion is in that, ignoring that the *Tàijíquán* abiding writings promote establishing harmony with opponents to make them no longer opponents, his descriptions refer to such as breaking bones and killing. And Yang Chengfu's 1931 book specifically forbids using malicious hand attacks.

And Dr. Yang explicitly denies or misrepresents other historical and religious and cultural facts also. And, while Yang Chengfu's references to Daoism and Buddhism are brief and oblique, Dr. Yang's 2010 book argues specifically against the relevance to *Tàijíquán* of both Buddhism and Daoism. Referring to Buddhism, Dr. Yang describes what he calls religious enlightenment as though it's a kind of temporary intoxication, and he says Daoism was secular until the influence of Buddhism made it religious after the writing of the *Dào Dé Jīng*, and that's contrary to secular historical fact.

Historical consensus' indicating that Lao Zi and the Buddha were at least approximately contemporaneous of course also indicates that the writing of the *Dào Dé Jīng* and the founding of Daoism in China and of Buddhism in India were also approximately contemporaneous.

And historians also agree that each of those developments was after the political development of the Zhōu Dynasty and that Buddhism didn't reach China until centuries after the beginning of promulgation of the *Yì Jīng* beyond the Zhōu empire.

So, beyond expressing opinions irrelevant to *Tàijíquán* and arguing them with *non sequitur*s, Dr. Yang misrepresents easily verifiable actuality. And another example is that, ignoring that "*bodhidharma*" is Sanskrit meaning "consciousness of the universal order" while "*dá mó*" is a Chinese appellation for Bodhidharma but literally means "attaining rubbing", Dr. Yang says in his 2010 book that the name Bodhidharma is a sort of alias for Da Mo. And part of the absurdity of that is in that Sanskrit was Bodhidharma's native language.

And Dr. Yang also mistranslates Chinese. And an example of that indicating the extremity of his preoccupation with violence is his translation of "*shuāng fēng guàn ěr*". It means "double winds through ears", and it's the name of one of the forms in the practice sequence Yang Chengfu's books describe, but Dr. Yang "translates" it "attack the ears with the fists".

And he also says in his 2010 book that, while the number of segments in the traditional Yang style *Tàijíquán* sequence varies from 81 to 150, the names of the forms and the order of them doesn't vary. But the practice sequence he describes in that book and calls classical Yang style Tai Chi Chuan varies from Yang Chengfu's books not only in the number of segments but also in the order of the forms and in their names and performance. And, while he correctly says in that book that the principal purpose of *qìgong* is physical health, he describes the movements he calls qigong as though their principal purpose is training for martial arts.

And he also says Bodhidharma instituted martial arts at the Shaolin Monastery because too much meditation was impairing the health of the monks. So, while some of the *non sequitur* opinions he presents correctly extend the electrical energy theory of acupuncture to *qìgong*, he ignores the fact that Buddhist scripture both describes what modern medical doctors call biofeedback and directs including it in meditation. The term "biofeedback" refers to sensing the operation of internal organs, and so the *Satipatthana Sutta*'s directing being mindful of various internal functions and components of the body makes plain the relationship of that function of *Tàijíquán* with Buddhism, as do the *Tàijíquán* abiding writings.

But Dr. Yang's book may serve a Buddhist purpose. Readers may use it as a Zen koan, an effort to find relevance in apparent irrelevance by seeking relationships in the absence of apparent relationships, effectually seeking *sequitur* in what logicians call *non sequitur*. The reasoning for that is that the process would be a step toward realizing that everything ultimately relates to everything in the way *tàijí* ultimately returns to *wújí*. So it's explicitly both Buddhist and Daoist.

"Koan" is a Japanese pronunciation of the Chinese phrase "*gōng àn*", which idiomatically refers to a judge's desk, while literally it means "public incident". And Zen koans are public incidents in that, while Zen monks ordinarily meditate alone, they share koans with one another and the public. And they share them with the public for the same reason *bodhisattva*s try to share *nirvana* with everyone.

That is, their reason for that is that, as the martial purpose of *Tàijíquán* is to end enmity by establishing unity with an opponent, fundamental to both Daoism and Buddhism and perhaps most explicitly to what the newest and largest of the two main sects of Buddhism calls *bodhisattva*s is acceptance that each is all. And the name of that sect is Mahayana Buddhism, and "*mahayana*" is Sanskrit for "large vehicle", and Zen is a subsect of that sect. So Zen monks offer koans to everyone, anyone, all.

But, be it sectarian or nonsectarian or secular, any book as well as any situation or condition can operate toward reconciliation as do Zen koans.

Hindus call trying to use intellect to understand how everything relates to everything *jnana yoga*. As *hatha yoga* is an effort to return to *wújí* by way of recognizing that the air and space inside what ostensibly is one's separate body is the same as the air and space apparently outside it, *jnana yoga* is an effort to return to *wújí* by way of recognizing that everything is ultimately *sequitur*, and "*jnana*" is a Sanskrit word meaning "knowledge". And the *Satipatthana Sutta* also proffers that method.

And comparing the *Satipatthana Sutta* and the *Diamond Sutra* and other Buddhist *suttas* and *sutra*s to the *Upanishad*s would tell you that the most substantial difference between Buddhism and Hinduism is that Buddhism is more directly yogic than are Hinduism's rituals or worship of symbols, and reconciling the variations in the *Upanishad*s' various deific personifications and then reconciling that reconciliation with the rituals the *Veda*s also describe also can act as a koan, making apparent that the rituals and symbolic personifications are metaphors for what the *Diamond Sutra* says more directly, less metaphorically.

That is, all Hindu scripture is but one complex metaphor for all differences being nothing other than imaginings of the one deific totality, while the *Diamond Sutra* is partly an effort to explain that metaphorical meaning by obliquely referring to rituals to which other Buddhist *sutra*s and *sutta*s refer while not saying the Buddha directed them. And comparing the *Diamond Sutra* to the *Dào Dé Jīng* would tell you that the most substantial difference between Buddhism and Daoism is that the *Dào Dé Jīng* refers both metaphorically and more directly to epistemological and political obstructions to returning to the primal unity. And, with the term "*shèng rén*" in the *Dào Dé Jīng* being effectually a synonym for "*bodhisattva*", that would explain Mahayana Buddhist Bodhidharma's synthesizing Daoism and Buddhism into Zen.

And further attention to the relationship between Hinduism and Buddhism would tell one how Bodhidharma synthesized Buddhism and Daoism into *Tàijíquán*. And comparing *hatha yoga* and *jnana yoga* to the *Satipatthana Sutta* would clarify that. And one could follow that cycle interminably.

But understanding all that doesn't require treating those scriptures or the *Tàijíquán* abiding writings or Dr. Yang's books as Zen koans. And another indication that Yang Chengfu was more attentive to the *Tàijíquán* abiding writings than is Dr. Yang is that Dr. Yang's sequence ends many yards aside from where it begins. The sequence Yang Chengfu's books describe, after meandering to the right and back to the left and then through various other turns, ends three steps forward from where it begins and both in its beginning posture and facing in the same direction.

So, with the significance of that being that both the symbolic and the actual purpose of *Tàijíquán* is advancing to returning to *wújí* after straying from it into *tàijí*, considering variations in motion also can act as a Zen koan.

But, while so can scriptures of the other three of the six most popular religions, the three dualistic Abrahamic religions Judaism and Christianity and Islam, none of that may seem reasonable in a society those dualistic religions dominate, in an epistemologically dualistic society.

The notion of God in those religions is of a person separate from his creation, a person who creates some persons more evil than others and punishes them for that, partly by demanding that one race he created annihilate nine or ten other races, rewarding them for that by giving them the other races' homeland, promising to help them accomplish that genocidal landgrab, and punishing them for failing in that endeavor.

But such, be it east or west or both, inherently presents a koan perhaps as dynamic as the *Vedas*, and it may be why we need *Tàijíquán*. It's why, instead of trying to unite east and west by arguing either for or against the *Torah* or the Gospels or the *Qur'an* or for or against the *Vedas* or the *Suttas* or *Sutras* or the *Dào Dé Jīng*, we need to end such as the notion of the Zhōu Dynasty, and of the approximately contemporaneous Israelites, that subjugation unifies. And one might also try to reconcile why the Christian part of the Bible says the person Christians call the Christ would say both that he didn't come to bring peace but to bring a sword to divide us against one another and that the first and great commandment is to love God with all one's heart and soul and mind, that the second is to love one's neighbor as one's self, and that the second is like the first. And one might also try to reconcile the *Qur'an*'s saying it confirms both the Torah and the Gospels and that God is merciful with its also saying God created the disparity between humans by determining who'd believe in him and who wouldn't. Dualism is essential to bigotry while monism is inherently peace.

And a current example of the relevance of that to *Tàijíquán* may be in the *de facto* alliance of Barbara Davis with Dr. Yang to subvert Zhang Sanfeng's effort to perpetuate Bodhidharma's *bodhisattva* purpose for what eventually acquired the designation *Tàijíquán*. Ms. Davis' heritage is Judaic, and her 2004 book *The Tàijíquán Classics: an Annotated Translation, Including Commentary by Chen Weiming* is mainly a pretentious hodgepodge of tritely pedantic nonsense and *non sequiturs*. And its bibliography, while including a 1991 book by Dr. Yang, omits any *upanishad* or *sutta* or *sutra* and the *Dào Dé Jīng* and anything by Bodhidharma. And, while she refers in her book to the *Dào Dé*

Jīng and the *Diamond Sutra,* those references are examples of her pedantic *non sequitur*s. And a quotation she says is "well known" and from the *Diamond Sutra* is a misquotation of the *Heart Sutra.*

And, while not attributing to Dr. Yang his assertion that Bodhidharma introduced martial arts at the Shaolin Monastery because too much meditation was impairing the monks' health, she repeats it in the "history" section of her book. And Chen Weiming's commentary on the five *Tàijíquán* abiding writings Yang Chengfu presents in his books dominates her book. And Chen Weiming's commentary extrapolates from those writings for martial arts purposes.

And indicative of Ms. Davis' general bellicosity is that, throughout her "translations" of those abiding writings in her book, she "translates" the *zì* meaning "human" to mean "opponent".

Of course Abrahamic bellicosity doesn't explain the Zhōu Dynasty or the *Yì Jīng* or why or how the Shaolin Monastery became an academy for what English-speaking people generally call kung fu. But, despite Judaic scripture's being most of Christian scripture and Islamic scripture's saying it confirms both Christian scripture and Judaic scripture, Israelite bellicosity effectually defines the current war among the three Abrahamic religions we the dominantly Christion people of the United States have come to call a war on terror while Muslims call it a struggle. And both Christian and Islamic imperialism by conquest extended all over Earth through centuries long after the fall of the Zhōu Dynasty to other Chinese and the fall of the Israelite occupation of the land of Canaan to Babylonians, events that also may have been approximately contemporaneous, and kung fu isn't nearly as murderous as any of that.

But one of Solomon's proverbs suggests that the bellicosity and greed in Judaic scripture is irony. The first proverb in the eighteenth chapter of the Book of Proverbs says that, "through desire a man, having separated himself, seeketh and intermeddleth with all wisdom," and accepting that would obviate not only all the bellicosity and greed in Abrahamic scripture but also all the futility in general and misogyny and child abuse in particular that Solomon effectually promotes not only in other proverbs in that book but also in his Book of Ecclesiastes, in which he calls himself the preacher. That one proverb succinctly expresses the fundamental premise of Hinduism, Buddhism, and Daoism.

And much of what the part of the Bible that's particular to Christianity says of Jesus suggests that he was more Hindu Buddhist Daoist than Christian. What the Gospels say Jesus said of loving neighbors expresses the basic principle of the *Metta Sutta*, and one of the Gospels also says Jesus said the kingdom of God is within us and that thus one shouldn't look for it in other places, as the *Dào Dé Jīng* directs not watching through windows to display the *dào* of the sky. And the *Chandogya Upanishad* says all, specifically including both the earth and the sky, is in the heart.

And the popularity of *Tàijíquán* in the United States could be a step toward reconciliation if we didn't have such as Dr. Yang and Ms. Davis promoting perverting it effectually into a denial of Kipling's assertion that east and west won't meet until they meet at God's great judgement seat, effectually that eventually they'll meet at God's great judgement seat because God's great judgement is reconciliation into unity, an assertion suggesting that dualism isn't entirely disjunct from monist epistemology.

And another occidental step in the direction of the oriental monism of Hinduism and Buddhism and Daoism is that definition of "intellect" in *Webster's New World College Dictionary* saying intellect is the ability to understand relationships and differences.

But a Hindu or a Buddhist or a Daoist might say a problem with that definition is that difference is a kind of relationship. While the basic tenet of Hinduism is that the way to bliss is by realizing the unity of all, the basic tenet of Buddhism is that the way to end suffering is by extinguishing the illusion of differences, and the basic tenet of Daoism is that the way to peace is by returning from the abstraction of words to accepting the absolute relationship of all to all. And each of those superficially different expressions is a way of saying we need to return from *tàijí* to *wújí*.

And the answer to one more question, the question of why all *Tàijíquán* practitioners should practice one sequence of motions, may provide a practical link between all of that and *Tàijíquán*. And one answer to that question is this quotation from Louis Swaim's translation of Yang Chengfu's introduction to his 1934 book: "There is only one school of taijiquan; there are not two ways of learning. One may not make a show of one's cleverness by rashly making additions or deletions. The former worthies developed these methods. If alterations or corrections could be made, the ancestors preceding me would already have put them into effect. Why wait for our generation?"

But, pertinent to that, in Swaim's commentary on his translation of that book, he says Yang Chengfu's student Fu Zhongwen, in a book Swaim also translated, describes "the received form". And he says, of differences between Yang Chengfu's descriptions and Fu Zhongwen's, that they may be because Yang Chengfu refined his forms during his decades of teaching them. But Fu Zhongwen doesn't say that.

And, while Yang Chengfu says in his introduction to his 1934 book that it's a refinement of his 1931 book and that he improved his performance of the forms during the decade preceding his publishing that book, he doesn't say he changed the forms. And another question, if the sequence Fu Zhongwen describes is the received form, is from whom Fu Zhongwen received it. And Fu Zhongwen was a student of Yang Chengfu's from his childhood until Yang Chengfu's death.

And, more specifically, his descriptions differ from Yang Chengfu's in no way other than in detail and numbering and in that he doesn't describe them in martial terms. And Yang Chengfu says in his introduction to his 1934 book that the applications in it are for people who are already proficient in *Tàijíquán* but wish to progress further. And Fu Zhongwen's omission of martial arts details was important enough to him for him to point it out in his preface to his book.

And he also says in that preface that 76 of the 251 drawings he used to illustrate his descriptions in his book are tracings by a Zhou Yuanlong of photographs of Yang Chengfu and that the others accord with the same principles. And the 76, which are among the 244 of the 251 I use to illustrate the descriptions in this book, are of photographs Yang Chengfu used to illustrate the descriptions in both of his books. And, incidentally, the only reason I omitted the other seven is that the point of view of the 244 is from the north while that of the other seven varies.

But also indicative is that a more particular difference between Yang Chengfu's descriptions and Fu Zhongwen's is that, while Fu Zhongwen describes all of what both say is the beginning segment of the sequence, Yang Chengfu's books describe only its closing. That may be because the beginning segment is only a stepping into the *wújí* stance before beginning the first segment Yang Chengfu numbers and thus has no martial purpose. But what English-speaking *Tàijíquán* practitioners generally call that next segment may also suggest the perversion of *Tàijíquán*.

A *zì* in the designation of that segment originally meant "arrow quiver cover". But Yang Chengfu says in his 1934 book that in *Tàijíquán* it has a variant meaning particular to *Tàijíquán*. And, while the *pīnyīn* spelling of the name of that *zì* is "*bīng*", every reference to it in English I've found spells it "peng" and translates it "ward-off". And the purpose of an arrow quiver cover isn't to deploy arrows but literally to protect a peaceful gathering of them. But using that term to refer to warding off doesn't contradict that.

It only provides to others a gateway to the perversion.

So the main shortcoming in Swaim's presentation is that, by calling Fu Zhongwen's description of the sequence the received form, he effectually ignores that Fu Zhongwen received it from Yang Chengfu.

That is, while in his commentary Swaim refers to the decades of Fu Zhongwen's receiving instruction from Yang Chengfu, he effectually ignores it. And, more important, by doing that he ignores the whole history of *Tàijíquán* to which his translations refer. And, still more important, he ignores that continuity is fundamental to *Tàijíquán*.

Not only is continuity the defining actuality of the flow from *wújí* to *tàijí* and back, but also it's essential to *Tàijíquán*'s use both as an alternative to martial arts and as *hatha yoga*, and it's also how biofeedback is fundamental to *Tàijíquán*.

Qì, breath, flows into the lungs, where oxygen in it transfers to the red corpuscles in blood, and the blood flows throughout the body. And, because otherwise few mammal's life would continue for more than a few minutes, *Tàijíquán* practitioners are correct in translating "*qì*" to mean "life breath". And, because energy is also essential to life, they also may be correct in translating it to mean "energy".

But, ordinarily, beyond the lungs, we don't directly sense that flow, and modern medical professionals, pointing out that we can control our lungs only because we can feel them and see our chest expanding and contracting, indicate why we ordinarily can't control the flow directly. And they also point out that, because neither the lungs nor the ribs are muscles, neither controls the lungs. They say the expansion and contraction of the diaphragm does that.

Yet that indirectness of control suggests validity of the *Tàijíquán* notion that we can learn to control the flow of *qì* by imagining that our concept of it controls it. That is, it suggests that, while complying with the *Tàijíquán* injunction to sink the *qì* to the *dāntián* may not be directly possible, it may be practical and hardly avoidable. Blood also flows to and from the pelvic region.

And, further, biophysicists say free flow of the medium of nutrition around cells makes them effectually immortal. They say single-cell organisms regenerate *ad infinitum* if air or water, the environment from which they receive their nutrients, flows freely around them. And that, in a multicell organism, would be *ad infinitum* regeneration of body tissue.

And the *Tàijíquán* abiding writing *Tàijíquán* practitioners call the Thirteen Potentialities Song ends by asking that *yì* and *qì* come to rule bones and administer flesh, and saying the wish of the song is to push how to use *yì* to end in beneficially living and prolonging years, a spring not aging.

So, if *Tàijíquán* can fulfill the promise of its abiding writings, a person with no legs can use it to regenerate new legs. And, whether or not that's physical actuality, the abiding writings of Hinduism and Buddhism and Daoism and also of *Tàijíquán* say it's universal actuality. And the abiding writings of Christianity say Jesus, the person they call the Christ and accordingly say defines Christianity, said our faith can make us whole. And "whole" is another word for "*wújí*". So it's the *quán* of *Tàijíquán*.

And nothing is to keep anyone from accomplishing both the biofeedback function and the *hatha yoga* function of *Tàijíquán* by using *yì* to imagine effecting the motion sequence in accordance with the *Tàijíquán* principles.

So another answer to the question of why all *Tàijíquán* practitioners should practice one sequence of motion is that doing that at least provides an aura of continuity reminding one of the whole purpose of *Tàijíquán* that some persons ostensibly practicing it apparently ignore or forget or deny.

But, be any of that as it may be, the other four sections of this book present the fundamentals of *Tàijíquán* that *Tàijíquán* practitioners generally accept. The second section summarizes the principals of *Tàijíquán* motion that both the *Tàijíquán* abiding writings and Yang Chengfu's books present, and the third section describes the sequence of forms that both Yang Chengfu's books and Fu Zhongwen's book describe. The fourth section is translations of the five *Tàijíquán* abiding writings Yang Chengfu and Fu Zhongwen present in their books, and the final section is a glossary of Chinese terms especially significant to all that writing.

The descriptions in the third section aren't translation. They detail the common core of Yang Chengfu's and Fu Zhongwen's descriptions, but they omit Yang Chengfu's references to hypothetical martial settings, and they omit some of Fu Zhongwen's details. And the omission of those details is only because human anatomy and the illustrations in that section and the principles in the second section make them obvious.

And, also in my detailing in the third section, I took advantage of the English language's having more specific ways of expressing time sequence than has the Chinese language. Of course part of that problem is that the Chinese language has no inflection for tense. But another is that it seldom deploys conjunctions and often omits relational adverbs.

And, for various reasons, I added some details not directly pertinent to the motion. But, unlike Yang Chengfu and Fu Zhongwen, I placed those comments not in the descriptions but below the illustrations. That's to avoid distracting you from the flow of the motion.

But I made the translation in the fourth section as literal as I could. I carefully read Swaim's translations of those writings, the translations of them by Benjamin Peng Jeng Lo and his collaborators in their 1979 book *The Essence of T'ai Chi Ch'uan: the Literary Tradition*, and those by Barbara Davis in her book. And I also carefully read Paul Brennan's translations of them in his 2011 translation of Yang Chengfu's 1931 book.

But I also compared those translations to one another and researched each word. And I found both that those translators contradicted each other and that none of those translations is nearly as literal as it easily might have been. And those translators indicated in their commentary with their translations that a reason may be that they "translated" some words as though they denote connotations particular to martial arts. So also, in my translation of those five abiding writings, I left some of those terms and others in Chinese. And I also left them in Chinese in other sections of this book.

But, for those terms, the first time I use each, I provide a literal translation of it and refer to its *Tàijíquán* use, and I also translate and define each in the fifth section of this book. And the reason I made it the final section is for you to find it easily. And I listed the terms alphabetically by their *pīnyīn* spelling.

The Chinese language has no alphabet of its own. So, in the middle of the twentieth century, the Chinese government developed what it calls *pīnyīn* to use the Roman alphabet to spell Chinese words. In the nineteenth century, two British sinologists whose names were Wade and Giles developed for that what we now call the Wade-Giles system, and that was an international standard for decades. But, however paradoxical it may seem, *pīnyīn* is much more like the English use of the Roman alphabet than is those British sinologists' system.

But it has some differences. So the last page of that last section of this book is a guide to approximate *pīnyīn* pronunciation. And that's for readers who wish to be able to pronounce what they read.

And, because the Chinese people use *zì* both to write and to read their words, I've also included in that glossary the *zì* for each word. And that's for readers who wish to see what the Chinese see or wish to research the terms for themselves. And "*zì*" is the last word in that glossary.

But, to close this introduction, let's consider a few more factors relevant to the problem of the perversion of an alternative to martial arts into a martial art and to Yang Chengfu's credibility.

Peace, in the Judaic scripture that's also fundamental to Christianity and Islam, is subjugating one's enemies. But claimants to at least two of the three ostensibly monistic of the six most popular religions also promote in the name of their religion the extreme polarity of bellicosity. And, in various ways, it's become doctrine in those two.

Hinduism's *Bhagavad-Gita* says that, because all being is one and eternal, no separate person kills or is killed. But it uses that notion to argue that members of the warrior caste should be grateful for opportunities to fulfil in war the "*karma*" that's their caste duty. And some claimants to Buddhism say people who lack the conscience that's fundamental to Buddhism don't deserve the absolute compassion the *Metta Sutta* dictates and that thus, as one should extinguish the illusion of differences, one may also extinguish those persons. So only Daoism, the one of those six religions that originated in the country in which *Tàijíquán* originated, presents no doctrine of extreme polarity.

And Dr. Yang may have made of himself a symbol of the ignorance perverting *Tàijíquán*. He says in his 2010 book that he studied various martial arts for decades and that he had at least two *Tàijíquán* teachers. But his books not only misrepresent Buddhism and Daoism and the *Tàijíquán* abiding writings but also are in polar opposition to what Yang Chengfu's introduction to his 1934 book says of continuity.

So, either Dr. Yang ignored his *Tàijíquán* teachers, or they also ignored the history and abiding writings of *Tàijíquán* and passed their ignorant misunderstanding on to Dr. Yang.

But pertinent to Yang Chengfu's credibility is that immediately following the list of succession of disciples in his

1931 book is this elaboration of the traditionally simple visual representation of *yīn* and *yáng*:

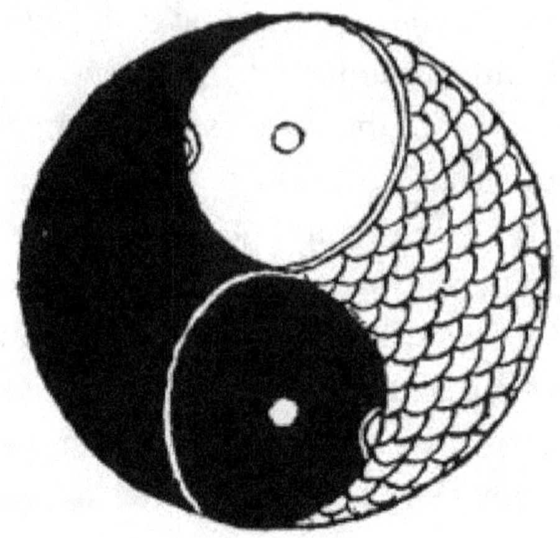

And the commentary on the *Tàijíquán Lùn* in that book refers to *Tàijí*'s *yīn* and *yáng* fish.

But, immediately following that diagram, that book says the genuine human Zhang passed on *Tàijíquán* and that his Daoist name was Sanfeng. So it doesn't say Zhang Sanfeng was Daoist but that he had a Daoist name, as many Chinese people receive various names as their lives progress as did Yang Luchan with "*lù chán*" literally meaning "revealer of Zen", and "*sān fēng*" means "three peaks". And that book doesn't say Zhang Sanfeng originated *Tàijíquán* but only that he passed it on.

And also in that biographical section, perhaps indicating how Zhang Sanfeng acquired the name Sanfeng, are assertions that he joined another monastery before traveling on to the Wudang Monastery and that he quickly learned scriptures.

And immediately after that biographical information is a fantastical story of Yang Luchan in which a Buddhist monk of large physical size who's a strong exponent of Shaolin seeks out Yang Luchan and attacks him with no provocation but fails and acquiesces and spends three days conversing with and learning from him.

But one may interpret that anecdote either to deprecate Buddhism or what some call *Shàolínquán* or to promote such as the reconciliation of that Buddhist monk and Yang Luchan with one another as the *Tàijíquán* abiding writings say one should reconcile *tàijí* into *wújí*.

And Yang Chengfu's books contain many other ambiguous references both to difference between Shaolin teaching and Wudang teaching and to particularity of the Yang teaching.

So the question of Yang Chengfu's credibility may be a result of the ambiguity resulting from the Chinese language being synthetic, a result of translators taking advantage of that to promote their extrapolations from *Tàijíquán*, or both.

But, whatever the relevance of any of that may be, a more succinct introduction to *Tàijíquán* would be this literal translation of the 68th segment of the *Dào Dé Jīng*:

> Good action mastering: One isn't violent.
> Good battling: One isn't angry.
> Good conquering opponents: One doesn't reciprocate.
> Good using humans: One acts as their below.
> That's called the *dé* of not contending.
> That's called using humans' strength.
> That's called connecting the sky's primal polarity.

And still more succinct would be simply pointing out that *tàijí* is disparity while *wújí* is unity.

Principles of Motion

Sōng is the most fundamental principle of *Tàijíquán* motion. 鬆, the *zì* of which *sōng* in that context is the name, originally was a picture of a tree and a human with their leaves and hair flowing in a breeze. And it means "loose", and in *Tàijíquán* all is *sōng*, both physically and mentally.

Physically, no straightening or opening ever locks, and no folding or closing ever clenches. And, most fundamentally, because breathing is the connection between air flowing through the space outside the body and oxygen flowing with the blood inside the body, *qì* is also *sōng*. So, because *sōng* is essential to that flow, neither inhaling nor exhaling is to the extent of straining the ribs or the diaphragm.

In *Tàijíquán* motion, inhaling is ordinarily while the hands are moving upward or toward the torso, and exhaling is ordinarily while the hands are moving downward or away from the torso, but assuring that the flow of the breath be smooth takes precedent over that, to keep the *qì* always *sōng*.

And the mouth is *sōng*, with the tip of the tongue lightly touching the roof of the mouth and the lower lip and teeth lightly touching the upper lip and teeth, and the jaws never clench as the fists never clench. And the shoulders never hunch, and the elbows generally sink into the position gravity gives them relative to the shoulders and the wrists, and each ankle is *sōng* when its knee rises. That is, every part of the body is *sōng*, until it supports weight or drives motion.

So, when a knee rises, the heel of its foot leaves the ground before its ball leaves the ground. And settling the weight onto a foot while it's flat on the ground never flexes the ankle to the extent of straining it. And neither does any other joint ever fully flex or extend.

So *xū líng dǐng jìn*, being a *sōng* means of being *sōng*, is in itself a principle both of *Tàijíquán* motion and of *Tàijíquán* in general. In *Tàijíquán*, that phrase's literally meaning "empty alert head-top strength" refers to balancing the spine from the *wěilú* through the neck in a position requiring no effort to keep it and the head erect, and its words refer to *Tàijíquán*'s being not only *sōng* but also alert and strong. And the abiding writing the Thirteen Potentialities Song, with the term "*wěilú*" literally meaning "tail gate" but idiomatically meaning "coccyx", directs keeping the spine in *xū líng dǐng jìn* from the *wěilú* through the neck.

And the word "*líng*", meaning "alert" in that phrase, refers to the relationship between the physical and the mental. So one maintains *xū líng dǐng jìn* during nearly all of the *Tàijíquán* motion sequence and, either during the same segment or at the beginning of the next segment, returns to it nearly immediately from any deviation from it. That is, *xū líng dǐng jìn* is at least symbolically *wújí*, while deviations from it are *tàijí*.

Translators and commentators have varied in their efforts to translate and explain that phrase. But it's in the *Tàijíquán Lùn*, and in Fu Zhongwen's book it's first in a list of ten principles with commentary he says Yang Chengfu dictated to Chen Weiming, and it's second in a list of ten body methods Yang Chengfu lists in his 1931 book. And, if one accepts the relationship between Buddhism and Daoism and *Tàijíquán*, all one must do to know what "*xū líng dǐng jìn*" means is to look at a Chinese imagining of the Buddha meditating.

And an example is on the cover of this book. So, in this book, excepting in the glossary in its fifth section, I don't translate or define "*xū líng dǐng jìn*" further. But, of course, the *Tàijíquán* abiding writings in the fourth section of this book define it further.

And following are the ten principles of motion Yang Chengfu presents in his 1931 book and calls body methods, and next are the ten principles of motion he lists with them and calls practice methods, and they also define "*xū líng dǐng jìn*" further.

And my comments following Yang Chengfu's designations for these principles he calls body methods and practice methods also refer to how they're pertinent to *xū líng dǐng jìn*.

Body methods:

1. Carry and raise fine spirit.

This principle expresses the purpose of "*xū líng dǐng jìn*".

2. *Xū líng dǐng jìn*.

Placing *xū líng dǐng jìn* between the first and third body methods effectually suggests that it links the spirit with the body.

3. Contain the breast, and draw the back.

Containing the breast is embracing it with *sōng* shoulders, and drawing the back is drawing up the spine to make it erect, for *xū líng dǐng jìn*.

4. *Sōng* the shoulders, and sink the elbows.

Sinking the elbows is letting them also be *sōng*.

5. Sink the *qì* to the *dāntián*.

While, in *Tàijíquán*, the term "*dāntián*" refers to the center of the pelvic region, more generally it refers to any of three regions of the human body. The upper *dāntián* is in the region of the brain, while the central *dāntián* is in the region of the heart and the solar plexus, and the lower *dāntián* is in the *yāo*. And "*yāo*", in that context, refers to the entire pelvic region, the region of the skeletal component of the human body that connects the lower body to the upper body. So each *dāntián* participates in actuating the flow of *qì* and other motion. And each is along the physical path defining *xū líng dǐng jìn*.

6. Link the hands and the shoulders.

This principle directs extending that unity of flow to the ends of what one calls` the upper extremities.

7. Link the hips and the knees.

And this principle directs extending that unity of flow from the *dāntián* to the lower extremities.

8. The buttocks are a path to carrying the above.

And this principle specifies muscles of the *yāo* in that linkage.

9. The *wěilú* is central and upright.

This principle, like the Thirteen Potentialities Song, specifically includes the bottom of the spine in *xū líng dǐng jìn*.

10. Inside and outside are mutually whole.

And this principle effectually says how *Tàijíquán* is essentially *hatha yoga*.

Practice methods:

1. Don't *lì* using *jìn*.

"*Lì*" here means "force". And this *jìn zì* is the one meaning "strength" in "*xū líng dǐng jìn*". So this principle effectually directs always being *sōng*.

2. By *yì* conduct *qì*.

This *yì zì* is the one meaning "intention". So this principle directs intentionally directing the flow of the breath. And directing doing that implies that it's possible.

3. Step as cats move.

Cats are famous for the *sōng* of their motion while they're also alert.

4. Upper and lower mutually follow.

This principle effectually directs that all parts of the body move together.

5. Exhaling and inhaling is certainly so.

This principle says breathing isn't an exception to the fourth practice method.

6. One thread strings completely.

This principle paraphrases the fourth and fifth practice methods.

7. Changes exchange in the *yāo*.

This principle says how the fifth body method relates to the fourth through sixth practice methods.

8. *Qì* conducts the four limbs.

This principle expresses the relationship between the second practice method and the seventh.

9. Discern clearly *xū* and *shí*.

This *xū zì* means "empty" or "void", and it's the *zì* meaning "empty" in "*xū líng dǐng jìn*", and "*shí*" here means "full" or "solid". And, in *Tàijíquán*, those two words refer to whether a part of the body has weight on it or otherwise isn't *sōng*. So discerning between *xū* and *shí* is knowing whether a part of the body is available for motion. Of course *xū líng dǐng jìn* bears the weight of the head. But balance makes it available for motion. So, effectually, it's *xū* because it's *sōng*.

10. Circular turning is purposeful.

This principle effectually directs extending the metaphorical meaning of "*tài jí quán*" from the primal actuality into its temporal physicality.

And the gaze is also song. The eyes generally follow the motion. But, to attend to all, they never focus on anything in particular.

But, while perhaps ultimately inevitable, complying with those methodic principles, and perhaps especially the final practice method, may seem difficult. And, in the beginning, memorizing the physical motions may be too frustrating to be mentally *sōng*. But it needn't be.

Practicing alternating the closings of the two Golden Bird Single Stand forms before trying to practice the whole sequence can be an effective transition preventing the frustration. Those forms, the 68th and 69th segments in the sequence, exemplify and require all of those principles and accordingly can improve one's ability to guide one's attention and respond accordingly. So, if one doesn't try to hurry, they can develop both mental *sōng* and physical *sōng* enough to prevent any frustration.

They require maintaining *xū líng dǐng jìn* while standing on one leg, and standing on one leg in accordance with those principles requires lifting one knee while keeping it and its ankle *sōng*, and all of that requires ease of balance. If balance is difficult, the effort to maintain the closing positions of those forms for more than a few seconds may require waving one's arms and the leg one lifts, and that would require deviating from both *xū líng dǐng jìn* and the peripheral elements of the forms. And none of that is conducive to being either physically or mentally *sōng*.

But that's how it can be a way to learn both. And it also can be a way to understand the *hatha yoga* function of *Tàijíquán*. It can improve one's ability to pay attention to every part of the body and to how each depends on all of the others.

One can pay attention to the waving to understand what purpose it serves, how it's both compulsive and useful, and how to respond productively.

And, of course, sinking the *qì* to the *dāntián* in the *wújí* stance would be an appropriate beginning to that effort and would also be an appropriate component of the approximation of the *wújí* stance linking those two segments.

And, also regarding mental *sōng*, treating the compulsive waving as a learning process and not as obstruction to learning can be an alternative to the ordinary response to frustration. Frustration has become effectually synonymous with anger, and anger is effectually antonymous with being mentally *sōng* and synonymous with being extremely polar, and welcoming learning can obviate the motive for that anger. But also important is recognizing that the Golden Bird Single Stand segments aren't separate from *Tàijíquán*.

Some teachers recommend learning each segment of the sequence separately. But that may lead to failing to recognize or feel the unity of motion that practically defines *Tàijíquán*. And one may argue that recommending practicing the Golden Bird Single Stand segments separately argues for that. But, with practicing the Golden Bird Single Stand forms separately serving a teaching purpose that, by permitting being *sōng* from the beginning of the sequence, is pertinent to every segment of the sequence, it practically defines that unity. And beginning the sequence with frustration would be fragmentation and thus antonymous to *wújí*.

So a practical way to begin learning the sequence may be to begin each effort by practicing the Golden Bird Single Stand, until one can keep both the left and the right stand *sōng* for several seconds, and following that by reading some or all of the form descriptions, while actuating as much of each as one can, while holding this book.

The attention that would require would both facilitate remembering and extend into each segment the attitude that practicing the Golden Bird Single Stand facilitates. And, beyond being an effective transition between the reading and the motion, developing that attitude could be an effective transition between the motion and one's quotidian life. And, of course, the most comprehensive way to learn those principles and the distinction between martial arts and the *Tàijíquán* alternative to martial arts would be to try to practice those principles in every motion of one's life.

And, regarding biofeedback, modern medical professionals anywhere tell us of the detrimental effect on physical health of frustration in one's daily activities. And realizing that is also a purpose and function of both the attentive detachment the *Satipatthana Sutta* directs and the unifying function of *hatha yoga*.

And, of course, all of that would serve the purpose of effectually making *Tàijíquán* always *wújí*.

So, of course, it would lead to making not only the *Tàijíquán* abiding writings but also much of the writing we call scripture that has abided through several millennia less obscure than some of its authors have said it is.

The essence of that obscurity is failure to accept the Hindu Buddhist Daoist notion that all eventually shall return to the primal unity anyway.

And the *Tàijíquán* abiding writings indicate that applying these principles in a martial situation is always moving with the opponent and never against him or her. That is, they effectually direct treating the opponent as though one's the opponent's shadow, essentially as though one's one with the opponent. And Yang Chengfu's books say that's the purpose of the two-person practice he calls pushing hands.

And his 1934 book, referring to the *Tàijíquán Lùn*'s saying that in *Tàijíquán* one reaches spiritual light by stepping, says studying pushing hands is learning how to sense strength.

And, regarding biofeedback, one needn't have either arms or legs to have both *yì* and *qì*. And recognizing that actuality, in order eventually to realize that all is all, is the most fundamental purpose of *Tàijíquán*. So, whether or not one accepts that principle in the beginning, abiding by the principles of *Tàijíquán* motion will move one in that direction.

So, fundamentally, that's the only principle of *Tàijíquán*. That is, essential is recognizing that the three functions are one, that neither are they an exception to either the eventuality or the actuality of *wújí*. And that's that, whether or not we recognize it, all is always *sōng*.

So that may also raise the question of why anyone should learn a particular sequence of motion, why one shouldn't only apply these principles either to random motions or to no motion, to be absolutely *sōng*.

But the answer to that question is inherent in the process. It's in that, because we've strayed from the primal unity into the stress of *tàijí*, we need to relearn the *sōng* of *wújí*. And deviating from the proven is inherently *tàijí*.

And learning to follow another's instructions is inherently extinguishing disparity to accept unity, and the variety of motions in the sequence Yang Chengfu has passed on is the method most likely to effect that relearning, if only because of the probability of its having abided longer than has any other.

And one can test that from the beginning of learning it. Initially, in that process, one is likely to find wending through its complexity of motion frustrating. But, eventually, if one keeps these principles in mind, one will find complexity can also be *sōng*, and that's its whole purpose. It's how "*tàijí* and one's *wújí*, while being life and *yīn* and *yáng*, are their mother also." And that principal principle is how *sōng* is the most fundamental principle.

So, ultimately, the only principle of *Tàijíquán* or anything else or all is that, either ultimately or eventually, no constraint constrains.

Forms

The names and numbering of these descriptions of the forms are those in Yang Chengfu's 1931 book *Tàijíquán Application and Use Methods*. The illustrations are 244 of the drawings of Yang Chengfu from north of him that Fu Zhongwen used to illustrate the descriptions in his book the Chinese government published in 1963 and called *Yang Form Tàijíquán*. And the descriptions are a synthesis of Fu Zhongwen's descriptions with Yang Chengfu's.

One may imagine for oneself whether *Yì Jīng* augurs' traditionally facing south during their augury process is relevant to the orientation of the photographs and drawings. But the practicality of the constant point of view is in that it permits describing the motions of each form relative to the motions of the other forms in the sequence. Left and right are relative only to the separate body moment by moment.

And reasons to use the drawings instead of the photographs that are their model are that the drawings include arrows indicating the direction of motion of the hands and feet between the positions they illustrate and that they also include shadows indicating whether the toes or heel or all of the foot is touching the ground.

And my process of synthesis was also methodical. After carefully reading all three books, I paraphrased the descriptions in Yang Chengfu's 1931 book into more complete descriptions of the 244 illustrations but with none of the martial arts references, and next I synthesized into that details his 1934 book adds that are essential to the motion but not obvious from the illustrations. And next I synthesized into that details from Fu Zhongwen's book that are neither obvious from the illustrations nor in either of Yang Chengfu's books.

And next, sequentially, I compared Fu Zhongwen's description of each segment to what I'd written. And next, to be sure I'd retained Yang Chengfu's details of motion through that process, I compared the results of that to Yang Chengfu's 1934 book. And next, in the same way and for the same purpose, I compared the results of that to Yang Chengfu's 1931 book.

And, finally, partly to be sure that what I described ends in alignment with its beginning and with the same orientation, I physically followed what I'd written.

And, in that process, further suggesting continuity and agreement over time, at least in regard to the motions of the solo practice sequence, I found none of the three books to contradict either of the other two, in any detail of the motion.

But a difference between this book and both Fu Zhongwen's and Yang Chengfu's books is repetition. After the first description of each form, instead of describing subsequent occurrences of each form, each of those books repeats the name of the form but not the description. But, for you to be able to learn the motions sequentially while holding the book in one hand and not needing to stop to find the earlier description, this book presents a full description of each form on each occurrence.

And, also to minimize the need to turn pages while learning the motions, each illustration in this book is on the page of its description. And I've used but one sentence to describe each illustration of a motion or repetition of that motion's illustration. That is, excepting for the gaze references, each period in each description is at the end of such a sentence.

But, for economy of language, and also for your convenience, this book doesn't fully repeat the five descriptions of components of more than one form that follow this paragraph. But also pertinent is that, like some of the names of the forms in the sequence, the names of at least the first two of these components originated from martial arts and have martial connotations. But, like "*quán*" in the designation *Tàijíquán*, those designations don't require their referents to be martial in *Tàijíquán*.

In *mǎ bù*, the horse stance, the feet are flat and approximately parallel. The knees are bent but not to the extent that keeping the feet flat strains the ankles. And the distance between the feet varies but ordinarily approximates the width of the shoulders. Presumably the name of this stance is because of its resemblance to straddling a horse.

In *gōng jiàn bù*, the bow and arrow stance, one foot is in front of the other while both feet are flat. The foot furthest to the rear angles, to the left if it's the left foot or to the right if it's the right foot, while the foot furthest to the front ordinarily points directly forward but may angle to either side. And, for most of the weight of the body to be on the front leg, the front knee bends forward over its instep while the rear leg is nearly straight. And, like Yang Chengfu's and Fu Zhongwen's books, the remainder of this book calls this component the bow stance.

In *zuò pán bù*, the tray setting stance, one foot is also in front of the other. But the rear heel in this stance is above the ground and ordinarily angles to the left if the left foot is in front or to the right if the right foot is in front. This posture is like setting a tray on a table while not bending the waist. And the remainder of this book calls it the tray stance.

Shí zì shǒu, ten *zì* hands, is crossing the wrists in front of the torso. *Shí Zì Shǒu* is also the name of the form that's the sixteenth and 53rd segments of the sequence and the beginning of the final segment, and in that form the palms are facing inward with the right hand furthest from the torso, but the relative positions of the hands vary in other instances of this component.

The reason for the name of this component and that form is the cross shape of the *zì* meaning "ten", and the remainder of this book calls this component crossing the hands, and each reference to it indicates any variance from the *Shí Zì Shǒu* form.

And *zuò wàn*, settling the wrists, is flexing the wrists as though one were about to use the palms to push an object.

But a component I mentioned in the introduction to this book has no name. It's turning one's palms toward one another in front of one's torso with one hand above the other. It's what both Yang Chengfu's 1931 book and his 1934 book say in descriptions is as if one's holding a sphere or a ball. And, considering the circular shape of the *yīn* and *yáng* diagram, I describe it that way in this book. And it occurs twenty times in the sequence.

And I've also otherwise tried to make the descriptions in this book a continuation of the standing tradition, not the deviating from it Yang Chengfu deprecates in his introduction to his 1934 book, and not a beginning of a presumptuous new style.

And the variation in the names within Yang Chengfu's descriptions of the sequence suggests that, however constant the sequence may have been through the centuries since the origination of this discipline, words for describing it may have developed along the way.

But, for those of you who wish to call the forms what Yang Chengfu called them, I've presented his designations not only in literal English translation but also in both *zì* and *pīnyīn*.

So you may verify them as you wish.

太極拳起勢預備
Tài jí quán qǐ shì yù bèi
Tàijíquán Beginning Potentiality, Advance Preparation.

Face south with the gaze song and levelly forward,
the feet parallel and shoulder-width apart,
and the legs nearly straight.
The spine, from the *wěilú* through the neck, is in *xū líng dǐng jìn*.
The shoulders and elbows are *sōng*
with the arms hanging *sōng* from the shoulders
and the hands and fingers hanging *sōng* from the wrists.
Then, with the *yāo* also *sōng*, sink the *qì* to the *dāntián*.

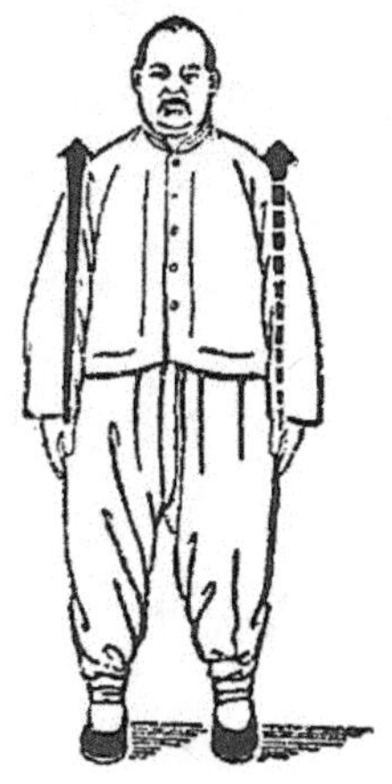

This is the *wújí* stance.

Then raise the hands toward the south to shoulder-level
while keeping the arms nearly straight
and turning the palms downward.
And then, while settling the wrists
to keep the palms facing downward,
push the hands downward until the arms are again *sōng*
with the right hand below and southwest of the *yāo*,
the left hand below and southeast of the *yāo*,
and the fingers of both hands pointing toward the south.
The gaze remains levelly toward the south.

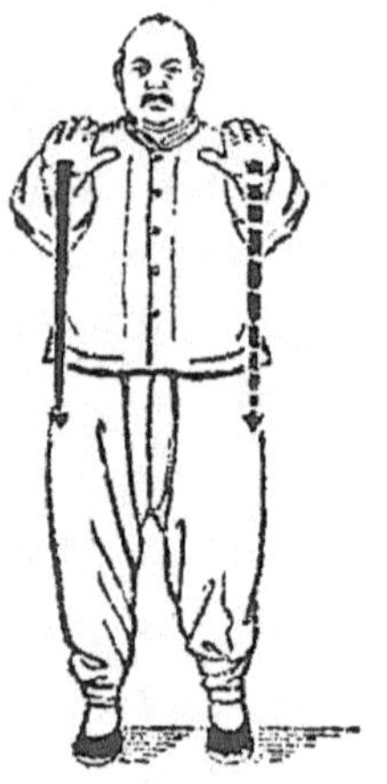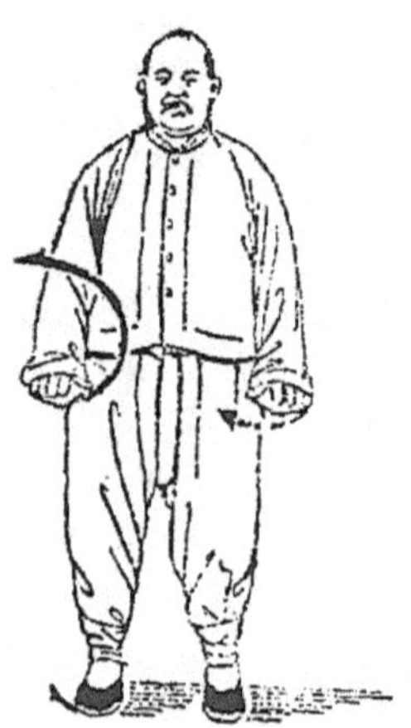

Yang Chengfu doesn't number this segment. But he says people
tend to neglect it and that the neglect is failure to recognize that
one can dissociate none of the applications from it. And he
expresses hope that readers or students give it both attention and
precedence.

1.

攬雀尾掤法

Lǎn què wěi bīng (peng) fǎ

Grasp Sparrow Tail: Arrow Quiver Cover (Ward-Off) Method.

Turning the right foot on its heel southwestward,
turn the torso southwestward
while circling the right hand eastward and upward
and then westward to southwest of the abdomen
for its palm to face downward and southeastward,
and shift the left hand westward and upward
to south of the left side of the *yāo.*
And then, bending the right knee to shift the weight to it,
lift the left knee to swing its foot toward the right ankle
and then to the south and then back toward the right ankle
while circling the right hand westward and upward
and then eastward to southwest of the sternum
and arcing the left hand westward
to turn its palm toward the right palm as if to hold a sphere.
The gaze shifts levelly with the turning of the body.

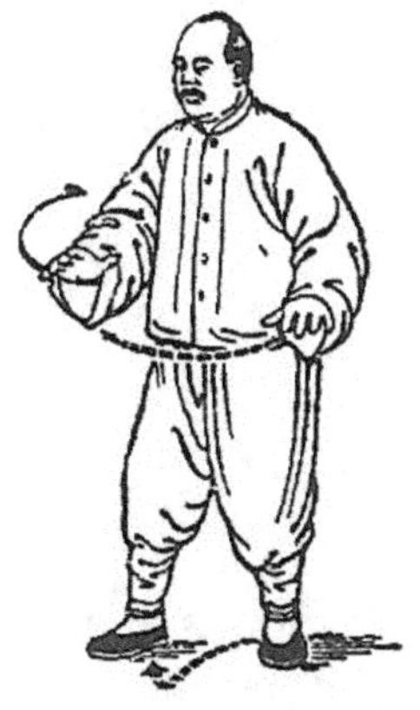 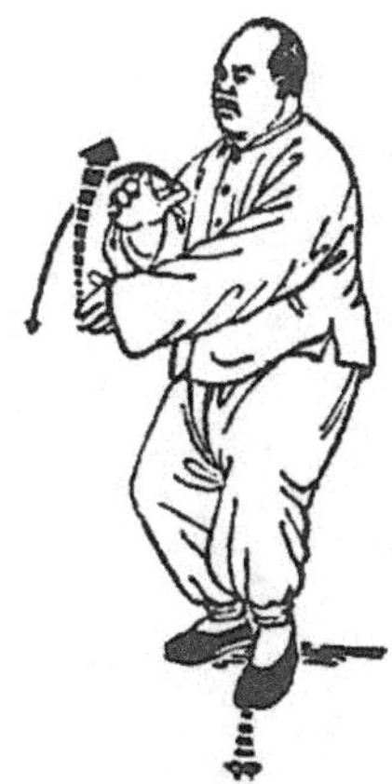

The second of these two illustrations, like other illustrations of as if
holding a sphere, isn't of the moment of the resemblance.

Then, stepping the left foot to the south
to shift into a left bow stance,
shift the left hand up to shoulder-level
while turning its palm upward and toward the north
and arcing the right hand westward and downward
for its palm to face downward from west of the *yāo*.
Then, shifting the left foot on its ball northeastward
and lifting the right knee
to circle the right foot toward the left foot and then westward,
circle the right hand downward and southeastward
and then upward to southwest of the abdomen
while turning its palm upward and southeastward
and sinking the left elbow to draw the left hand eastward
while turning its palm toward the right palm as if to hold a sphere
with the left hand at the level of the sternum
and the right hand at the level of the left wrist.
The gaze remains levelly southwestward.

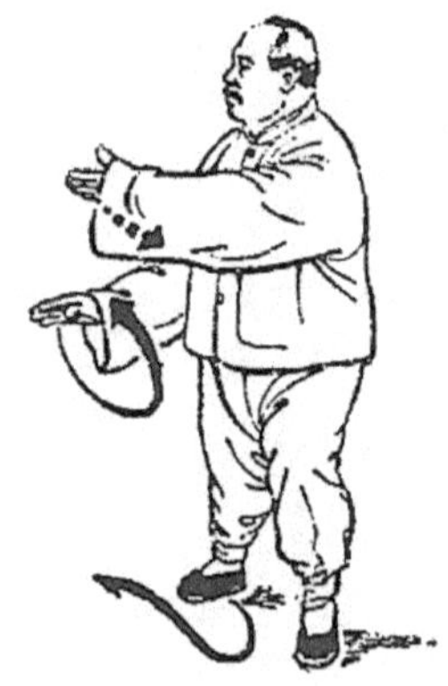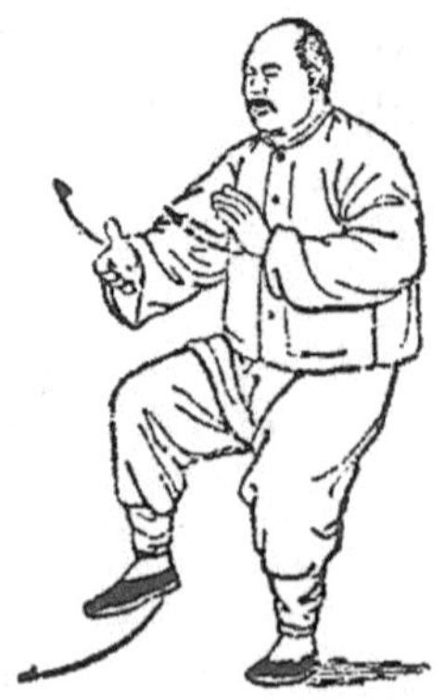

The instructions regarding the gaze with these descriptions, mainly
only serving as reminders that the gaze generally follows the
motion, are neither precise nor comprehensive.

Then step the right foot westward
to touch its heel to the ground *xū*
while shifting the right hand westward and upward
and shifting the left hand levelly westward
for its fingers to point upward toward the right wrist.
And then, shifting the weight westward into a right bow stance
while shifting the right hand further westward and upward
to west of the face for its palm to face the face,
shift the left hand with the right hand
while settling its wrist for its fingertips to point further upward.

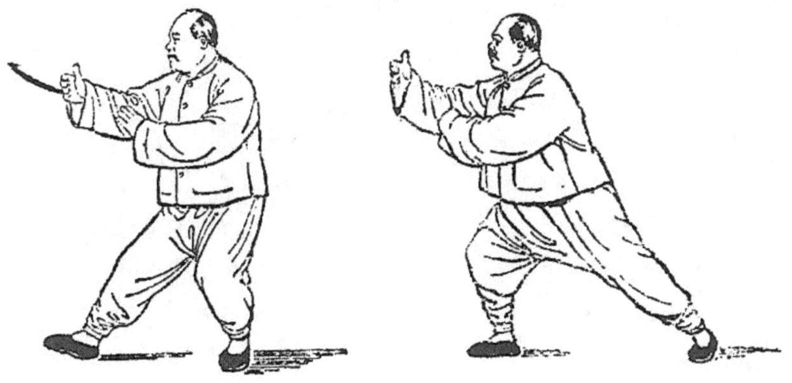

Yang Chengfu says the Grasp Sparrow Tail form is the main hand application of the essence and application of *Tàijíquán*.

2.

攬雀尾抒法

Lǎn què wěi lǚ fǎ

Grasp Sparrow Tail: Stroke (Rollback) Method.

Turning the right palm downward and westward
while turning the left palm upward and toward the north,
begin to roll the hands downward and eastward.
Then, to continue rolling the hands downward and eastward,
bend the left knee to straighten the right leg
to shift the weight eastward onto the left leg.

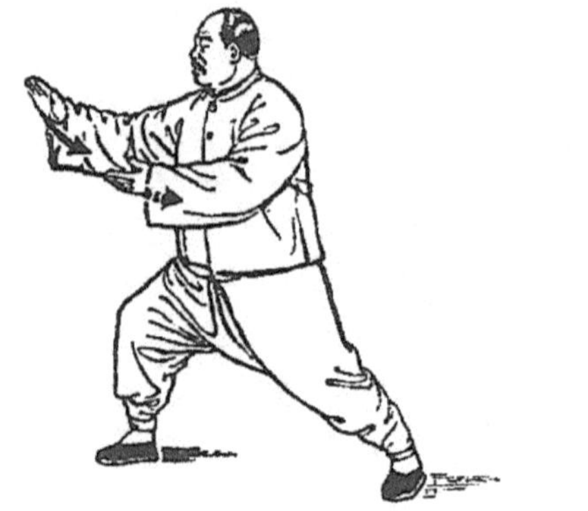 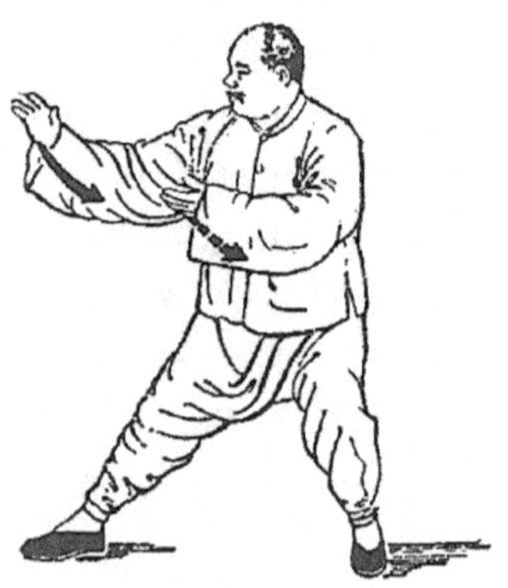

Yang Chengfu also says the *Tàijíquán* use of the designation for
this component of the Grasp Sparrow Tail form differs from its
original meaning for reasons particular to both *Tàijíquán* and
martial arts. But pointing that out leaves to each practitioner's
discretion the question of whether to call these first two
components of the Grasp Sparrow Tail form Arrow Quiver Cover
and Stroke or call them Ward-Off and Rollback. And the
differences aren't extremely polar.

And then, keeping the elbows at least a fist's width from the torso,
continue rolling the hands downward and eastward
while turning the right palm southeastward.
The gaze follows the right hand.

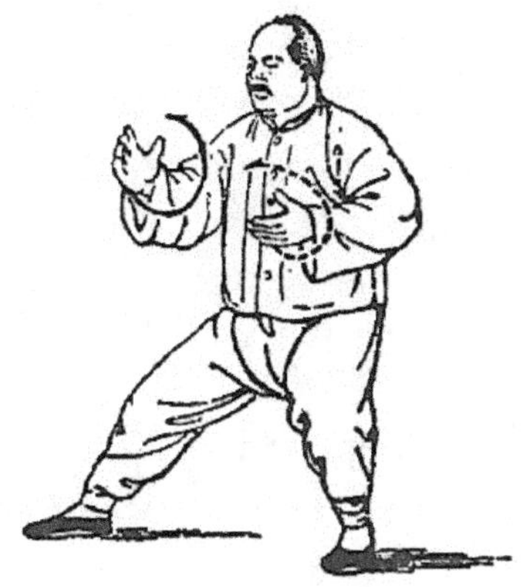

3.
攬雀尾擠法
Lǎn què wěi jǐ fǎ
Grasp Sparrow Tail: Press Method.

Beginning to shift the weight westward,
circle both hands downward and southeastward
and then upward and westward
to turn the left palm downward and westward
while turning the right palm eastward.
And then, completing the shift of the weight westward
to shift into a right bow stance,
press the back of the right hand westward and upward
for its palm to face the face,
and push the left hand westward and upward
while settling its wrist
to press the right forearm further westward.
The gaze is toward the right wrist.

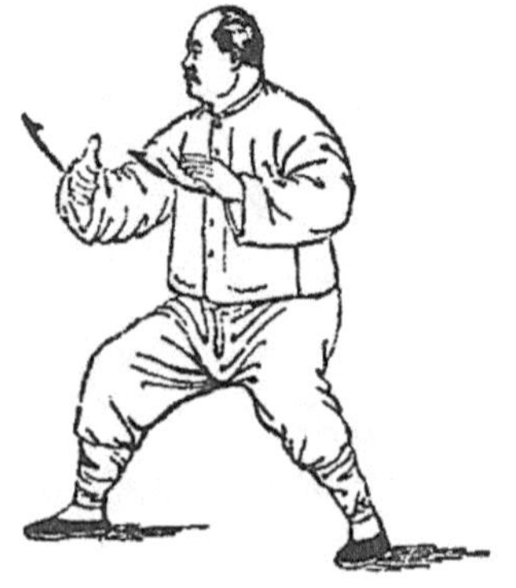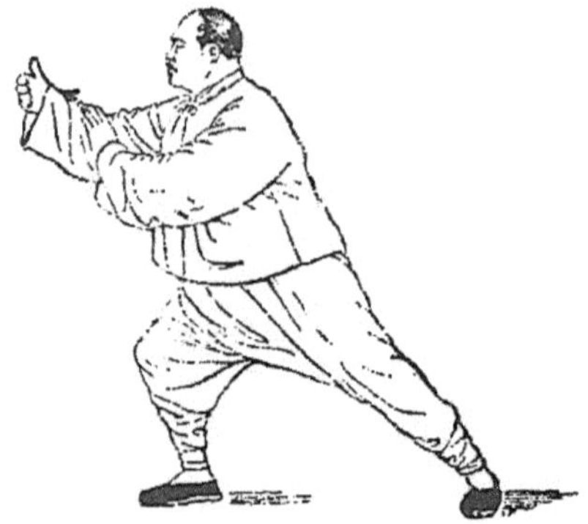

4.

攬雀尾按法
Lǎn què wěi àn fǎ
Grasp Sparrow Tail: Push Method.

Turning the torso westward,
shift the right hand down to shoulder-level,
and pass the left hand over the right wrist
while turning both palms downward
to spread them shoulder-width apart.
Then, turning the palms to face one another
with their fingers pointing upward and westward,
sink the elbows to draw the hands eastward toward the sternum
while bending the left knee to straighten the right leg
to shift the weight to the left leg.
The gaze is level and westward.

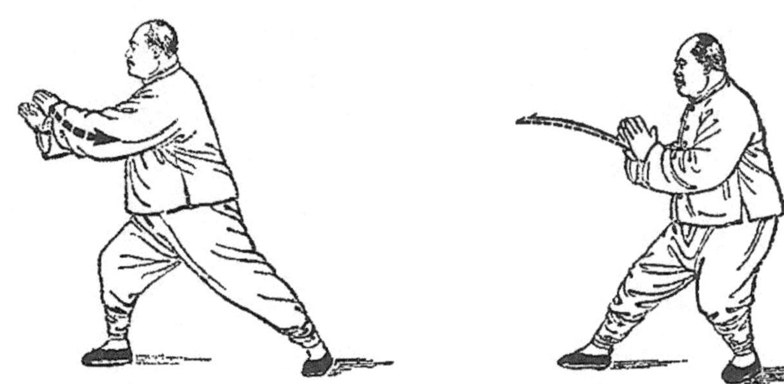

And then quickly straighten the wrists
to turn the palms downward
to push them upward and forward while settling their wrists
and shifting the weight westward again into a right bow stance.
The gaze remains level and forward.

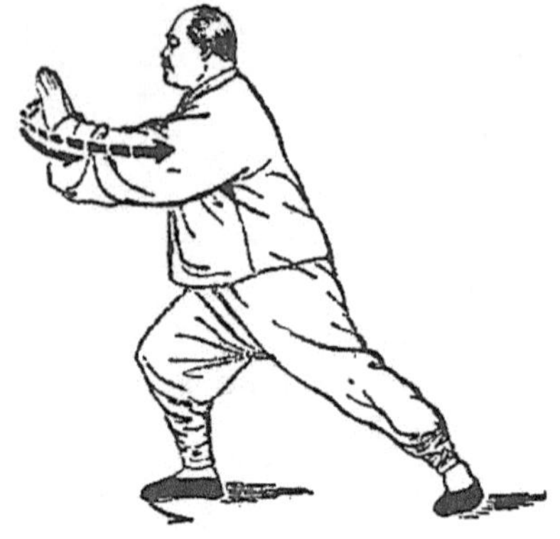

"Quickly", "promptly", and "swiftly" here and in other
descriptions in this book are translation specific to Yang Chengfu's
instructions but must never be jerking or otherwise not *sōng*.

5.
單鞭
Dān biān
Solitary Whip.

Bending the left knee and straightening the right leg
to shift the weight to the left leg, turn the torso southwestward,
and turn the right foot on its heel southwestward
while swinging the hands with the turn
and beginning to turn the palms downward.
And then, turning the torso southeastward
while swinging the arms with the turn
and continuing to turn the palms downward,
turn the left foot on its ball northwestward,
and turn the right foot on its ball also northwestward
while bending the right knee while straightening the left knee
to shift the weight to the right leg.
The gaze levelly shifts with the turn.

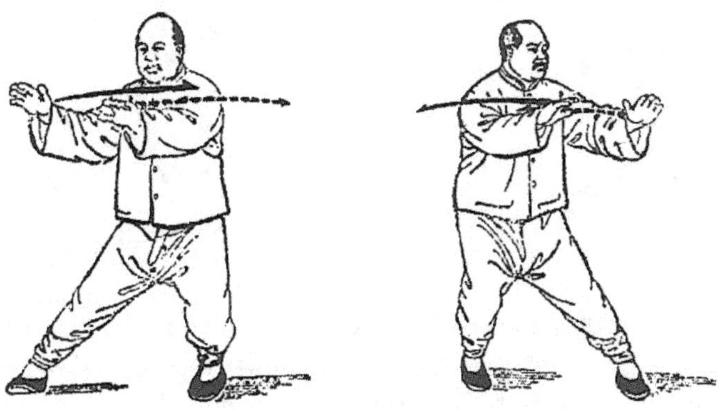

Turning the torso or a palm in a direction is facing it in that
direction. Turning a foot on its heel in a direction is pointing its
toes in that direction. Turning a foot on its ball in a direction is
pointing its heel in that direction.

Then, keeping the weight on the right leg,
turn the torso again southwestward
while swinging the arms with the turn
and shifting the gaze with the turn.
And then, again turning the torso southeastward
while shifting the left hand
upward and eastward to southeast of the chin
to turn its palm toward the chin,
lift the left knee eastward,
and *sōng* the right wrist while extending its hand westward
and gathering its fingers and thumb to each other
for the hand to hang downward
to form a hook shape with its wrist.
The gaze shifts levelly with the turn.

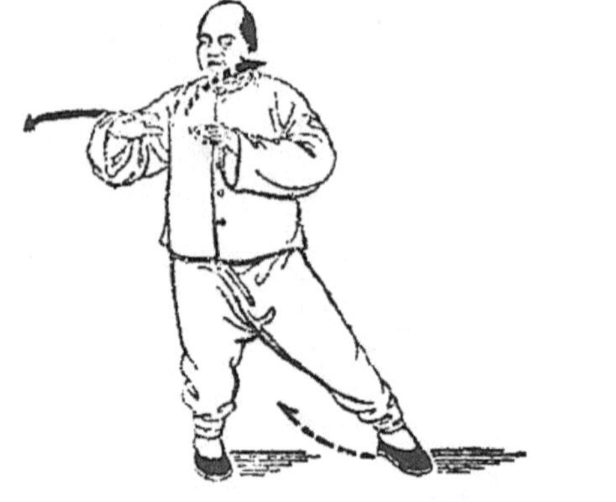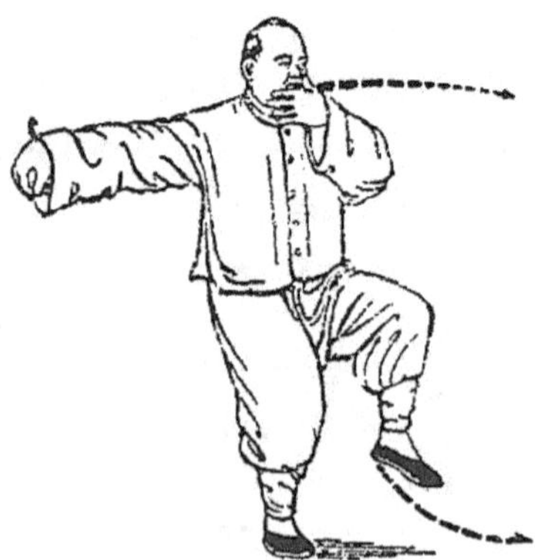

Lifting a knee in a direction doesn't necessarily move the knee in
that direction. Designating the direction of the lifting only
indicates that the knee is pointing in that direction at the
completion of the motion. And an example is that, because of the
beginning position of the leg and the turning of the torso and the
yāo, this lifting of the knee is nearly directly vertical.

Then, shifting the right hand up to shoulder-level
and stepping the left foot eastward into a left bow stance,
extend the left hand eastward while turning its palm downward
before settling its wrist and turning its palm southeastward.
The gaze shifts levelly with the motion of the left hand.

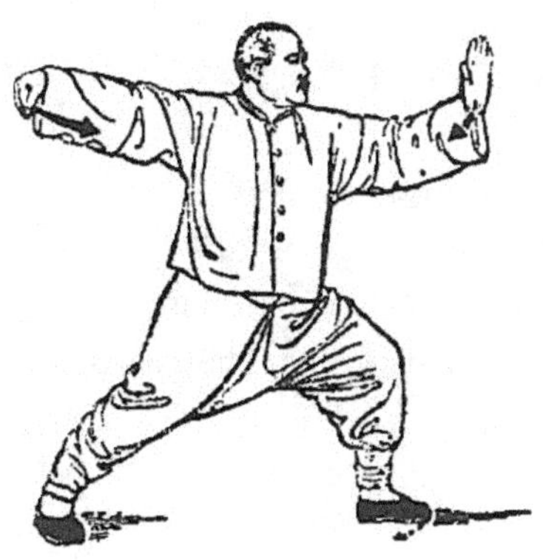

6.
提手上式
Tí shǒu shàng shì
Raise Hands Up Form.

Shifting the right foot on its ball northeastward
to turn the torso toward the south,
sōng the right hand while straightening its wrist
and turning its palm toward the south,
and then, turning the left foot on its heel southeastward,
sink both elbows, and turn the left palm toward the south
for the fingers of the left hand to point upward and eastward
while the fingers of the right hand point upward and westward.
Then swing the right foot southeastward
to touch its heel to the ground *xū* with its toes upward
while drawing the left hand downward and southwestward
to southeast of the sternum for its palm to face the sternum
and arcing the right hand upward and southeastward
to above and to the south of the right shoulder
for its palm to face eastward at the level of the face
with its fingers pointing upward and toward the south.
The gaze is toward the right palm.

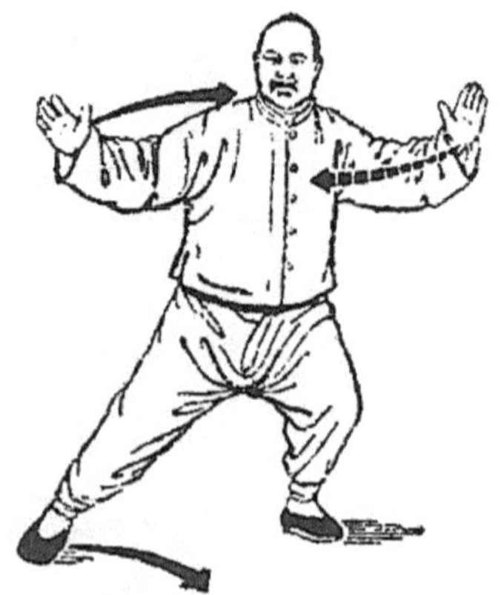 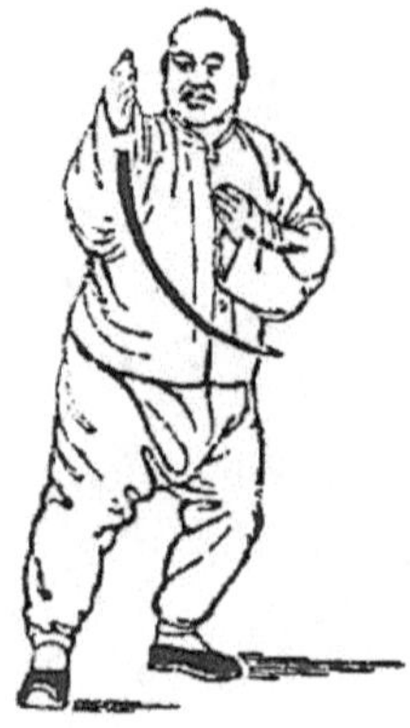

7.

白鶴亮翅

Bái hè liàng chì
White Crane Shines Wings.

Turning the torso southeastward,
arc the right hand downward and eastward
to southeast of the abdomen
while turning its palm downward and northeastward
and shifting the left hand southeastward
to turn its palm downward and northwestward.
And then turn the palms toward one another
as if to hold a sphere
while beginning to lift the right knee to the south
to shift the right hand eastward and upward
while turning its palm northeastward.
The gaze follows the right hand
before shifting toward the left elbow
before leveling toward the south.

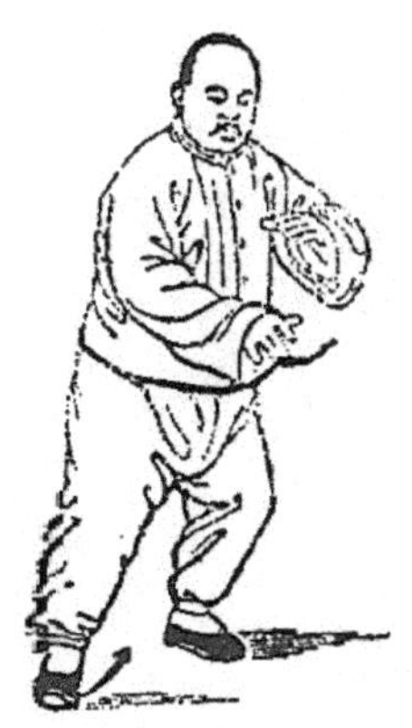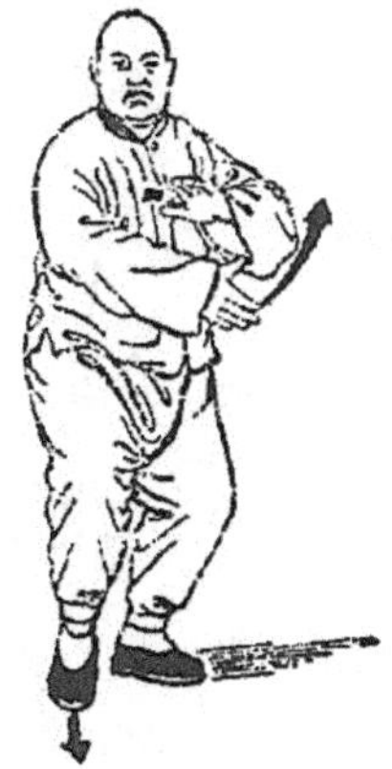

The leaning of the torso in the first of these illustrations and in
illustrations of other forms is contrary to Yang Chengfu's
injunctions against swaying and against the general injunction in
the *Tàijíquán Lùn* not to lean or incline. So the reader may decide
whether that leaning is intentional or accidental deviation from *xū
líng dǐng jìn*. But, whichever, *sōng* remains the first principle.

Then, stepping the right foot to the south
into a right bow stance with the right toes pointing southeastward,
turn the torso further southeastward
while continuing the arc of the right hand eastward and upward
to east of the right shoulder
and swinging the left hand with the turn
to point its fingers upward and over the right elbow.
The gaze follows the motion of the right forearm and hand.
And then, turning the torso eastward,
step the left foot southeastward to east of the right heel
to set it on the ground *xū,*
and arc the left hand downward and toward the north
to above and to the north of the left knee
while settling its wrist to keep its palm downward
and arcing the right hand southwestward and upward
to above and to the southeast of the forehead
while turning its palm eastward.
The gaze levelly shifts to the east with the turn.

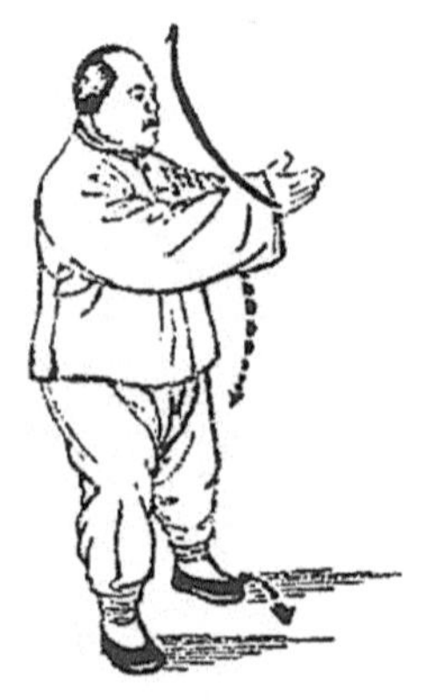
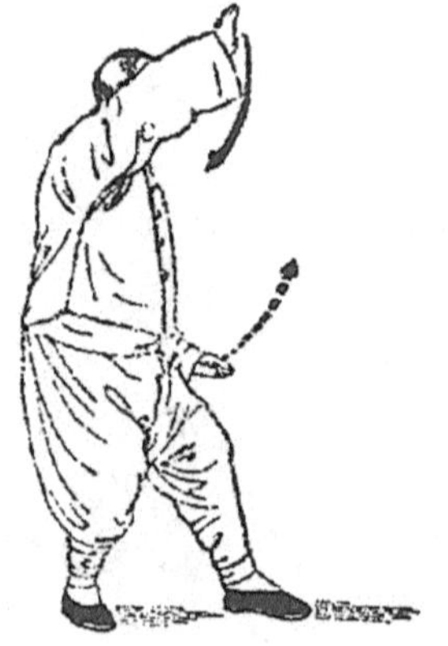

8.

摟膝拗步用法

Lǒu xī ǎo bù yòng fǎ
Draw and Bend Knee to Step Use Method.

Turning the torso southeastward,
sink the right elbow to draw the right hand downward
while turning its palm toward the face
and arcing the left hand southeastward and upward
for its fingers to point upward and toward the south.
And then arc the right hand downward and westward
to south of the right side of the *yāo*
while turning its palm toward the abdomen
and drawing the left hand westward toward the sternum.
The gaze follows the right palm.

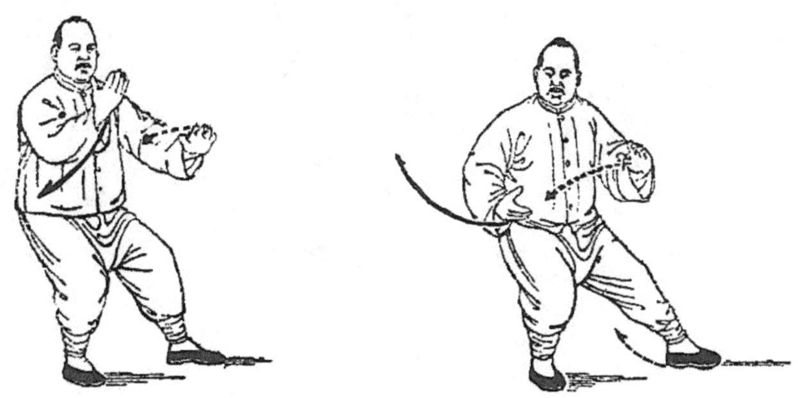

The *zì* meaning "use", in this phrase meaning "use method" some
translate "usage", is an adjective modifying the *zì* meaning
"method" and not a verb of which the *zì* meaing "method" is an
object.

Then, lifting the left knee eastward,
arc the right hand westward and upward
while turning its palm upward and southeastward
and arcing the left hand southwestward and downward
to south of the abdomen.
The gaze continues to follow the right palm.
And then, arcing the right hand upward and eastward
to southwest of the right ear
while turning its palm downward and northeastward,
step the left foot eastward to touch its heel to the ground *xū*,
and arc the left hand downward and eastward
to southeast of the *yāo* while turning its palm downward.

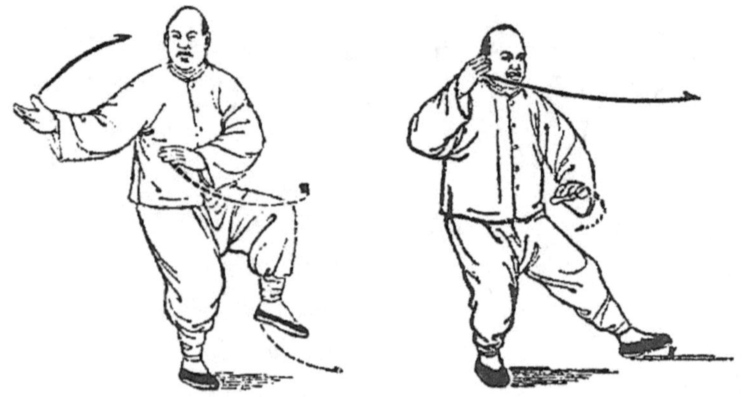

And then, turning the torso eastward,
shift the weight eastward into a left bow stance
while pushing the right hand eastward while settling its wrist
for its palm to face northeastward
and brushing the left hand eastward and downward
and then northwestward to above and to the north of the left knee
while keeping its palm facing downward.
The gaze continues to follow the right hand.

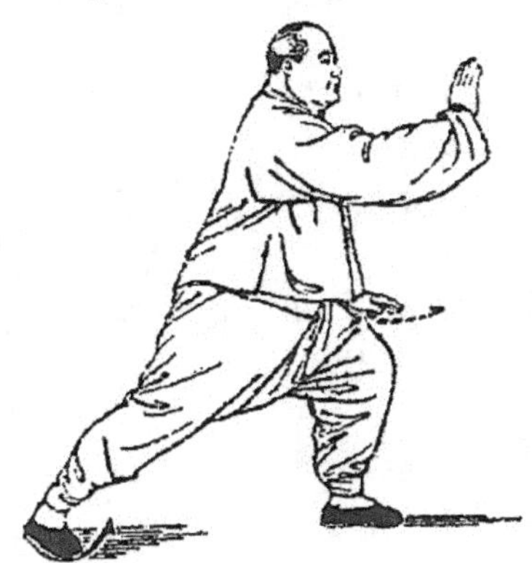

9.
手揮琵琶
Shǒu huī pí pá
Hand Strums Pipa.

Lifting the right heel to begin to draw the right foot eastward,
begin to arc the left hand eastward and upward
while straightening both wrists.
And then, turning the torso southeastward,
draw the right foot eastward to south of the left foot
to shift it on its ball northwestward to settle it flat
to shift the weight to it to step the left foot eastward
to touch its heel to the ground *xū*
while continuing the arc of the left hand eastward and upward
to east of the face while turning its palm toward the south
for its fingers to point upward and eastward
and drawing the right hand downward and westward
to east of the sternum
while turning its palm downward and northwestward
for its fingers to point toward the left elbow.
The gaze is past the left hand.

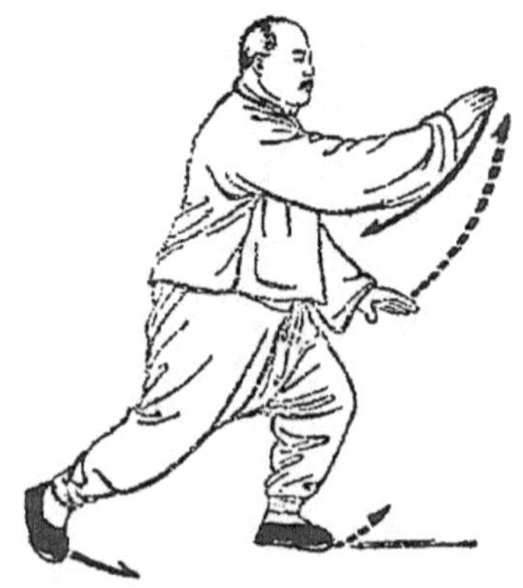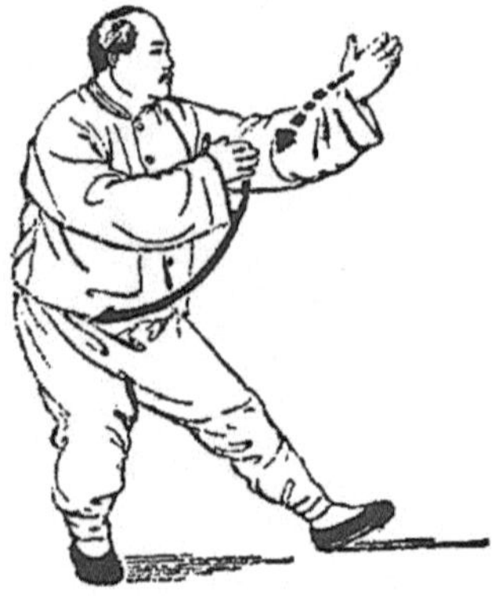

A pipa is like a lute.

10.

搂膝拗步用法

Lǒu xī ǎo bù yòng fǎ

Draw and Bend Knee to Step Use Method.

Turning the torso further southeastward,
draw the left hand westward and downward toward the sternum
while turning its palm downward and southwestward
and arcing the right hand downward and southwestward
to south of the right side of the *yāo*
for its palm to face the *yāo*.
The gaze, remaining level, shifts with the turn.
Then, lifting the left knee eastward,
arc the right hand westward and upward
while turning its palm upward and southeastward
and arcing the left hand southwestward and downward
to south of the abdomen.
The gaze continues to follow the right palm.

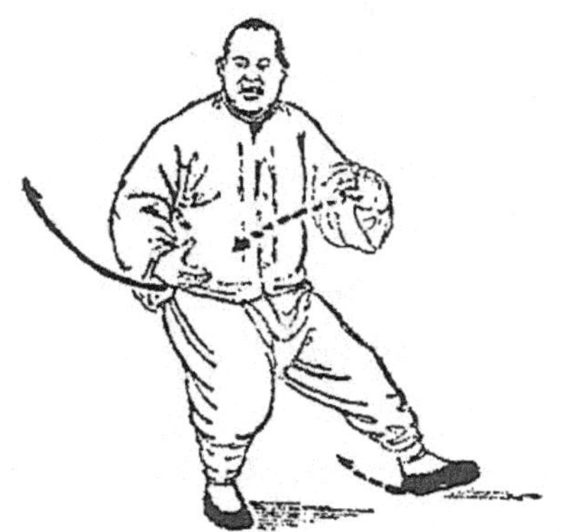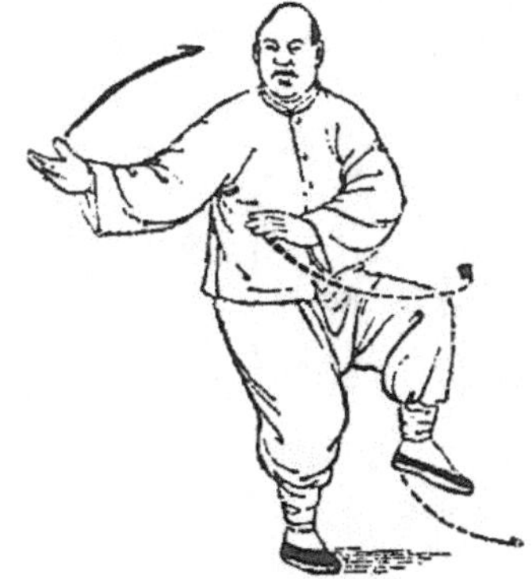

And then, arcing the right hand upward and eastward
to southwest of the right ear
while turning its palm downward and northeastward,
step the left foot eastward to touch its heel to the ground *xū*,
and arc the left hand downward and eastward
to southeast of the *yāo* while turning its palm downward.
Then, turning the torso eastward,
shift the weight eastward into a left bow stance
while pushing the right hand eastward while settling its wrist
for its palm to face northeastward
and brushing the left hand eastward and downward
and then northwestward to above and to the north of the left knee
while keeping its palm facing downward.
The gaze follows the right hand.

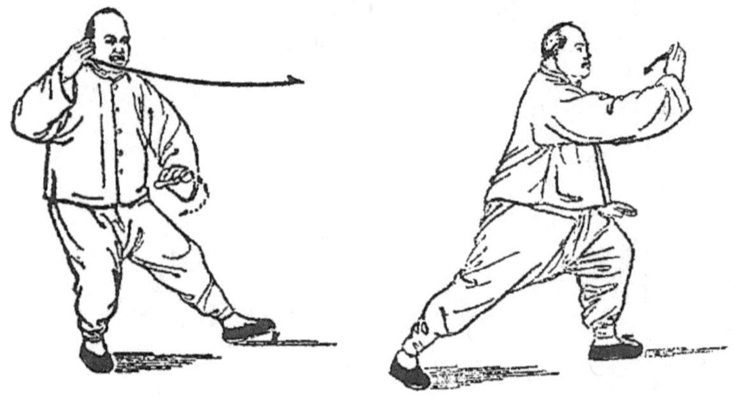

11.
右摟膝
Yòu xī ǎo
Right Drawing Knee.

Turning the left foot on its heel northeastward,
lift the right heel to shift into the tray stance
while turning the torso northeastward
and swinging the hands with the turn
while sinking the right elbow until its forearm is horizontal
with its palm facing downward and northwestward.
And then, lifting the right knee eastward,
arc the left hand westward and upward to northwest of the left ear
while turning its palm upward and eastward
and arcing the right hand upward and northwestward
and then downward to east of the abdomen
while turning its palm downward.
The gaze shifts from the right hand toward the left hand.

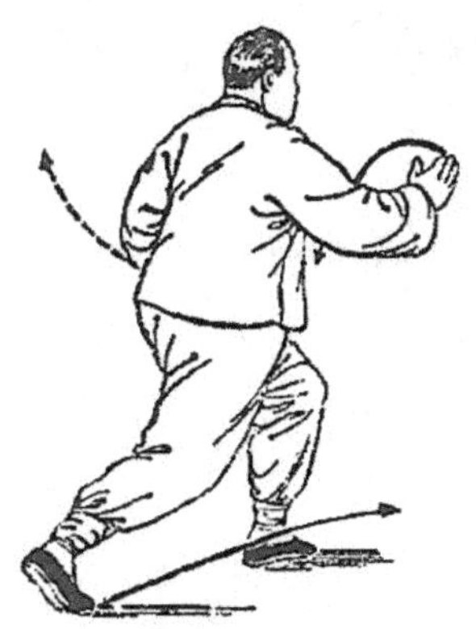
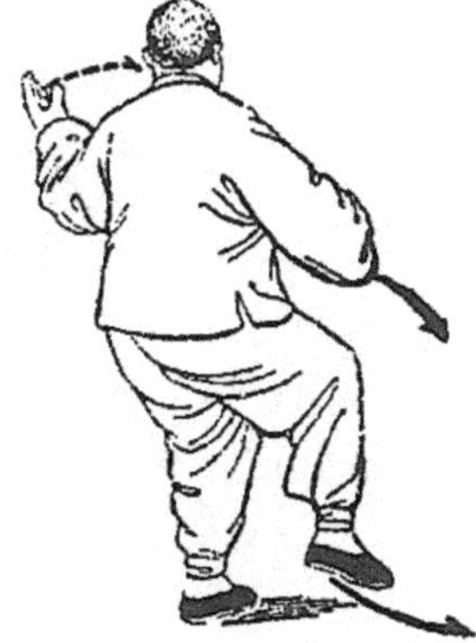

And then, stepping the right foot eastward
to touch its heel to the ground *xū*,
shift the right hand southeastward to above the right knee,
and push the left palm eastward to north of the left ear
while settling its wrist to keep it facing eastward.
And then, shifting the weight eastward into a right bow stance,
turn the torso eastward
while pushing the left palm further eastward
and further settling its wrist to keep it facing eastward
while brushing the right hand southeastward and downward
and then westward to above and to the south of the right knee
while keeping its palm downward.
The gaze follows the left hand pushing forward.

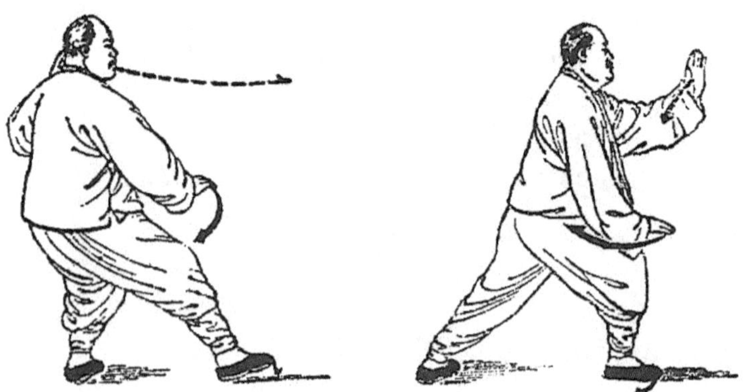

What makes this and other forms left or right is which foot is
furthest forward at the end of the segment.

12.

左摟膝

Zuǒ xī ǎo

Left Drawing Knee.

Shifting the right foot on its heel southeastward
to turn the torso southeastward,
draw the left hand southwestward and downward
to southeast of the sternum
while turning its palm southwestward
and shifting the right hand westward
to south of the right side of the *yāo*
while turning its palm toward the *yāo*.
The gaze shifts levelly with the turn.
Then, lifting the left knee eastward,
arc the right hand westward and upward
while turning its palm upward and southeastward
and arcing the left hand westward and downward
to south of the abdomen
while turning its palm downward and northwestward.
The gaze follows the right palm.

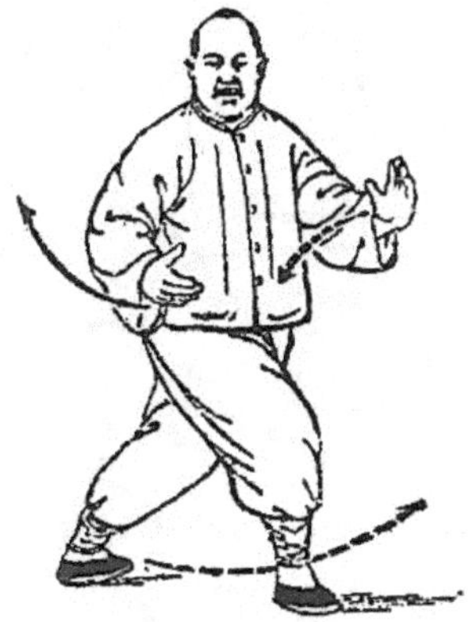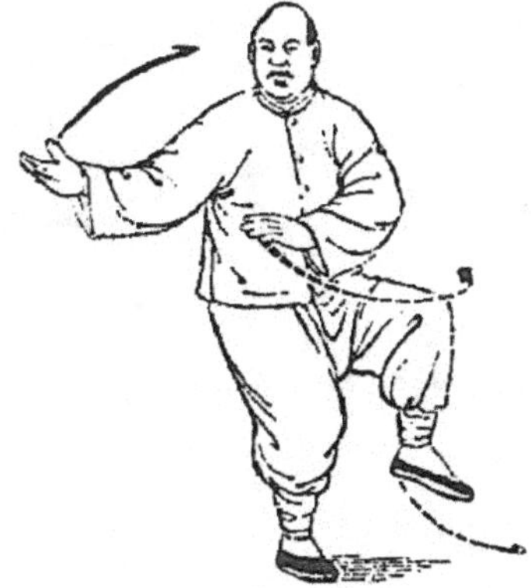

Then, arcing the right hand upward and eastward
to southwest of the right ear
while turning its palm downward and northeastward,
step the left foot eastward to touch its heel to the ground *xū*,
and arc the left hand downward and eastward
to southeast of the *yāo*
while turning its palm downward.
And then, turning the torso eastward,
shift the weight eastward into a left bow stance
while pushing the right hand eastward while settling its wrist
for its palm to face northeastward
and brushing the left hand eastward and downward
and then northwestward to above and to the north of the left knee
while keeping its palm facing downward.
The gaze follows the right hand.

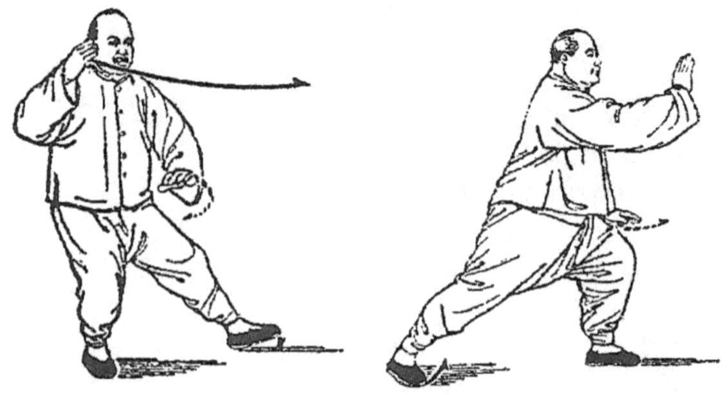

13.
手揮琵琶
Shǒu huī pí pá
Hand Strums Pipa.

Lifting the right heel to begin to draw the right foot eastward,
begin to arc the left hand eastward and upward
while straightening both wrists.
And then, turning the torso southeastward,
draw the right foot eastward to south of the left foot
to shift it on its ball northwestward to settle it flat
to shift the weight to it to step the left foot eastward
to touch its heel to the ground *xū*
while continuing the arc of the left hand eastward and upward
to east of the face while turning its palm toward the south
for its fingers to point upward and eastward
and drawing the right hand downward and westward
to east of the sternum
while turning its palm downward and northwestward
for its fingers to point toward the left elbow.
The gaze is past the left hand.

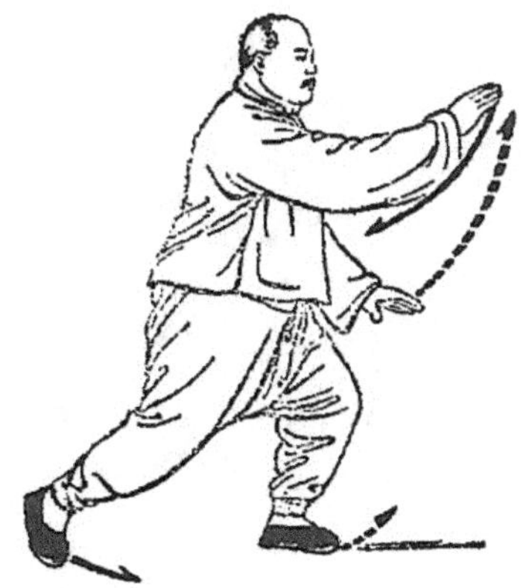 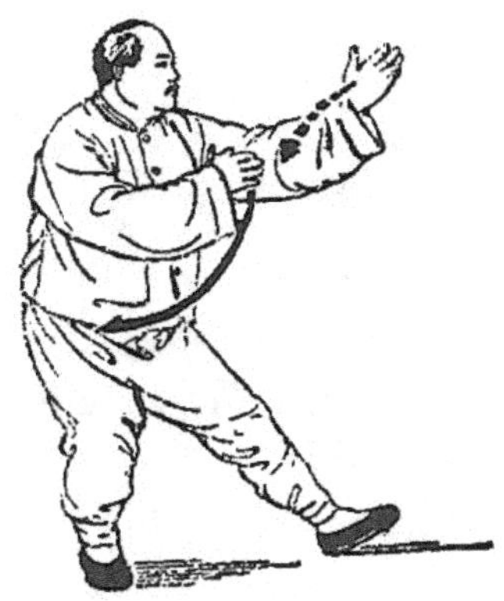

Transitional Draw and Bend Knee to Step Use Method repetition.

Drawing the left hand
westward and downward toward the sternum,
turn its palm downward and southwestward,
and arc the right hand downward and southwestward
to south of the right side of the *yāo*
for its palm to face the *yāo*.
The gaze, remaining level, shifts with the turn.
Then, lifting the left knee eastward,
arc the right hand westward and upward
while turning its palm upward and southeastward
and arcing the left hand southwestward and downward
to south of the abdomen.
The gaze continues to follow the right palm.

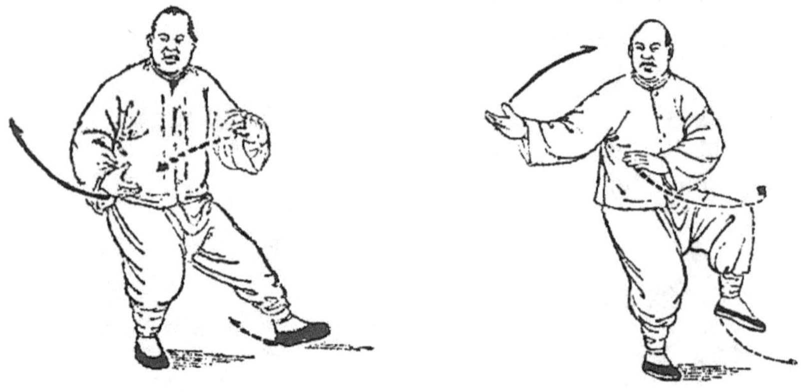

Neither Yang Chengfu's books nor Fu Zhongwen's book specifies
this repetition. But, as with the previous Hand Strums Pipa form,
it's essential to the flow of motion into the next form. And the
illustrations indicate that.

And then, arcing the right hand upward and eastward
to southwest of the right ear
while turning its palm downward and northeastward,
step the left foot eastward to touch its heel to the ground *xū*,
and arc the left hand downward and eastward
to southeast of the *yāo* while turning its palm downward.
Then, turning the torso eastward,
shift the weight eastward into a left bow stance
while pushing the right hand eastward while settling its wrist
and brushing the left hand eastward and downward
and then northwestward to above and to the north of the left knee
while keeping its palm facing downward.
The gaze follows the right hand.

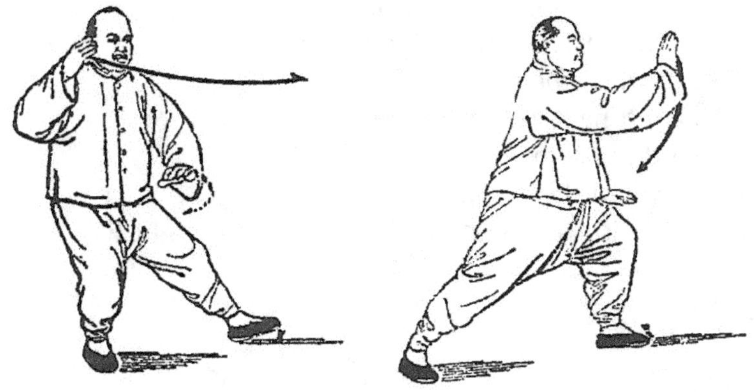

14.

進步搬攔捶用法

Jìn bù bān lán chuí yòng fǎ
Advance Step Shift Block Cudgel Use Method.

Turning the left foot on its heel northeastward
and lifting the right heel to shift into the tray stance,
turn the torso northeastward
while swinging the left hand with the turn
and arcing the right hand downward and northwestward
while closing it into a fist
for its heart to face downward from east of the *yāo*.
The gaze shifts levelly with the direction of the right hand.
And then, lifting the right knee eastward,
coil the right fist northwestward and upward
to northeast of the abdomen
while arcing the left hand westward and upward
and then eastward to northwest of the left ear
for its palm to face northeastward.
The gaze continues to shift with the direction of the right fist.

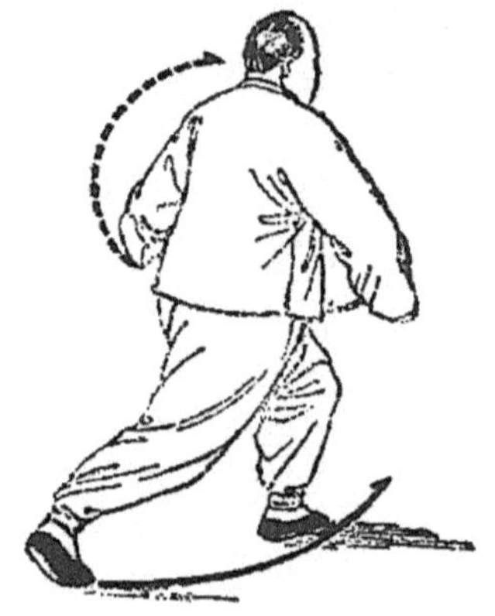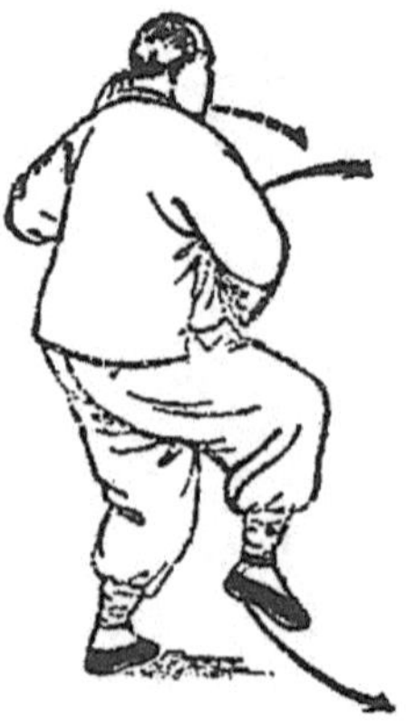

The heart of a fist is the palm of the hand while it's in a fist.

Then, turning the torso eastward,
step the right foot southeastward
to touch its heel to the ground *xū*
to turn it southeastward with its toes upward
while arcing the right fist upward and eastward
and arcing the left hand southeastward and downward
to cross the hands in front of the sternum
with the left palm facing south with its fingers pointing upward
and the right fist on the outside with its heart northwestward.
And then, turning the torso southeastward
and settling the right foot flat and *shí* pointing southeastward,
bend the right knee to settle the weight onto the right leg
to lift the left knee eastward
while arcing the right fist downward and southwestward
to south of the abdomen
and beginning to extend the left hand eastward.
The gaze is over the left hand.

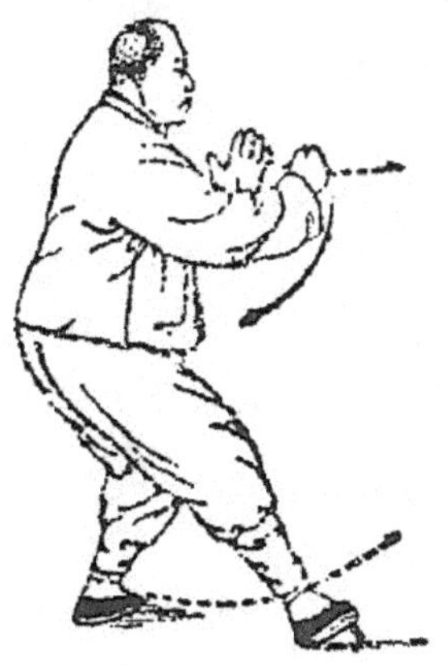 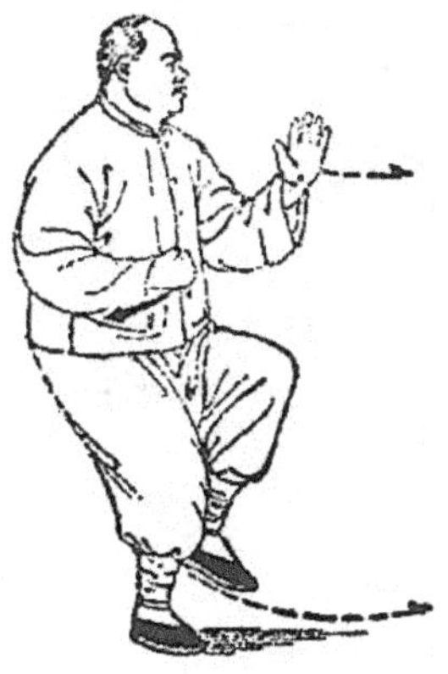

Then step the left foot eastward
to touch its heel to the ground *xū*
while continuing to extend the left hand eastward
and continuing the arc of the right fist westward.
And then, turning the torso eastward
while shifting the weight eastward into a left bow stance,
cudgel the right fist upward and eastward
while drawing the left hand southwestward
toward the right shoulder
as the right forearm glides eastward past it
until the right arm is nearly straight
with the left palm facing the right forearm
with its thumb nearly touching the right elbow.
The gaze follows the left palm before shifting to the right fist.

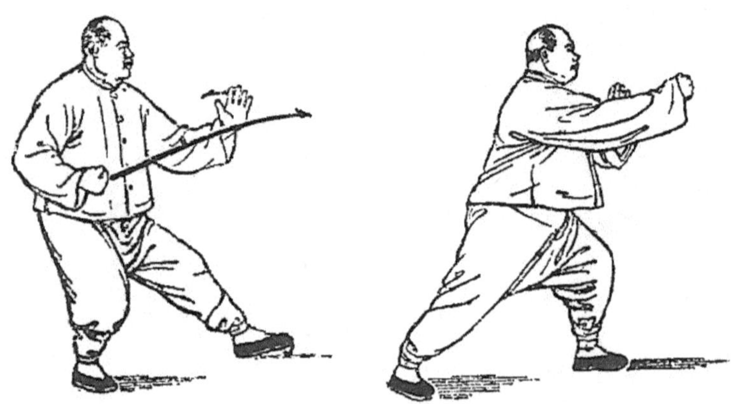

15.

如封似閉

Rú fēng shì bì

As Sealing Like Closing.

Thread the left hand beneath the right elbow
and to the southeast of it to turn the left palm southwestward
while opening the right hand
to turn its palm upward and northwestward.
Then, bending the right knee to shift the weight westward onto it,
sink the right elbow to draw its hand westward toward the clavicle
while shifting the left hand upward to cross the hands
for both palms to face the clavicle with the left hand on the outside
with its fingers pointing upward and toward the south
while the right fingers point upward and toward the north.
The gaze includes the palms.

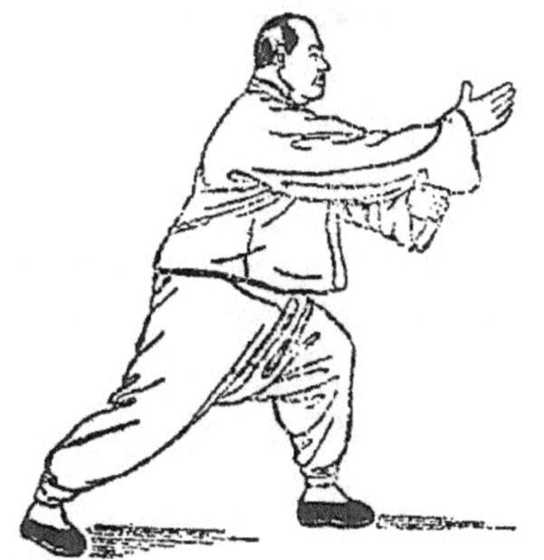 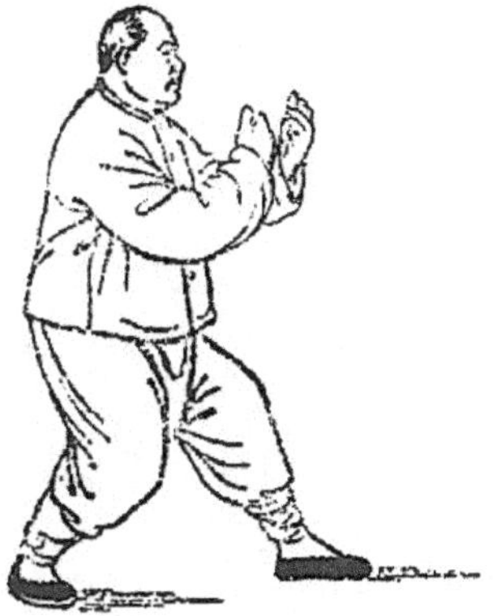

Then, shifting the left hand downward and northwestward while shifting the right hand downward and southeastward, turn the palms to face one another at the level of the sternum. And then, shifting the weight eastward into a left bow stance, push both hands upward and eastward to east of the clavicle while settling their wrists and turning their palms eastward. The gaze is levelly eastward.

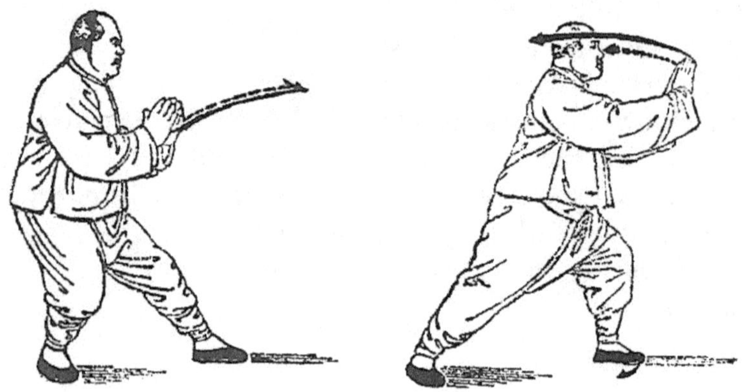

16.

十字手

Shí zì shǒu
Ten *Zì* Hands.

Keeping the weight on the left leg
while turning its foot on its heel to the south,
quickly turn the torso to the south
while swinging the hands with the turn
and turning the right foot on its heel southwestward
while spreading the elbows apart
for the right fingers to point upward and eastward
while the left fingers point upward and westward.
The gaze is through the space between the palms.
Then arc the hands upward and away from one another
and then downward to shoulder-level
for the right fingers to point upward and westward
while the left fingers point upward and eastward.

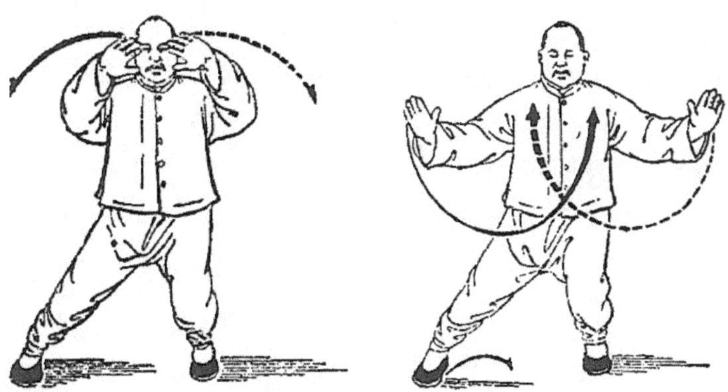

And then, stepping the right foot toward the left foot
into the horse stance,
arc the hands downward and toward one another and then upward
to cross them in front of the clavicle
with the palms facing inward and the right hand on the outside.
The gaze is over the intersection of the wrists.

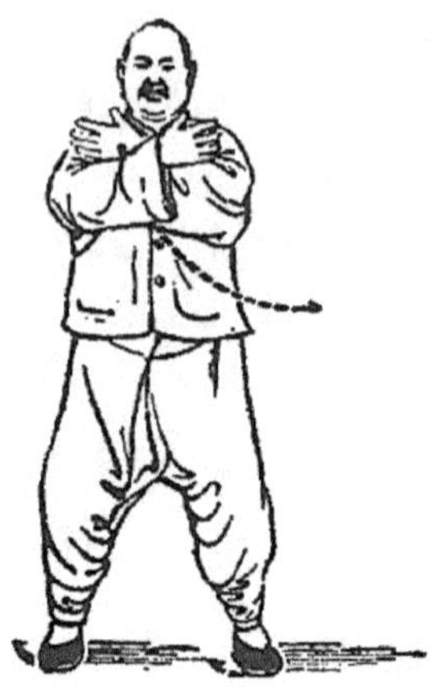

17.

抱虎歸山

Bào hǔ guī shān

Embrace Tiger and Return to Mountain.

Right drawing knee.

Turning the right foot on its heel westward,
promptly turn the torso southwestward
while swinging the right hand with the turn
and turning the left foot on its heel southwestward
while arcing the left hand downward and eastward
to southeast of the *yāo* while turning its palm northwestward.
Then, continuing the southwestward turn of the torso,
lift the right knee westward
while arcing the right hand downward and westward
to southwest of the abdomen while turning its palm downward
and arcing the left hand up to shoulder-level
while turning its palm upward and westward.
The gaze follows the left hand.

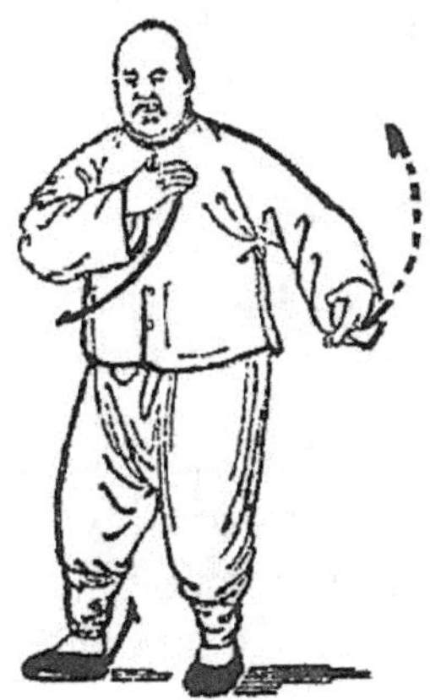
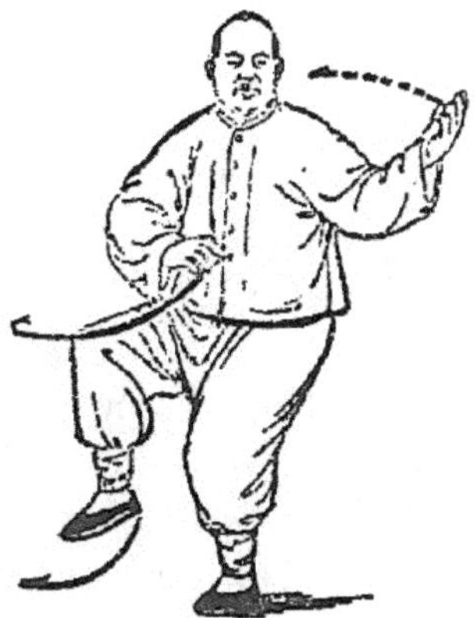

Then, continuing the southwestward turn of the torso
and stepping the right foot northwestward
to touch its heel to the ground *xū*,
arc the left hand upward and westward to southeast of the left ear
while turning its palm downward and northwestward
and shifting the right hand downward and northwestward
to west of the *yāo*
And then, drawing the right hand northeastward
to north of the *yāo*,
shift the weight northwestward into a right bow stance
while turning the torso northwestward
and pushing the left hand northwestward while settling its wrist.
The gaze shifts levelly with the turn
to follow the left hand pushing forward.

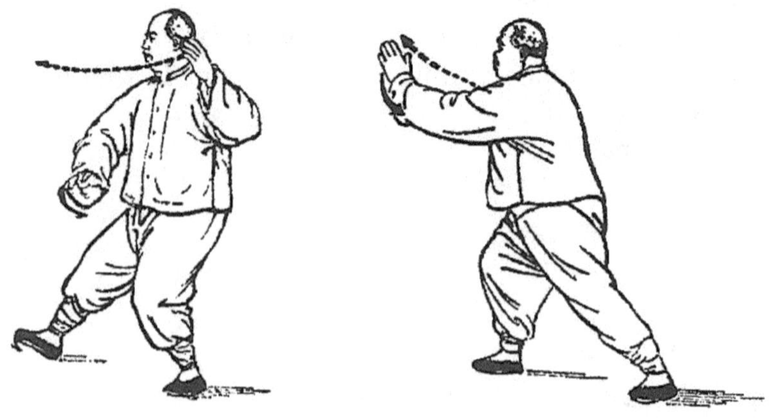

Neither Fu Zhongwen's book nor either of Yang Chengfu's books explains how this repetition of the Right Drawing Knee form with the following repetition of the second through fourth components of the Grasp Sparrow Tail form constitute the Embrace Tiger and Return to Mountain form.

18.

抱虎歸山內之三式

Bào hǔ guī shān nèi zhī sān shì
Embrace Tiger and Return to Mountain:
Its included Three Forms.

Stroke (Rollback).

Sinking the left elbow
to shift its hand down to the level of the sternum,
arc the right hand westward and upward
for its palm to face downward and westward
from west of the right shoulder.
And then, turning the torso southwestward,
straighten the right leg to bend the left knee
to shift the weight southeastward onto the left leg
to roll the right hand downward and southeastward
to the level of the sternum
while sinking the left elbow to roll the left hand southeastward
while turning its palm toward the north.

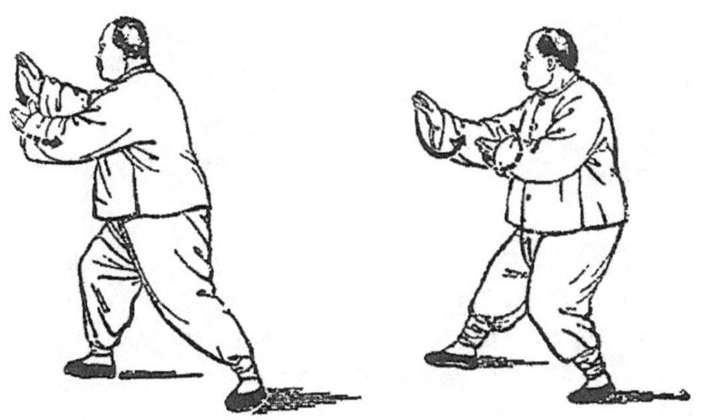

Press.

Turning the torso westward
while beginning to shift the weight again northwestward,
circle both hands downward and southeastward and then upward
for the left palm to face downward and northwestward
at shoulder-level with the right palm facing the left wrist
from northwest of the left forearm.
And then, turning the torso again northwestward
while completing the shift of the weight again northwestward
into a right bow stance,
press the back of the right hand northwestward and upward,
and push the left hand northwestward while settling its wrist
to press the right forearm further northwestward.
The gaze is toward the right forearm.

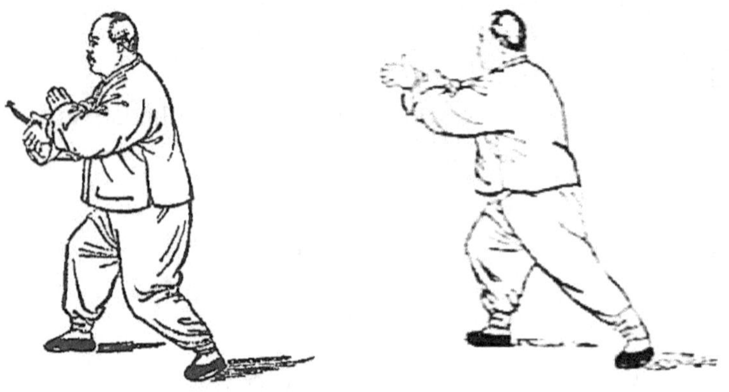

Yang Chengfu specifies that this Press and the following Push are the same as in the Grasp Sparrow Tail form but in a different direction. The difference in direction is that their orientation in this form is northwestward. Their Grasp Sparrow Tail form orientation is westward.

Push:

Pass the left hand over the right wrist
while turning both palms to face downward,
and then spread the hands
to shoulder-width apart at shoulder level.
Then, bending the left knee while straightening the right leg
to shift the weight southeastward to the left leg,
sink the elbows to draw the hands southeastward
for the left palm to face northwestward
while the right palm faces westward,
The gaze is level and westward.

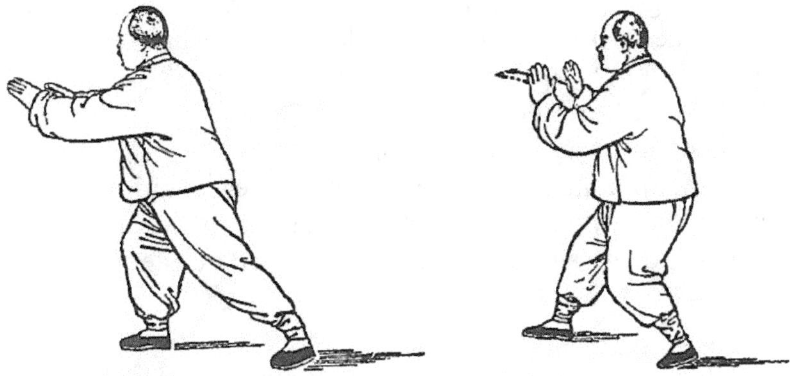

And then, quickly pushing the palms
upward and northwestward while settling their wrists,
again shift the weight northwestward into a right bow stance.
The gaze remains level and forward.

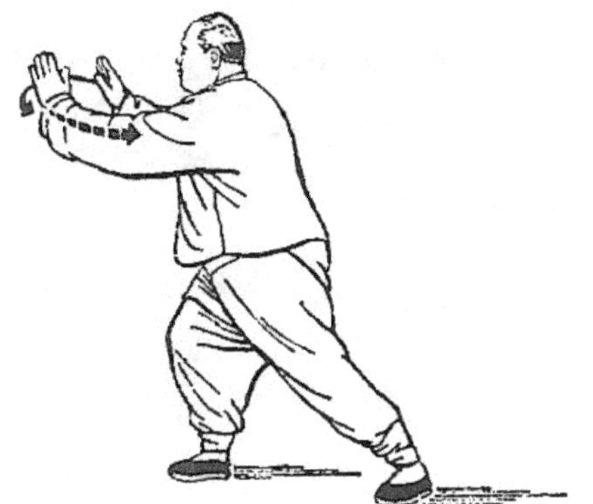

19.

肘底看錘

Zhǒu dǐ kàn chuí

Elbow Bottom Hammer Look

Bending the left knee and straightening the right leg
to shift the weight to the left leg, turn the torso southwestward
while swinging the hands with the turn
and shifting them down to shoulder-level
while straightening the left wrist
and somewhat straightening the right wrist
to turn its palm southwestward.
Then turn the right foot on its heel toward the south,
and bend its knee while straightening the left knee
to return the weight to the right leg
to turn the torso toward the south
while swinging the arms with the turn
and turning the right palm downward and southeastward
while turning the left palm downward and southwestward
and sinking the elbows to draw the hands toward the sternum.

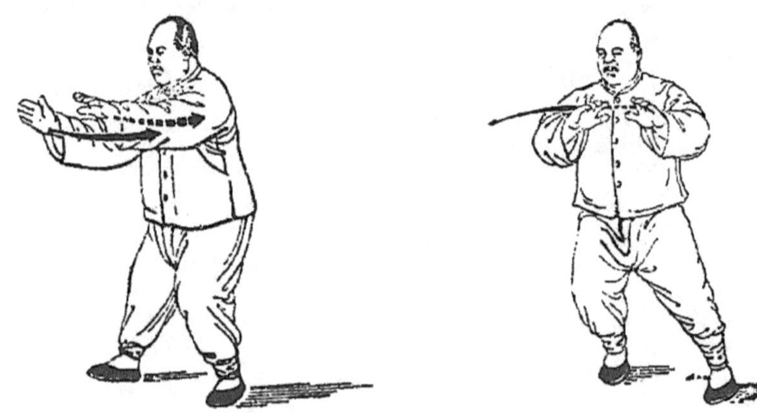

Then, turning the torso again southwestward
to begin lifting the left heel
while again swinging the arms with the turn,
turn the left palm toward the north,
and complete the turn of the right palm downward.
And then, lifting the left knee to swing its foot eastward
to turn the torso again toward the south,
swing the left hand with the turn
while shifting it up to shoulder-level
and turning its palm toward the right shoulder
while extending the right hand westward
while turning its palm toward the south.

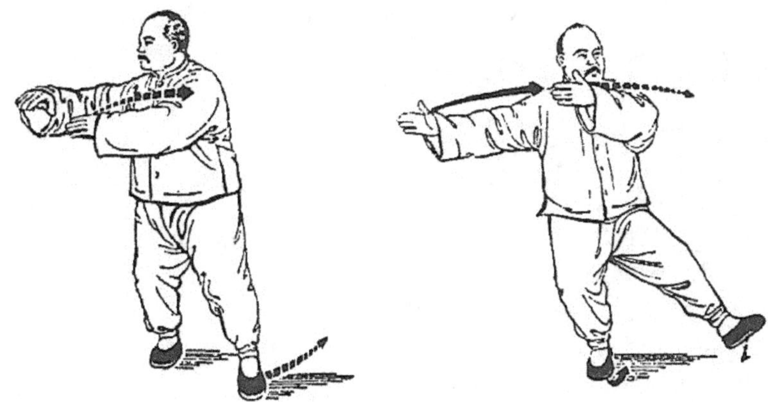

Then, pivoting the right foot on its heel southeastward
to turn the torso southeastward,
complete the eastward swing of the left foot
to set it on the ground pointing eastward
to bend its knee to shift the weight to its leg
to lift the right heel to shift into the tray stance
while arcing the left hand eastward to east of the clavicle
while turning its palm southwestward
and arcing the right hand eastward to south of the right shoulder
while turning its palm downward and southeastward.
The gaze follows the left palm.
And then, turning the torso eastward,
promptly draw the right foot a quarter step eastward
to southwest of the left foot
to set it on the ground *shí* with its heel northwestward
to shift the weight to the right leg
while extending the right hand eastward
to turn its palm toward the north
while shifting the left hand down to the level of the abdomen
to turn its palm downward.
The gaze continues to follow the left hand
until the right hand rises above it,
and then it shifts toward the right hand.

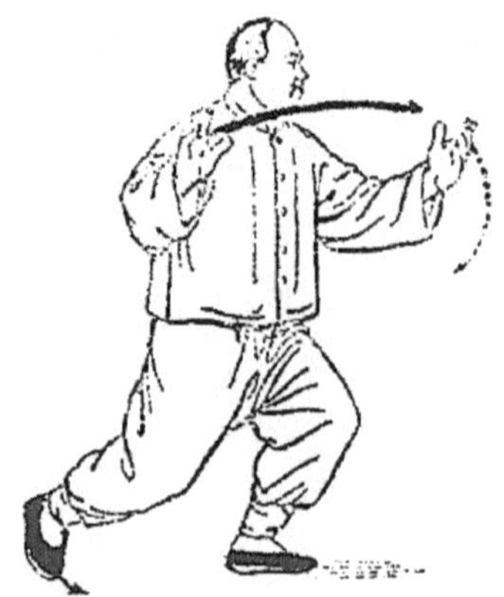
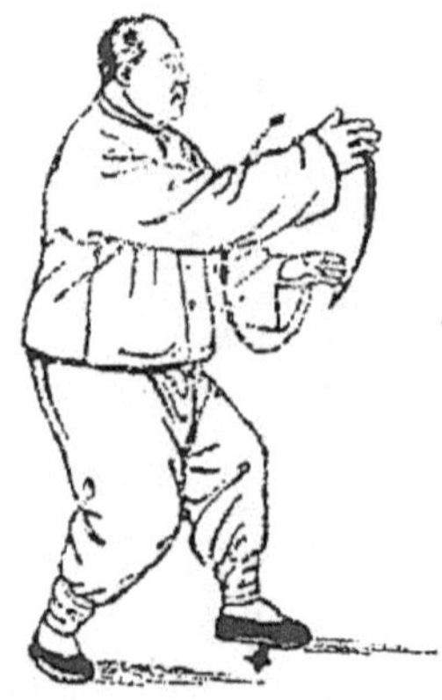

And then, settling the weight more fully onto the right leg,
shift the left heel to east of the right heel,
and straighten the left knee to lift the left toes
to shift them to east of their heel
while circling the left hand downward and southwestward
and then upward and northeastward to east of the face
while turning its palm toward the south
and arcing the right hand downward and northwestward
to below the right elbow
while closing it into a fist with its heart northwestward.
The gaze follows the motion of the right palm
but shifts forward as the left palm passes the inside of the right arm
in its upward motion.

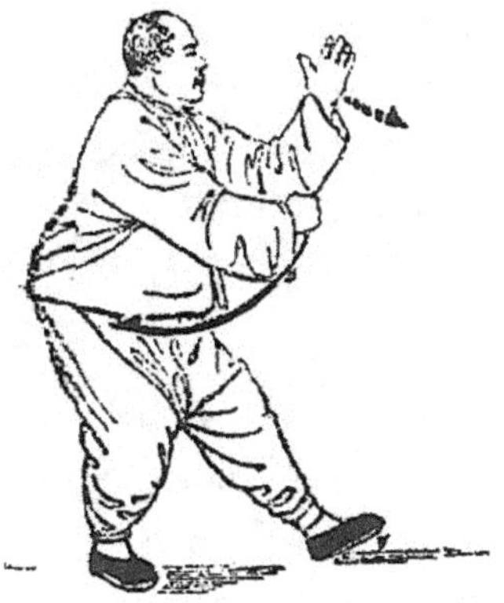

This shift of the left foot, whatever may be its purpose, results in
verticle alignment of the left heel with the right fist and the left
thumb.

20.

倒輦猴左

Dào niǎn hóu zuǒ

Invert Monkey Carriage, Left.

Turning the torso toward the south, settle the left foot flat,
and promptly shift the left hand downward and eastward
while arcing the right hand downward and southwestward
to below and to the south of the right side of the *yāo*
while opening it and turning its palm upward.
The gaze is toward the left hand extending forward.
And then, turning the torso southeastward,
arc the right hand southwestward and upward
while turning its palm upward and southeastward
and shifting the left hand down to the level of the sternum
while turning its palm toward the south and lifting the left knee
to begin to swing the left foot westward past the right ankle.
The gaze shifts toward the arcing right hand.

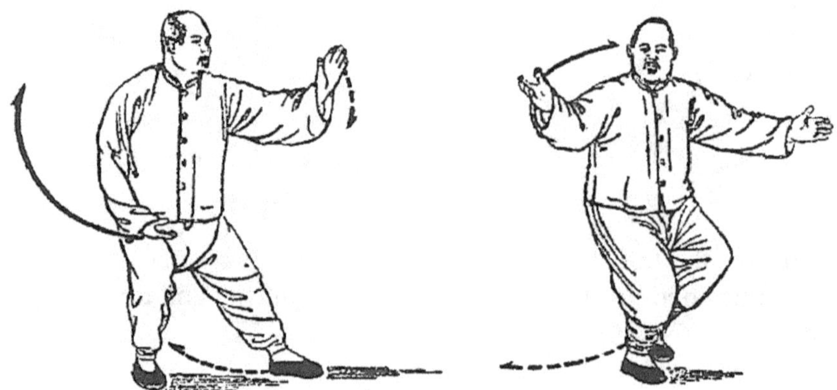

Then, turning the right foot on its heel eastward
to begin to turn the torso eastward,
complete the swing of the left foot westward
to set its toes on the ground to shift into the tray stance
while pushing the right palm eastward to south of the right ear
while turning its palm eastward and turning the left palm upward
while shifting it westward.
And then, completing the turn of the torso eastward
while pushing the right hand eastward
and settling its wrist while turning its palm northeastward,
arc the left hand downward and westward to north of the *yāo*
while bending the left knee and straightening the right leg
to turn the left foot on its ball southwestward to settle it flat
to shift the weight from the right foot to the left foot.
The gaze is toward the right hand pushing forward.

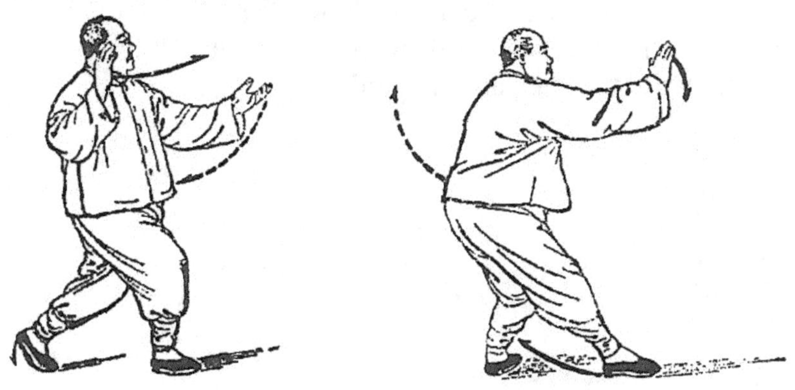

For this form, because of its stepping backward, what makes the
difference between designating it left and designating it right is
which foot is furthest to the rear at the end of the segment. But,
while Fu Zhongwen ends each of his descriptions of it with a
drawing of a photograph Yang Chengfu uses for his descriptions of
it, he calls this left form right and its right form left. So,
apparently, Fu Zhongwen preferred to designate by the general
convention of designating by the foot furthest forward.

21.

倒輦猴右

Dào niǎn hóu yòu
Invert Monkey Carriage, Right.

Turning the torso northeastward,
arc the left hand northwestward and upward
while turning its palm northeastward
and shifting the right hand down to east of the sternum
while turning its palm northwestward and lifting the right knee
to swing the right foot westward past the left ankle.
The gaze shifts toward the arcing left hand.
Then, swinging the right foot southwestward
to set its toes on the ground into the tray stance,
push the left palm southeastward to north of the left ear
while turning its palm eastward and sinking the right elbow
to begin arcing the right hand downward and southwestward
while beginning to turn its palm upward.

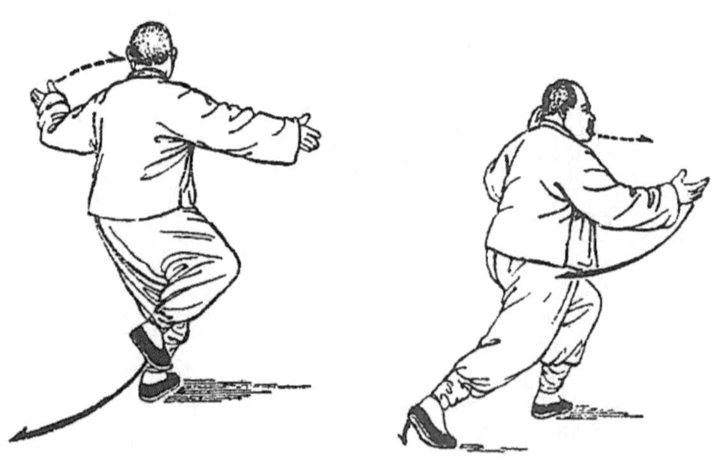

And then, turning the torso toward the south
while pushing the left hand eastward and settling its wrist
while turning its palm southeastward,
turn the left foot on its heel eastward,
and turn the right foot on its ball to the north to settle it flat
while arcing the right hand downward and westward
to south of the right side of the *yāo* while turning its palm upward
and bending the right knee while straightening the left leg
to shift the weight to the right leg.
The gaze is toward the left hand pushing forward.

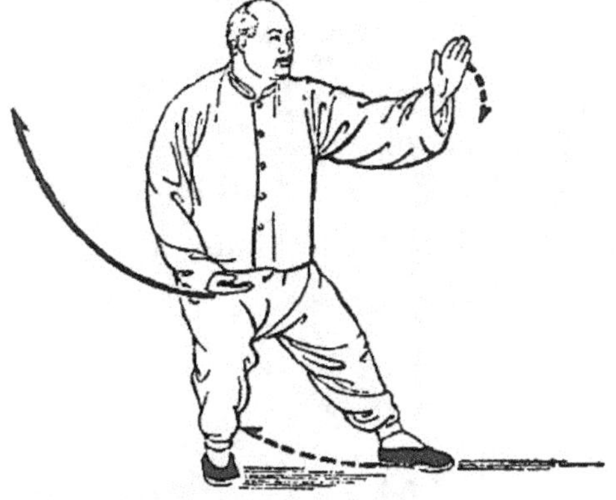

The remainder of this segment is one of several instances of Yang
Chengfu's following a form with a repetition of a variation of the
form but not naming it or numbering it separately.

Left.

And then, turning the torso southeastward
and shifting the right foot on its ball northwestward,
arc the right hand southwestward and upward
while turning its palm upward and eastward,
and shift the left hand down to the level of the sternum
while turning its palm toward the south and lifting the left knee
to begin to swing the left foot westward past the right ankle.
The gaze shifts toward the arcing right hand.
Then, turning the right foot on its heel eastward
to begin to turn the torso eastward,
complete the swing of the left foot westward
to set its toes on the ground to shift into the tray stance
while pushing the right palm eastward to south of the right ear
while turning its palm eastward and turning the left palm upward
while shifting it northwestward.

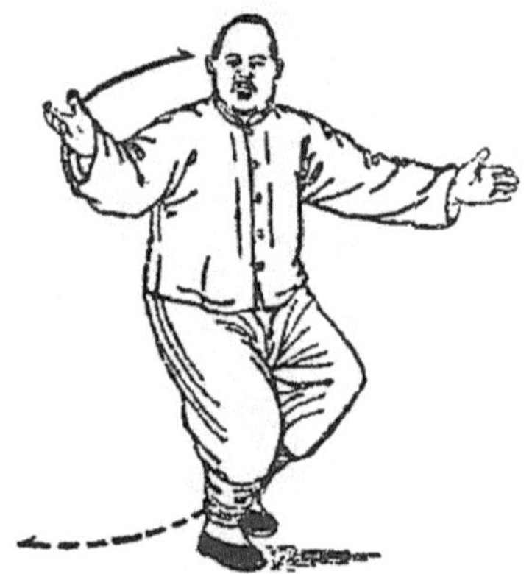
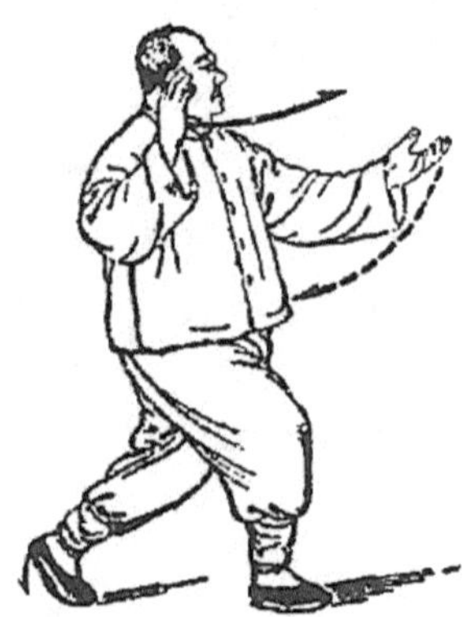

And then, completing the turn of the torso eastward
while pushing the right hand eastward
and settling its wrist while turning its palm northeastward,
arc the left hand downward and westward to north of the *yāo*
while bending the left knee and straightening the right leg
to turn the left foot on its ball southwestward to settle it flat
to shift the weight from the right foot to the left foot.
The gaze is toward the right hand pushing forward.

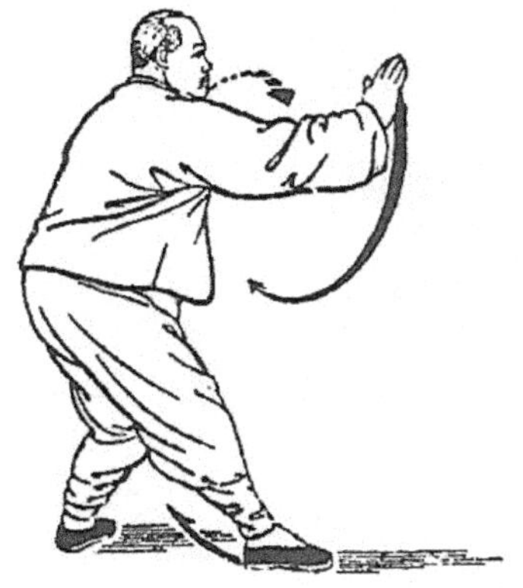

Yang Chengfu says one may repeat the Invert Monkey Carriage
forms three or five or seven times but that the series must end with
the right hand forward. But, of course, that would put the *wújí*
stance at the end of the sequence in a place west of in front of the
position of the beginning *wújí* stance. And Yang Chengfu doesn't
say how to compensate.

22.
斜飛式
Xié fēi shì
Oblique Flying Form.

Continuing the arc of the left hand northwestward and upward
and then promptly southeastward and downward
to east of the sternum
while turning its palm toward the south,
arc the right hand downward and then quickly northwestward
to east of the *yāo* while turning its palm upward
and beginning to lift the right knee.
The gaze is over the left hand.
Then, pivoting the left foot on its heel eastward
while turning the torso southeastward
and swinging the arms with the turn,
lift the right knee southeastward
to swing the right foot southwestward
to set its heel on the ground *xū*
with its toes upward and southwestward
while drawing the hands toward one another
to turn their palms toward one another as if to hold a sphere.

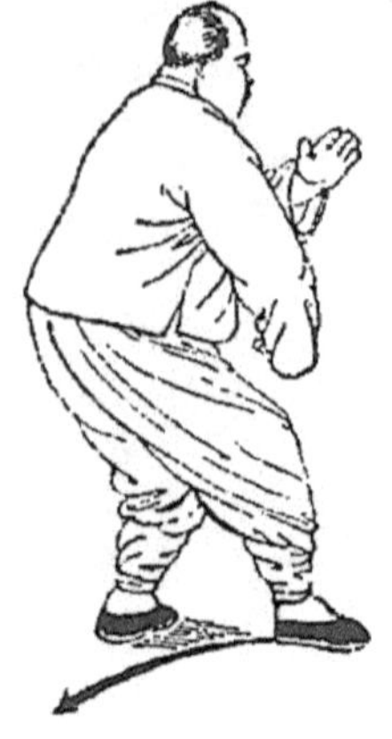
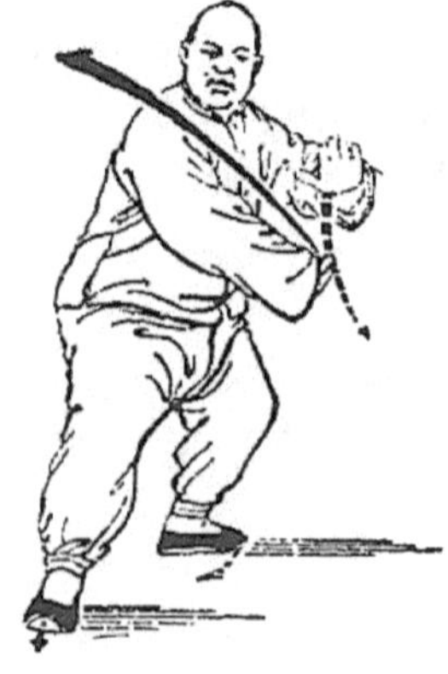

And then, turning the torso to the south
while shifting the left foot on its heel southeastward,
shift the weight southwestward into a right bow stance
while arcing the right hand upward and southwestward
for its palm to face eastward
with its fingers pointing upward and toward the south
from southwest of the face
and arcing the left hand downward to southeast of the *yāo*
for its palm to face downward with its fingers toward the south.
The gaze follows the motion of the right hand.

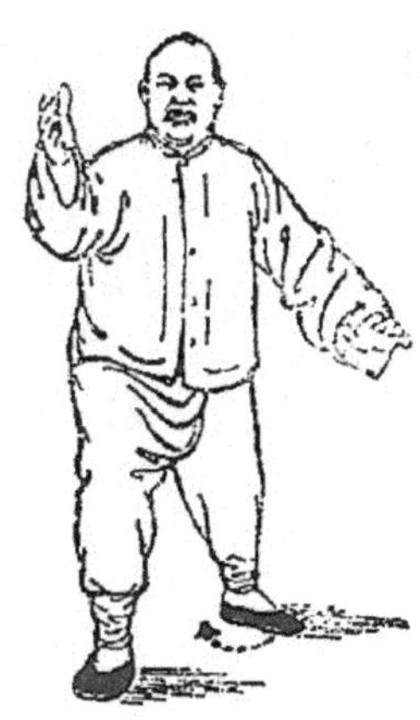

23.

提手上式
Tí shǒu shàng shì
Raise Hands Up Form.

Shift the left foot on its heel toward the south
to lift its heel to shift the weight fully to the right leg
while shifting the right fingers downward and southwestward.
And then turn the left foot on its ball northwestward
to settle it flat to bend the left knee
to straighten the right leg to lift its toes
to shift the weight to the left leg
while arcing the left hand southwestward and upward
for its fingers to point upward and southwestward
from south of the sternum
and shifting the right hand eastward and upward
to above and directly to the south of the right shoulder
for its fingers again to point upward
and more directly toward the south.
The gaze continues to follow the right palm.

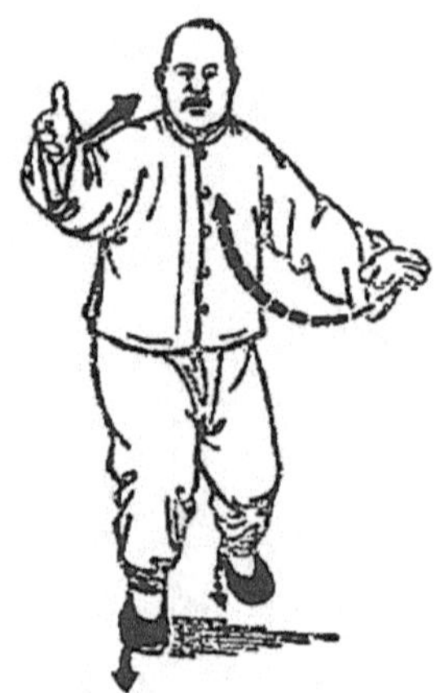 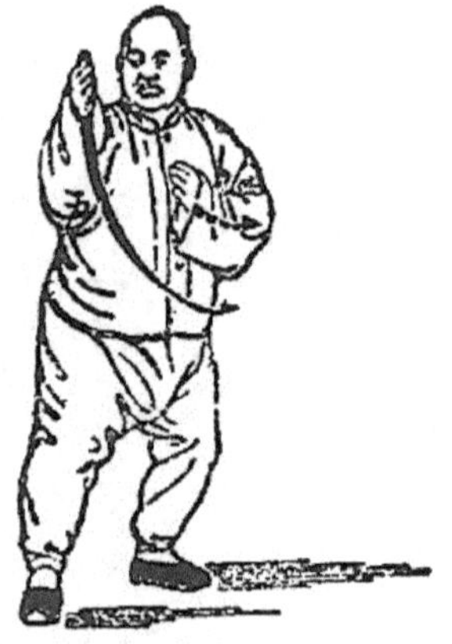

24.
白鶴亮翅
Bái hè liàng chì
White Crane Shines Wings.

Turning the torso southeastward,
arc the right hand downward and eastward
to southeast of the abdomen
while turning its palm downward and northeastward
and beginning to turn the left palm downward.
And then turn the palms toward one another
as if to hold a sphere
while beginning to lift the right knee to the south
to shift the right hand eastward and upward
while turning its palm northeastward.
The gaze follows the right hand
before shifting toward the left elbow
before leveling toward the south.

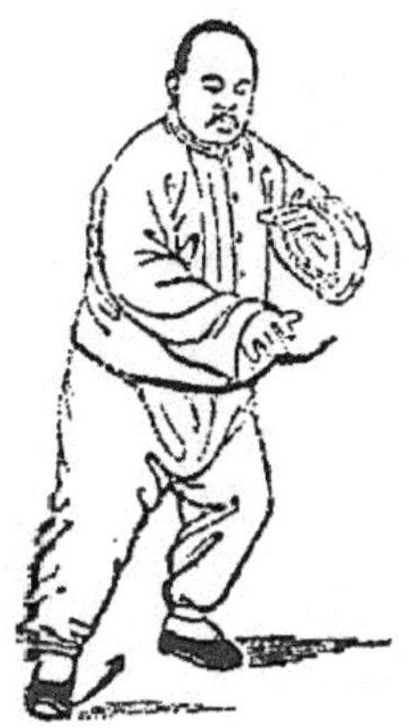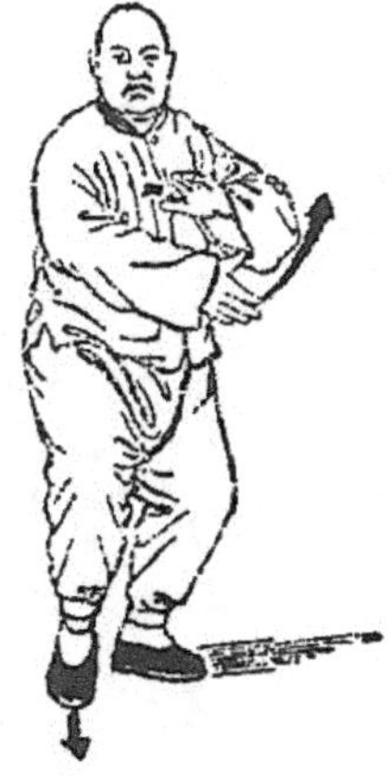

Then, stepping the right foot to the south
into a right bow stance with the right toes pointing southeastward,
turn the torso further southeastward
while continuing the arc of the right hand eastward and upward
to east of the right shoulder
and swinging the left hand with the turn
to point its fingers upward and over the right elbow.
The gaze follows the motion of the right forearm and hand.
And then, turning the torso eastward,
step the left foot southeastward to east of the right heel
to set it on the ground *xū*,
and arc the left hand downward and toward the north
to above and to the north of the left knee
while settling its wrist to keep its palm downward
and arcing the right hand southwestward and upward
to above and to the southeast of the forehead
while turning its palm eastward.
The gaze levelly shifts to the east with the turn.

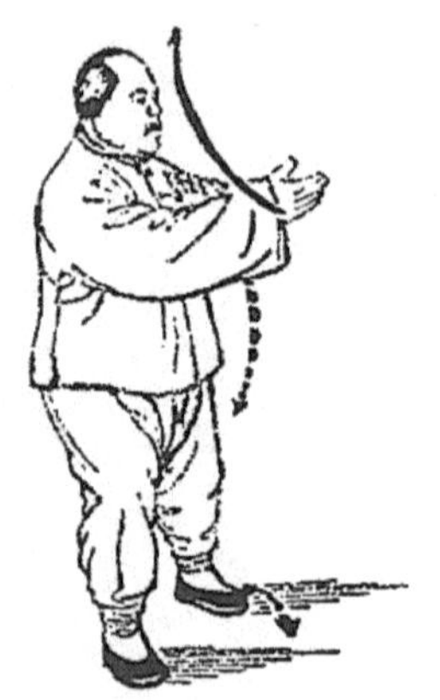
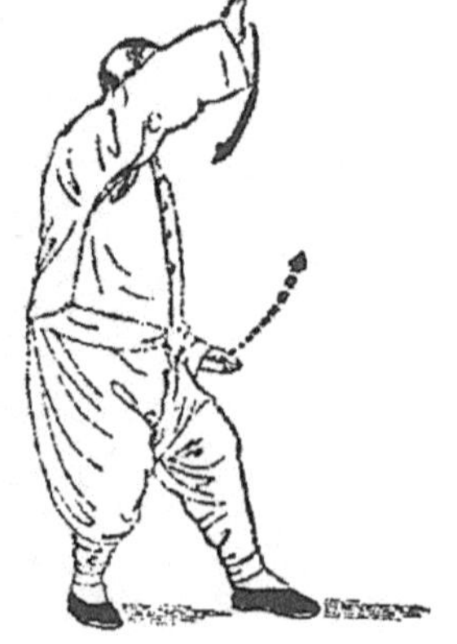

25.

搂膝拗步用法

Lǒu xī ǎo bù yòng fǎ
Draw and Bend Knee to Step Use Method.

Turning the torso southeastward, sink the right elbow
to draw the right hand down to southeast of the clavicle
while turning its palm northwestward toward the face
and arcing the left hand southeastward and upward
for its fingers to point upward and southeastward
from east of the abdomen.
And then arc the right hand downward and westward
to south of the right side of the *yāo*
while turning its palm toward the abdomen
and shifting the left hand westward toward the sternum
for its fingers to point upward and southwestward.
The gaze follows the right palm.

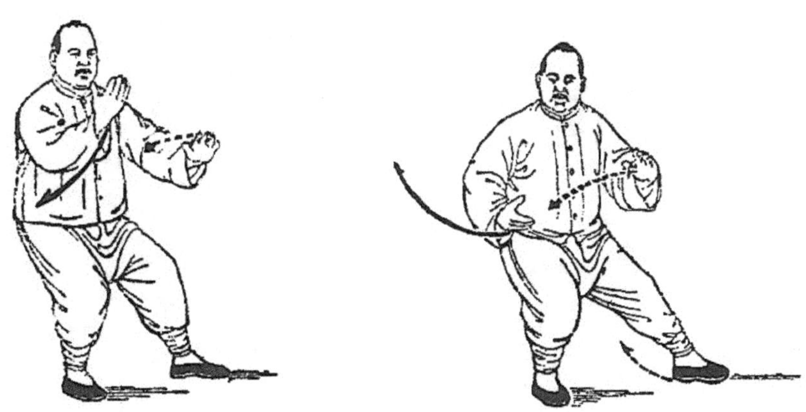

Then, lifting the left knee eastward,
arc the right hand westward and upward
while turning its palm upward and southeastward
and arcing the left hand southwestward and downward
to south of the right side of the abdomen.
The gaze continues to follow the right palm.
And then, arcing the right hand upward and eastward
to southwest of the right ear
while turning its palm downward and northeastward,
step the left foot eastward to touch its heel to the ground *xū*,
and arc the left hand downward and eastward
to southeast of the *yāo* while turning its palm downward.

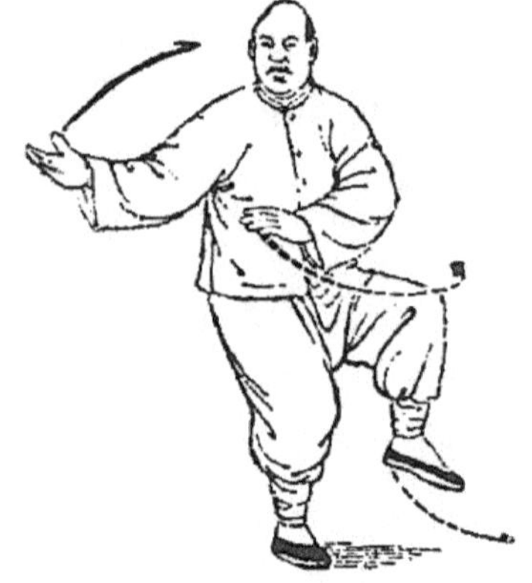 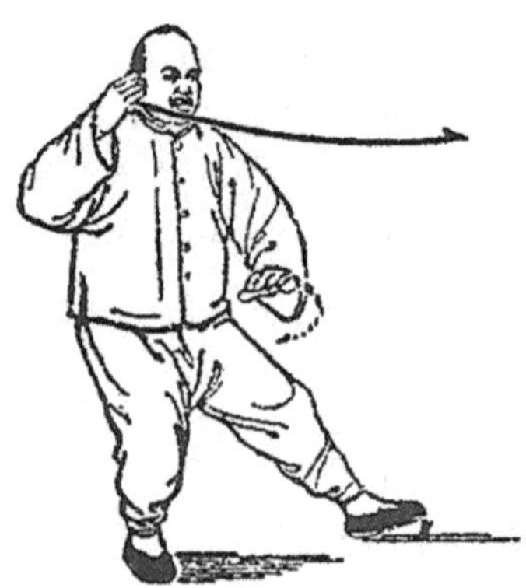

And then, turning the torso eastward,
shift the weight eastward into a left bow stance
while pushing the right hand downward and eastward
while settling its wrist for its palm to face eastward
and brushing the left hand eastward and downward
and then northwestward to above and to the north of the left knee
while keeping its palm facing downward.
The gaze follows the right hand.

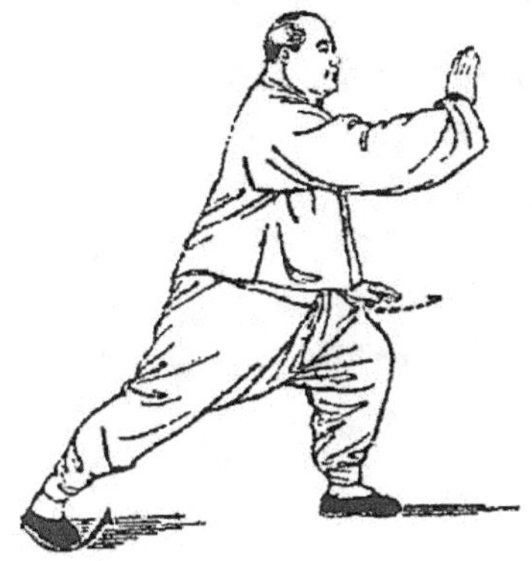

26.
海底針
Hǎi dǐ zhēn
Sea Bottom Needle.

Lifting the right heel to shift into the tray stance
while shifting the left hand eastward,
extend the right hand further eastward while straightening its wrist
and turning its palm toward the north.
And then step the right foot eastward to south of the left foot
to settle it *shí* with its toes pointing southeastward,
and lift the left knee eastward
while promptly sinking the right elbow
to draw the right hand toward the right shoulder
while flexing its wrist to shift the fingers downward
to point them more levelly eastward
while shifting the left hand upward
to above and to the west of the left knee
for its palm to face the left knee.

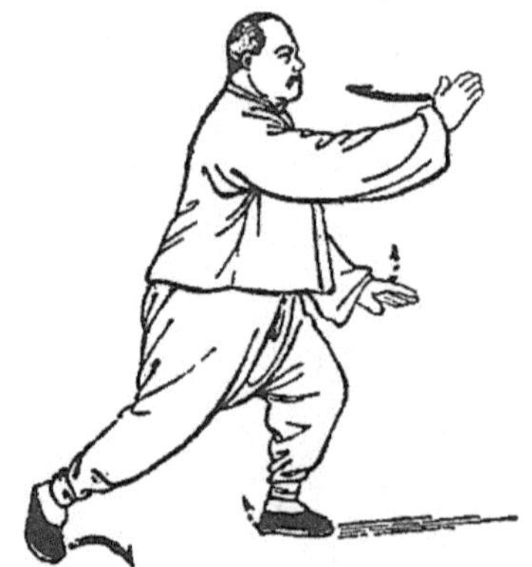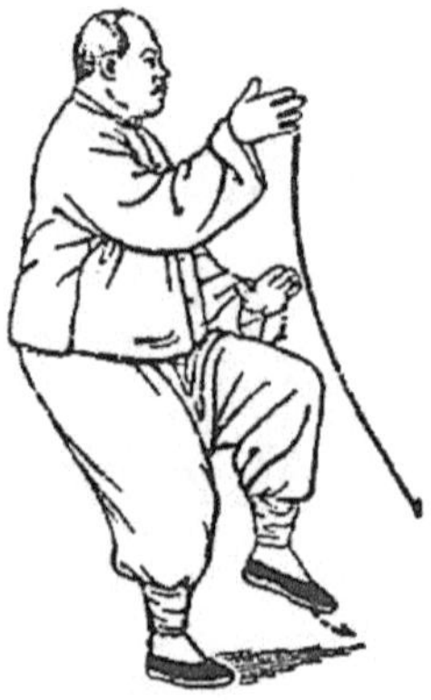

And then set the ball of the left foot on the ground
a half step east of the right heel,
and, bending the torso eastward and downward
while brushing the left hand northwestward
to above and to the northwest of the left knee, *sōng* the right wrist,
and promptly arc the right hand downward and southeastward
to scoop it toward the north.
The gaze is toward the right hand as it arcs toward the ground.

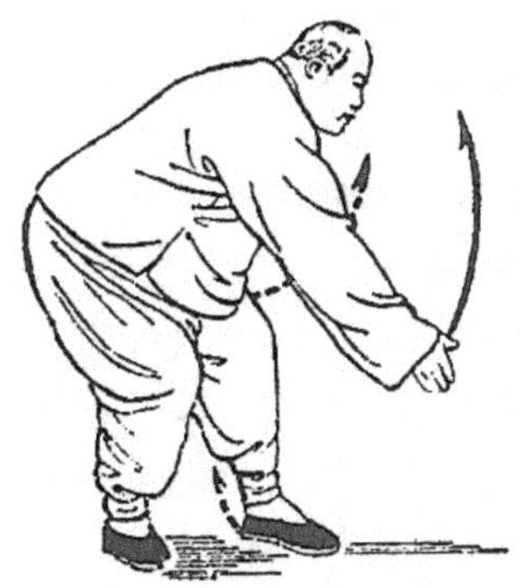

27.

扇通臂
Shàn tōng bì
Fan Through Arms.

Returning the torso to *xū líng dǐng jìn*,
lift the left knee eastward,
and quickly arc the right hand upward to east of the right shoulder
while turning its palm downward and southeastward
and arcing the left hand southeastward and upward
to north of the right forearm and east of the sternum
for its fingers to point upward and southeastward
toward the right forearm.
The gaze continues to follow the right hand.
Then, turning the torso toward the south,
step the left foot eastward into a left bow stance,
and extend the left hand eastward and upward
to east of the clavicle while settling its wrist
for its palm to face downward and southeastward
and arcing the right hand upward and westward
to south of the top of the head
while turning its palm toward the south.
The gaze is toward the left hand.

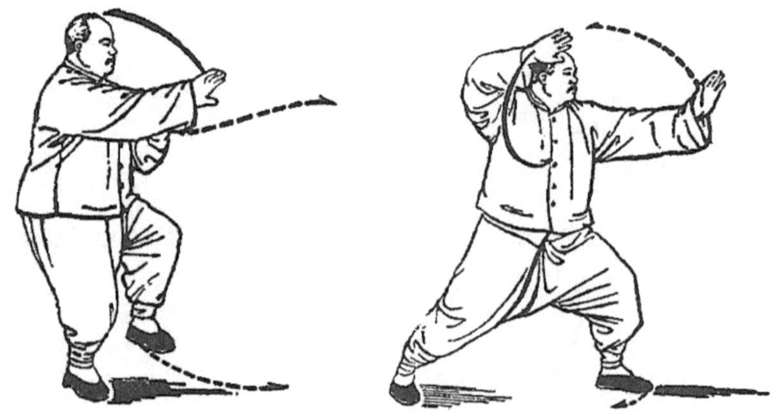

28.

撇身捶

Piē shēn chuí

Cast Body to Cudgel.

Turning the left foot on its heel toward the south
and turning the right foot on its heel southwestward,
circle the right hand southwestward and downward
and then northeastward to south of the sternum
while closing it into a fist with its heart downward
and arcing the left hand upward and southwestward
to south of the top of the head while turning its palm to the south.
The gaze shifts with the turn to follow the arc of the left hand
before following the arc of the right hand
and shifting levelly to the south.
And then, pivoting the left foot on its ball northeastward
to turn its knee southwestward
to turn the torso also southwestward,
promptly lift the right knee westward
while shifting the right fist upward with the turn
to turn its heart toward the sternum
while arcing the left hand downward with the turn
for its palm to face downward and northwestward
from below and to the west of the right fist.
The gaze includes the motion of the hands.

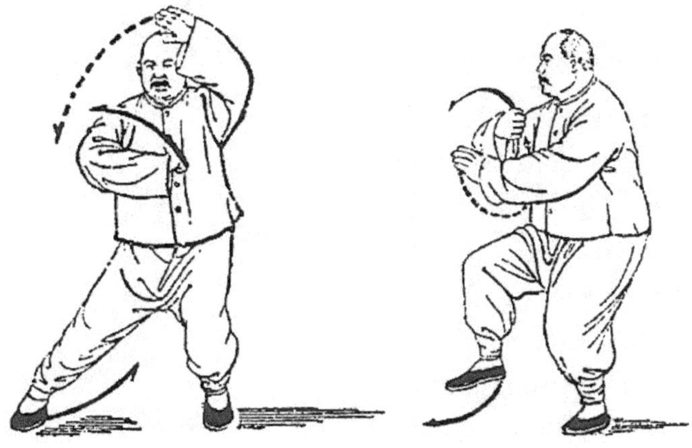

Then, stepping the right foot westward
to touch its heel to the ground *xū,*
press the back of the right fist upward and westward
and then downward
while circling the left hand downward and northeastward
and then upward and westward
for its fingers to point upward and westward toward the right wrist.
And then, turning the torso westward
while shifting the weight westward into a right bow stance,
arc the right fist downward and northeastward to north of the *yāo*
while extending the left hand upward and westward.

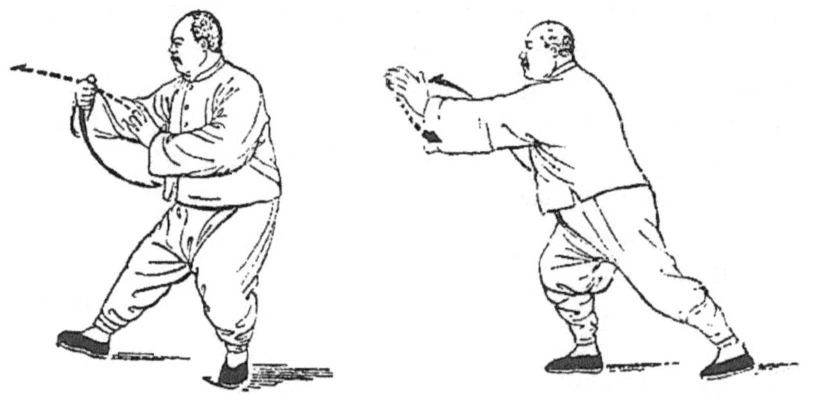

29.
進步搬攔捶
Jìn bù bān lán chuí
Advance Step Shift Block Cudgel.

Turning the torso southwestward,
bend the left knee while straightening the right leg
to shift the weight eastward onto the left leg
while arcing the right fist upward and southwestward
to turn its heart downward and toward the south
while sinking the left elbow
to shift the left forearm downward and southeastward
for its palm to face north from beneath the right fist.
The gaze is across the top of the right fist.
Then, turning the torso further southwestward,
shift the right fist down to the level of the sternum
while sinking the left elbow
to draw the left hand eastward to south of the abdomen.
The gaze shifts levelly toward the southwest.

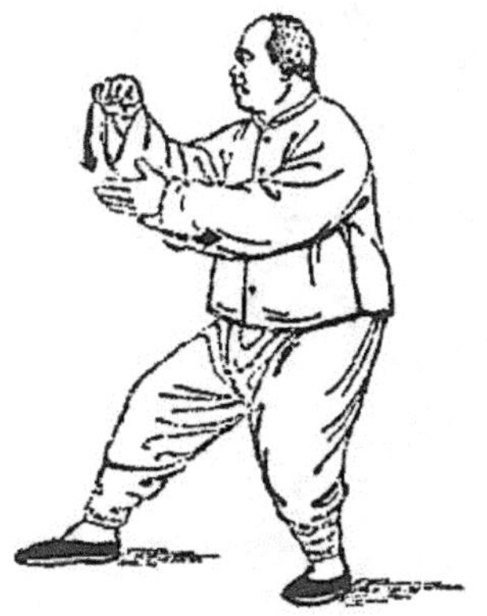
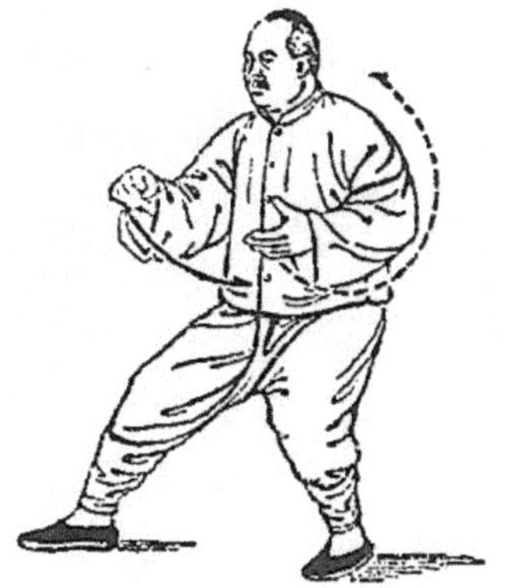

And then, lifting the right knee westward,
coil the right fist downward and eastward to south of the abdomen
while arcing the left hand downward and eastward
and then upward and westward to southeast of the face
while turning its palm westward.
The gaze follows the hands
before returning levelly southwestward.
Then, turning the torso westward,
step the right foot westward to touch its heel to the ground *xū*
while arcing the right fist upward and westward
and shifting the left hand northwestward and downward
to cross the hands with the left palm facing north
and the heart of the right fist facing southeastward.

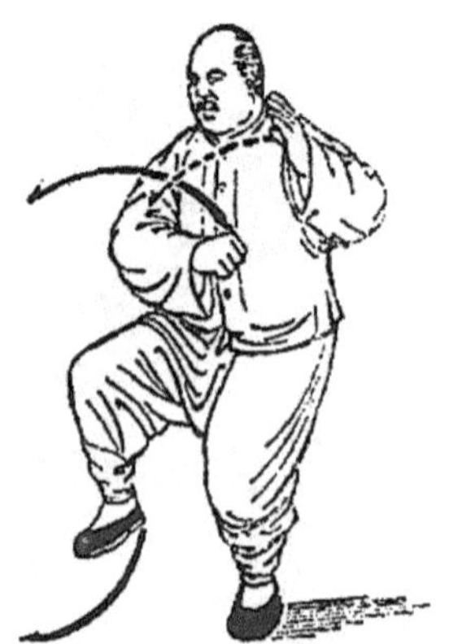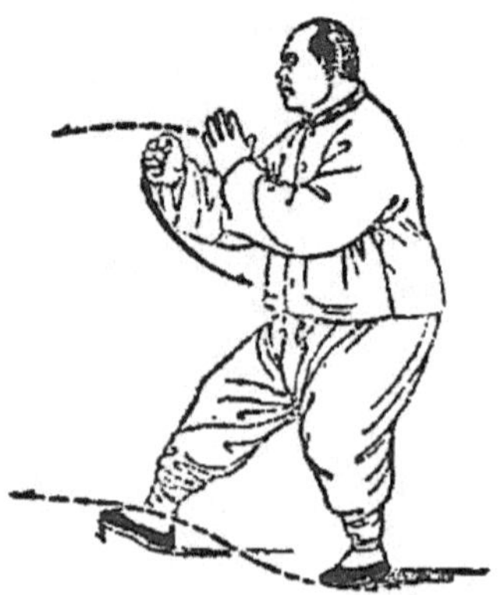

And then turn the right foot on its heel northwestward,
and settle it flat to shift the weight to it
to lift the left knee westward
while turning the torso northwestward
and shifting the left hand further westward
while arcing the right fist downward and northeastward
to north of the *yāo*.
Then, settling lower onto the right leg,
step the left foot eastward to touch its heel to the ground *xū*
while continuing to extend the left hand westward
and continuing to draw the right fist eastward.

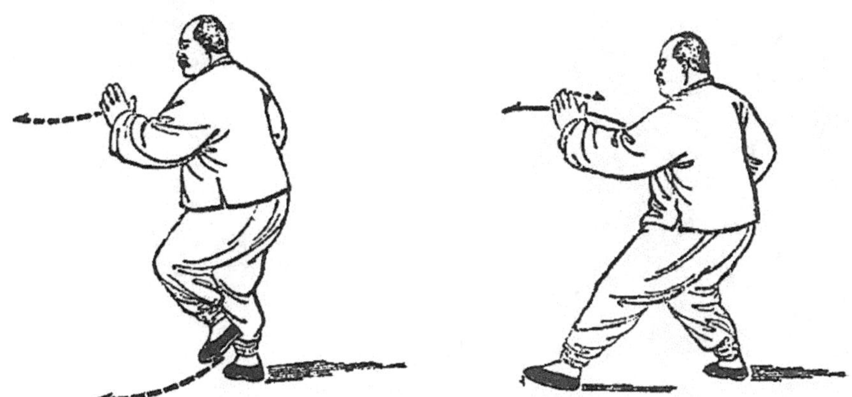

And then, turning the torso westward
while shifting the weight westward into a left bow stance,
cudgel the right fist upward and westward
while drawing the left hand northeastward
toward the right shoulder
as the right forearm glides westward past the left palm
until the right arm is nearly straight
with the left palm facing the right elbow and nearly touching it.
The gaze follows the left palm before shifting to the right fist.

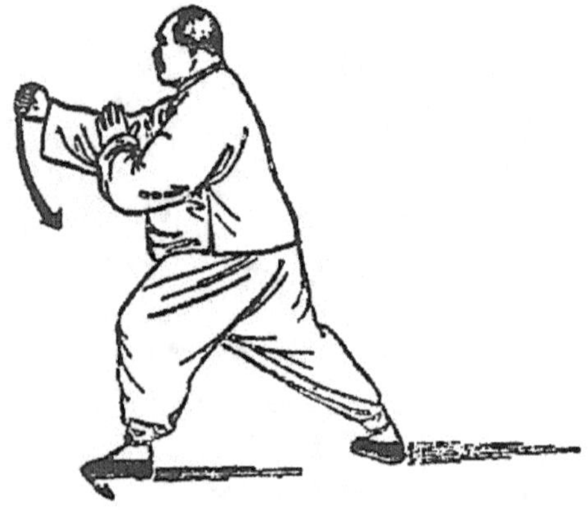

30.

上步攬雀尾

Shàng bù lǎn què wěi

Up Step Grasp Sparrow Tail.

Turning the left foot on its heel southwestward
to turn the torso southwestward,
shift the right hand downward to the level of the abdomen
while opening it and turning its palm downward
and shifting the left hand southwestward
while turning its palm downward and westward.
And then, shifting all of the weight to the left leg
to lift the right knee westward,
circle the right hand downward
and southeastward and then upward
to turn the palms toward one another as if to hold a sphere.
The gaze is briefly toward the left forearm
before shifting toward the right arm
and then returning levelly southwestward.

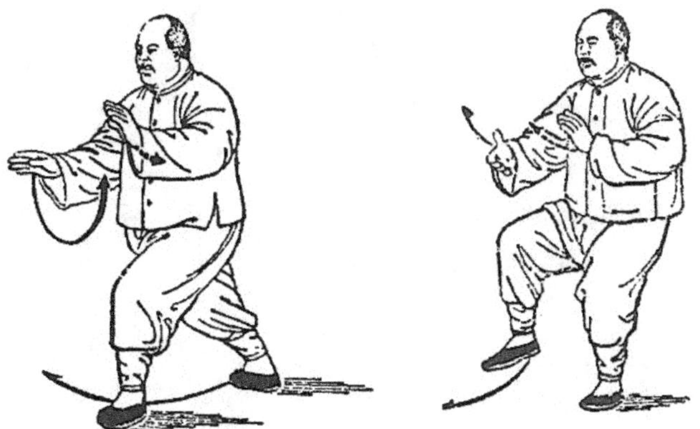

Fu Zhongwen doesn't explain why the orientation of the first of
these two illustrations is further southwestward than the orientation
of the final illustration of the previous segment. But the next two
illustrations return the orientation directly westward. So, whatever
may be the reason, the flow is easy to follow.

Arrow Quiver Cover (Ward-Off).

Then step the right foot westward
to touch its heel to the ground *xū*
while shifting the right hand westward and upward
and shifting the left hand levelly westward
for its fingers to point upward toward the right wrist.
And then, shifting the weight westward into a right bow stance
while shifting the right hand further westward and upward
to west of the face for its palm to face the face,
shift the left hand with the right hand
while settling its wrist for its fingertips to point further upward.

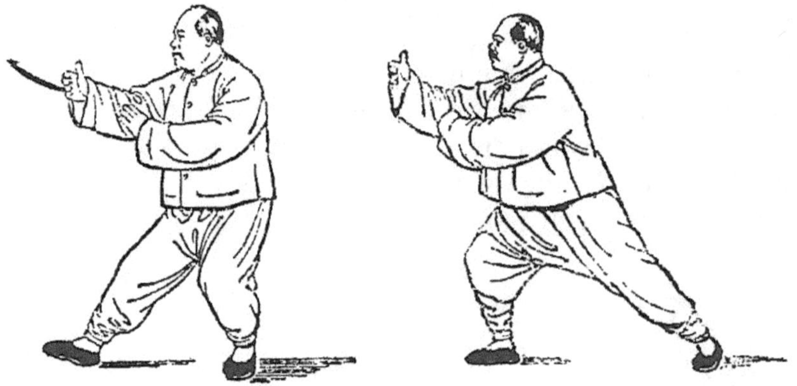

Yang Chengfu doesn't number separately this or other repetitions
of the components of the **Grasp Sparrow Tail form.**

Stroke (Rollback).

Turning the right palm downward and westward
while turning the left palm upward and toward the north,
begin to roll the hands downward and eastward.
Then, to continue rolling the hands downward and eastward,
bend the left knee to straighten the right leg
to shift the weight eastward onto the left leg.

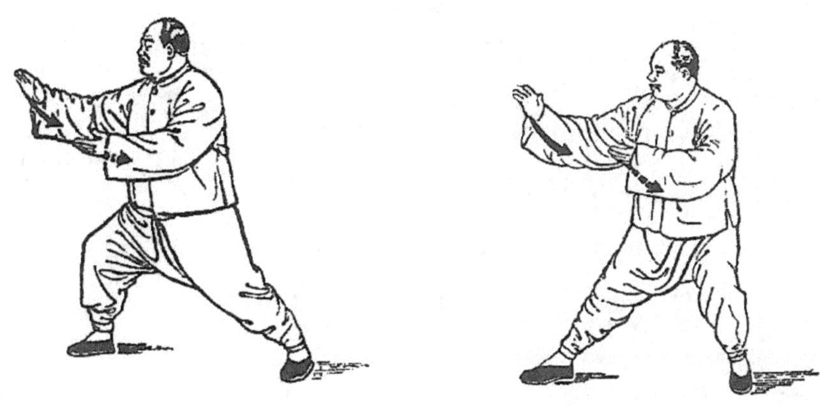

And then, keeping the elbows at least a fist's width from the torso,
continue rolling the hands eastward
while turning the right palm southeastward.
The gaze attends to the left hand before following the right hand.

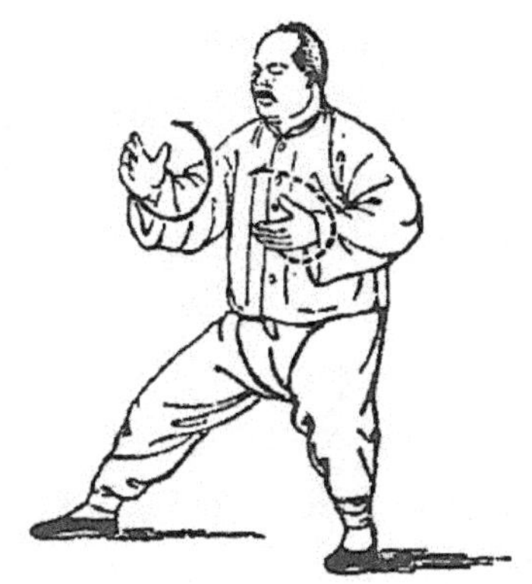

Press.

Beginning to shift the weight westward,
circle both hands downward and southeastward
and then upward and westward
to turn the left palm downward and westward
while turning the right palm eastward.
And then, completing the shift of the weight
westward again into a right bow stance
press the back of the right hand westward and upward
for its palm to face the face,
and push the left hand westward and upward
while settling its wrist to press the right forearm further westward.
The gaze is toward the right forearm.

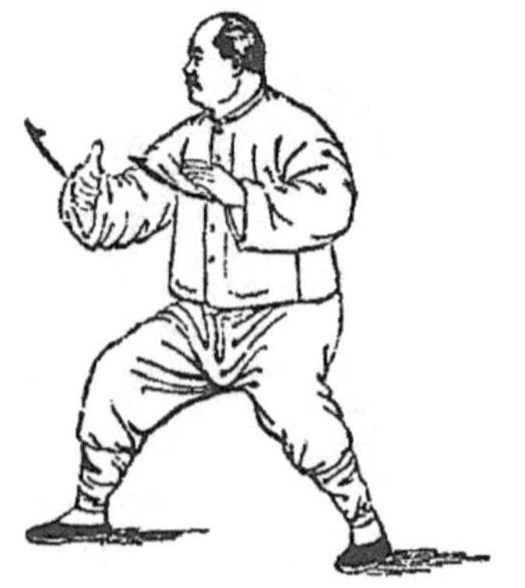 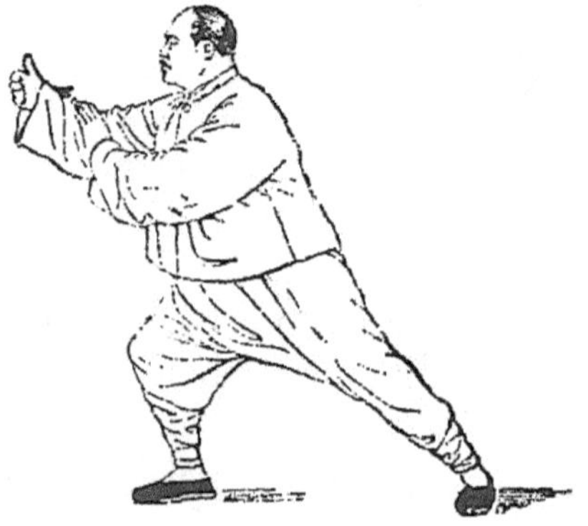

Push.

Turning the torso westward,
shift the right hand down to shoulder-level,
and pass the left hand over the right wrist
while turning both palms downward
to spread them shoulder-width apart.
Then, turning the palms to face one another
for their fingers to point upward and westward,
sink the elbows to draw the hands eastward toward the sternum
while bending the left knee to straighten the right leg
to shift the weight to the left leg.
The gaze is level and westward.

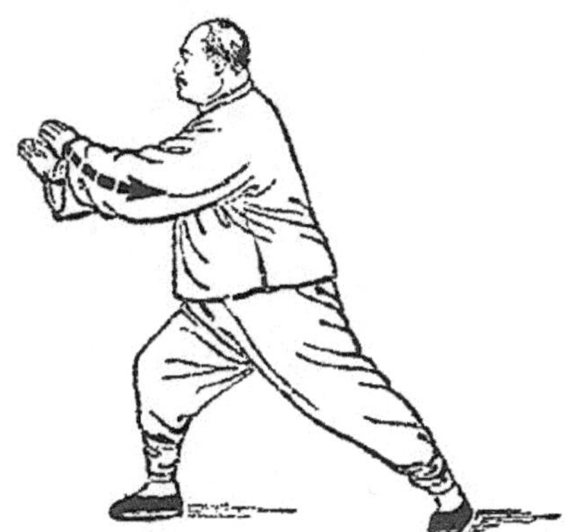 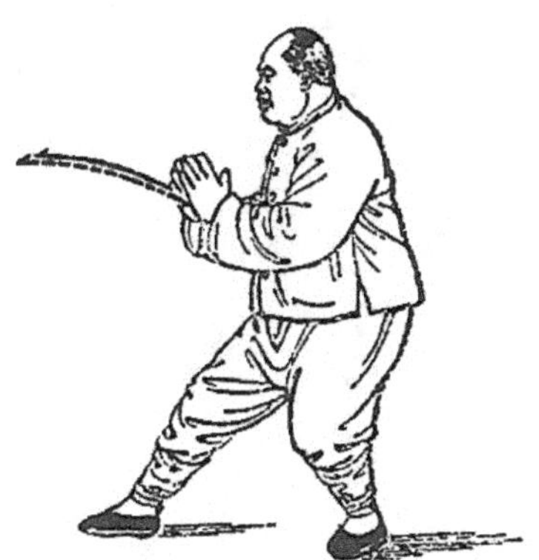

And then quickly straighten the wrists
to turn the palms downward
to push them upward and forward while settling their wrists
and shifting the weight westward again into a right bow stance.
The gaze remains level and forward.

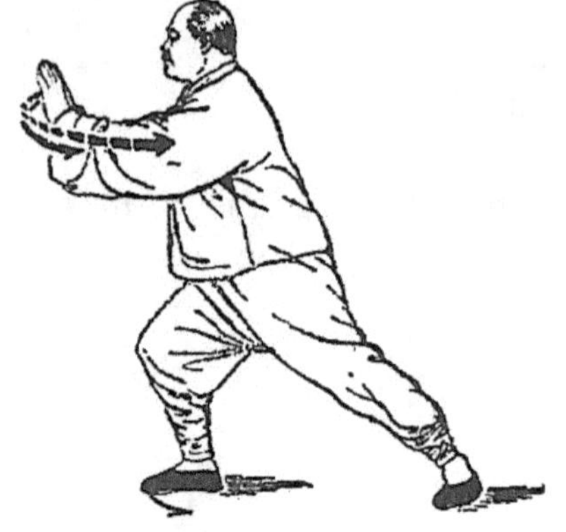

31.

單鞭式

Dān biān shì

Solitary Whip Form.

Bending the left knee and straightening the right leg
to shift the weight to the left leg, turn the torso southwestward,
and turn the right foot on its heel southwestward
while swinging the hands with the turn
and beginning to turn the palms downward.
And then, turning the torso southeastward
while swinging the arms with the turn
and continuing to turn the palms downward,
turn the left foot on its ball northwestward,
and turn the right foot on its ball also northwestward
while bending the right knee while straightening the left knee
to shift the weight to the right leg.
The gaze levelly shifts with the turn.

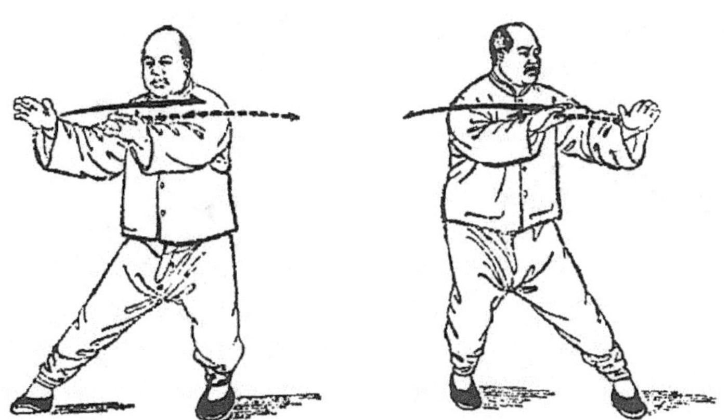

Then, keeping the weight on the right leg,
turn the torso again southwestward
while swinging the arms with the turn
and shifting the gaze with the turn.
And then, again turning the torso southeastward
while shifting the left hand
upward and eastward to southeast of the chin
to turn its palm toward the chin,
lift the left knee eastward,
and *sōng* the right wrist while extending its hand westward
and gathering its fingers and thumb to each other
for the hand to hang downward
to form a hook shape with its wrist.
The gaze shifts levelly with the turn.

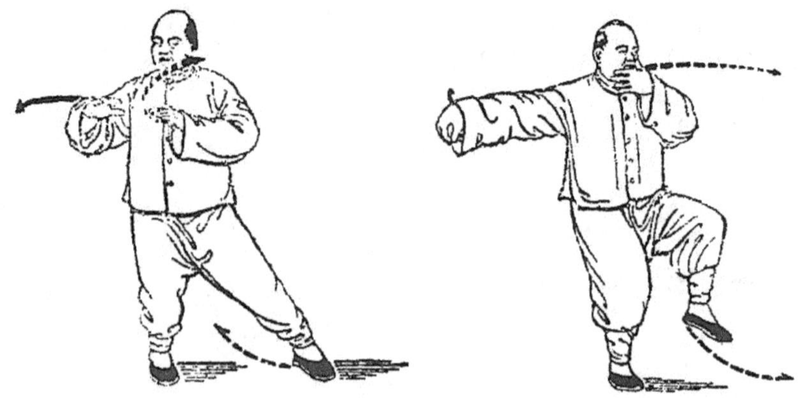

Then, shifting the right hand upward
until its fingertips are at shoulder-level,
step the left foot eastward into a left bow stance
while extending the left hand eastward
while turning its palm downward
before settling its wrist and turning its palm southeastward.
The gaze shifts levelly with the motion of the left hand.

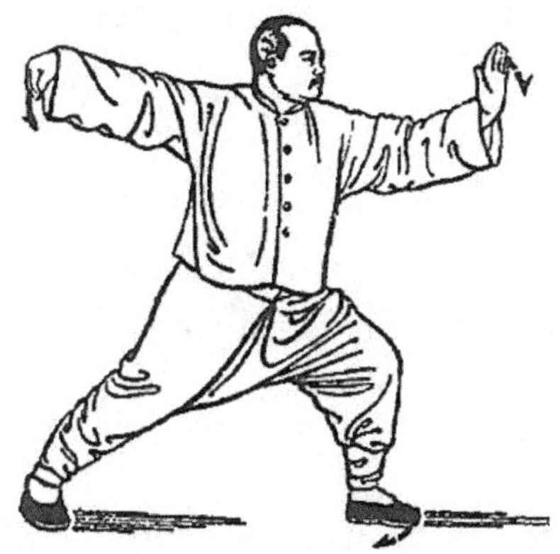

32.

�手右

Yŭn shŏu yòu
Cloud Hands, Right.

Lifting the left toes
to turn the left foot on its heel toward the south,
sōng the right hand while turning the left palm toward the south,
and begin to arc both hands downward.
Then, settling the left foot flat,
lift the right heel northeastward
to shift all the weight onto the left leg
while turning the torso to the south
and promptly arcing the right hand downward and eastward
while settling its wrist
for its palm to face downward and northeastward
from southwest of the *yāo*
and shifting the left hand down to southeast of the upper abdomen
while turning its palm downward for its fingers to point south.
The gaze shifts levelly to the southwest.

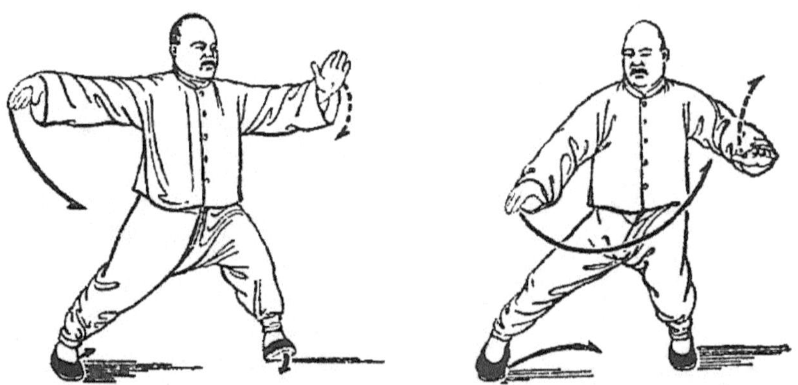

Yang Chengfu says this form is like clouds moving across the sky,
but that may not be apparent until one can do it by memory, for it
to flow *sōng*. And such is also true of the transition from all of the
fragmentary words and pictures to the unity of practice. But that
can also be an effective metaphor for returning from *tàijí* to *wújí*.

Then, lifting the right knee toward the south
while turning the torso southeastward,
shift the left hand up to shoulder-level for its palm to face south
with its fingers upward and eastward,
and continue the arc of the right hand downward and eastward
and then upward for its palm to face north with its fingers eastward
and its thumb at the level of the right elbow.
The gaze follows the right hand.
And then, turning the torso again to the south,
set the right foot on the ground flat to settle into the horse stance
while arcing the right hand upward and westward
for its palm to face the face from southwest of the face
and arcing the left hand downward and westward
for its palm to face the abdomen from south of it.
The gaze continues to follow the right hand.

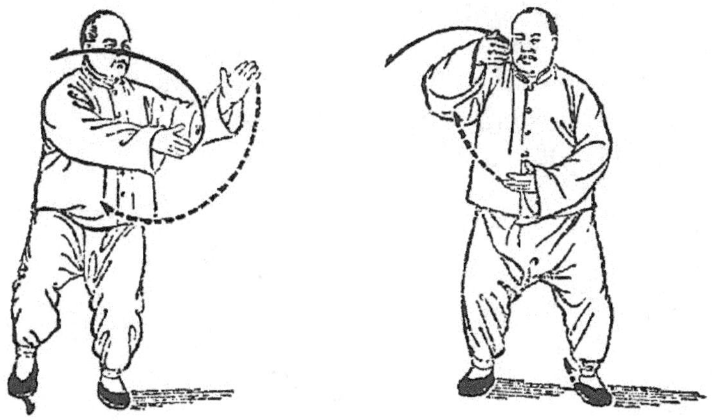

What makes the Cloud Hands form right or left is which hand is
higher at the end of the form.

33.
扽手左
Yŭn shŏu zuŏ
Cloud Hands, Left.

Lifting the left knee to the south
while turning the torso southwestward,
arc the right hand westward for its palm to face south
with its fingers pointing upward and westward,
and arc the left hand westward and upward
to southwest of the sternum
while turning its palm downward and northwestward.
The gaze continues to follows the right hand.
And then, turning the torso again to the south,
step the left foot eastward into a wide horse stance,
and, arcing the left hand upward and eastward
for its palm to face the face from southeast of the face,
arc the right hand downward and eastward and upward
for its palm to face the abdomen from south of it.
The gaze shifts to the left hand.

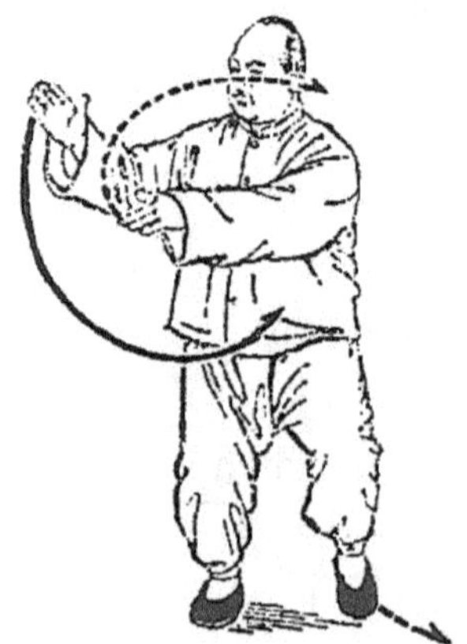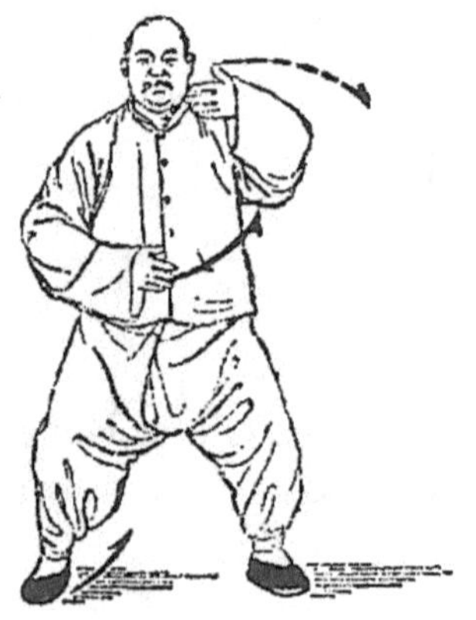

Yang Chengfu doesn't specify the following cloud hands
repetitions, but they're necessary for the closing *wújí* stance to be
directly south of the opening *wújí* stance, and Fu Zhongwen
specifies them.

Right.

Lifting the right knee toward the south
while turning the torso southeastward,
arc the left hand eastward
while turning its palm toward the south
to point its fingers upward and eastward,
and arc the right hand eastward and upward
for its fingers to point eastward
with its thumb south of the left elbow.
The gaze continues to follow the left hand.
And then, turning the torso again to the south,
set the right foot on the ground flat to settle into the horse stance
while arcing the right hand upward and westward
for its palm to face the face from southwest of the face
and arcing the left hand downward and westward
for its palm to face the abdomen from south of it.
The gaze shifts to the right palm.

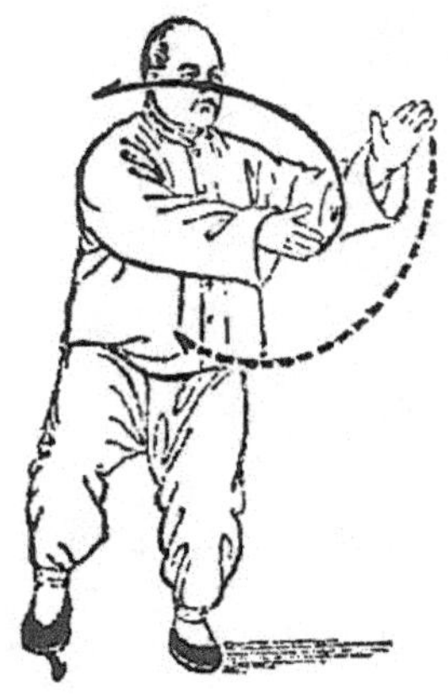 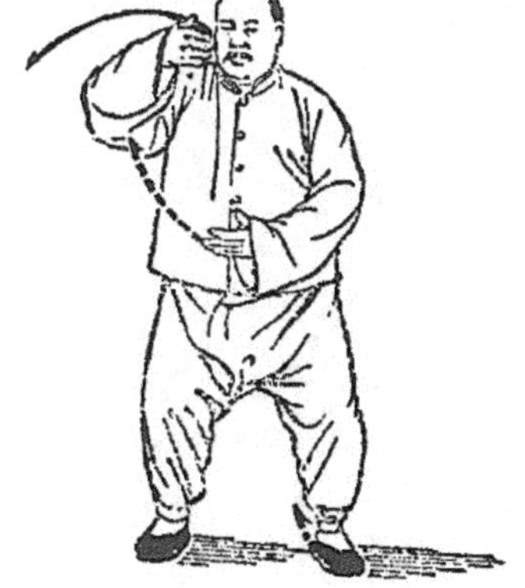

Left

Lifting the left knee to the south
while turning the torso southwestward,
arc the right hand westward for its palm to face south
with its fingers pointing upward and westward,
and arc the left hand westward and upward
while turning its palm downward and northwestward.
The gaze continues to follow the right palm.
And then, turning the torso again to the south,
step the left foot eastward into a wide horse stance,
and, arcing the left hand upward and eastward
for its palm to face the face from southeast of the face,
arc the right hand downward and eastward and upward
for its palm to face the abdomen from south of it.
The gaze shifts to the left palm.

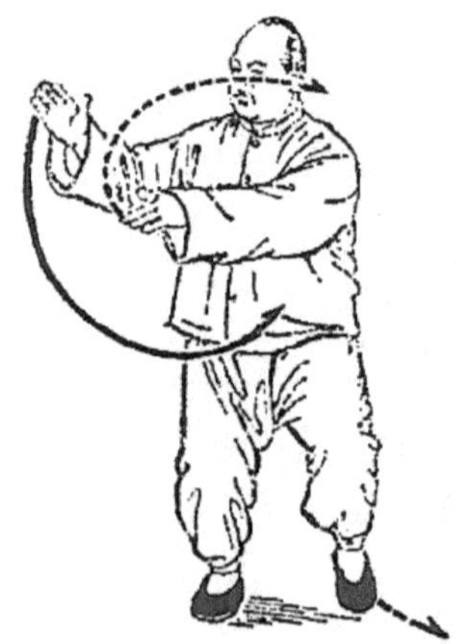 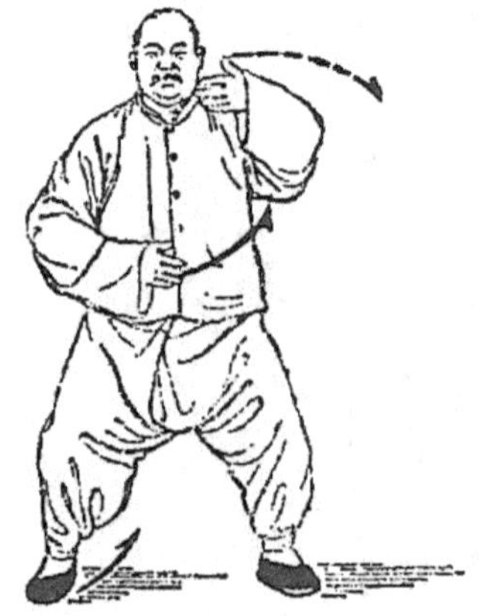

Right.

Lifting the right knee toward the south
while turning the torso southeastward,
arc the left hand eastward
while turning its palm toward the south
to point its fingers upward and eastward,
and arc the right hand eastward and upward
for its fingers to point eastward
with its thumb south of the left elbow.
The gaze continues to follow the left hand.
And then, turning the torso again to the south,
set the right foot on the ground flat to settle into the horse stance
while arcing the right hand upward and westward
for its palm to face the face from southwest of the face
and arcing the left hand downward and westward
for its palm to face the abdomen from south of it.
The gaze shifts to the right palm.

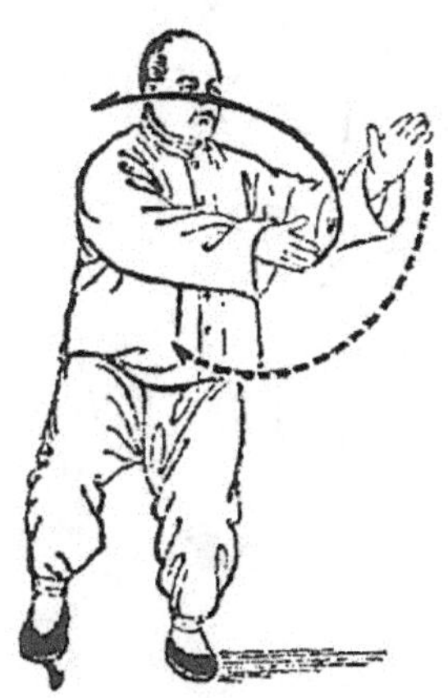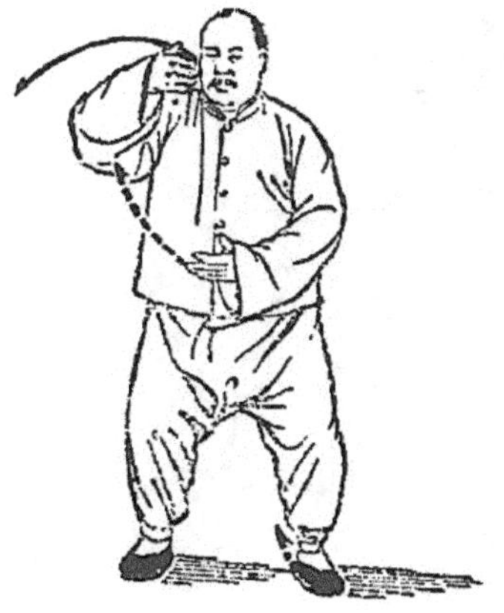

Left

Lifting the left knee to the south
while turning the torso southwestward,
arc the right hand westward for its palm to face south
with its fingers pointing upward and westward,
and arc the left hand westward and upward
while turning its palm downward and northwestward.
The gaze continues to follow the right hand.
And then, turning the torso again to the south,
step the left foot eastward into a wide horse stance,
and, arcing the left hand upward and eastward
for its palm to face the face from southeast of the face,
arc the right hand downward and eastward and upward
for its palm to face the abdomen from south of it.
The gaze shifts to the left palm.

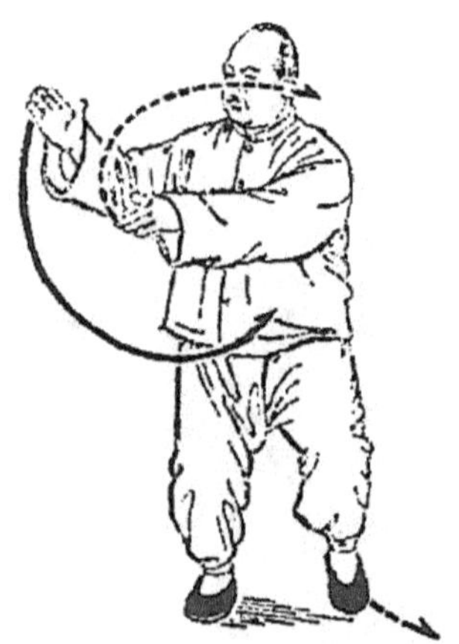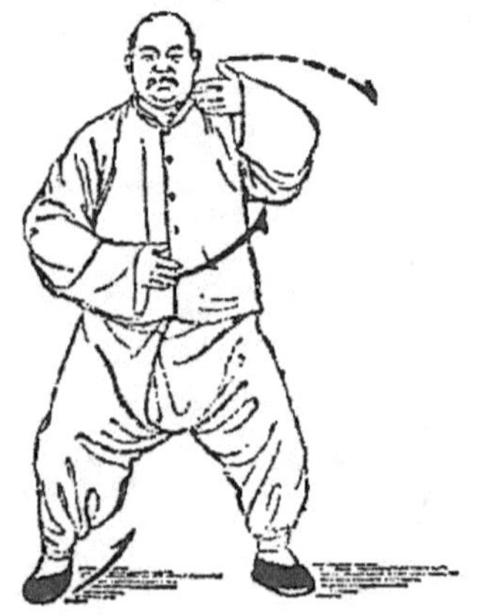

Right.

Lifting the right knee toward the south
while turning the torso southeastward,
arc the left hand eastward
while turning its palm toward the south
to point its fingers upward and eastward,
and arc the right hand eastward and upward
for its fingers to point eastward
with its thumb south of the left elbow.
The gaze continues to follow the left hand.
And then, turning the torso again to the south,
set the right foot on the ground flat to settle into the horse stance
while arcing the right hand upward and westward
for its palm to face the face from southwest of the face
and arcing the left hand downward and westward
for its palm to face the abdomen from south of it.
The gaze shifts to the right palm.

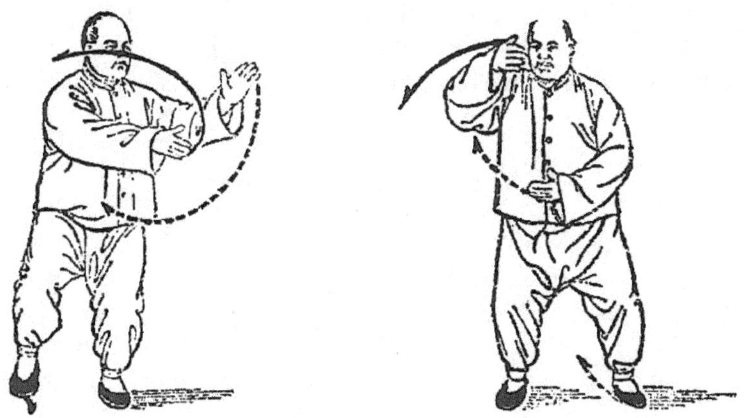

Varying the number of repetitions of the Cloud Hands form can compensate for varying the number of repetitions of the Invert Monkey Carriage form.

34.

單鞭

Dān biān

Solitary Whip.

Shifting the right foot on its ball northwestward
to shift the weight to the right leg
to lift the left knee southeastward
while turning the torso southwestward,
sōng the right wrist while arcing it westward and downward
to the level of the sternum
and arcing the left hand westward and upward
while turning its palm downward and toward the north.
And then, turning the torso southeastward,
extend the right arm fully westward
while gathering its fingers and thumb to each other
for the hand to form a hook shape with its wrist
and arcing the left hand upward and eastward
to southeast of the chin while turning its palm toward the chin.
The gaze, after following the movement of the right hand,
shifts southeastward over the left hand.

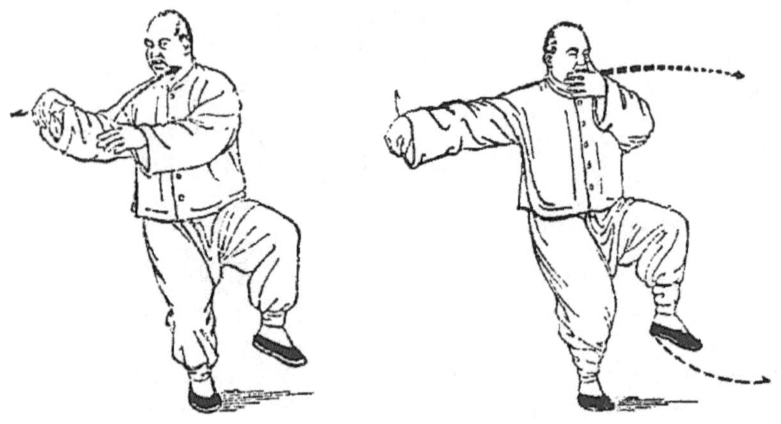

And then, shifting the right hand up to shoulder-level
while stepping the left foot eastward into a left bow stance,
extend the left hand eastward while turning its palm downward
before settling its wrist and turning its palm southeastward.
The gaze shifts levelly with the motion of the left hand.

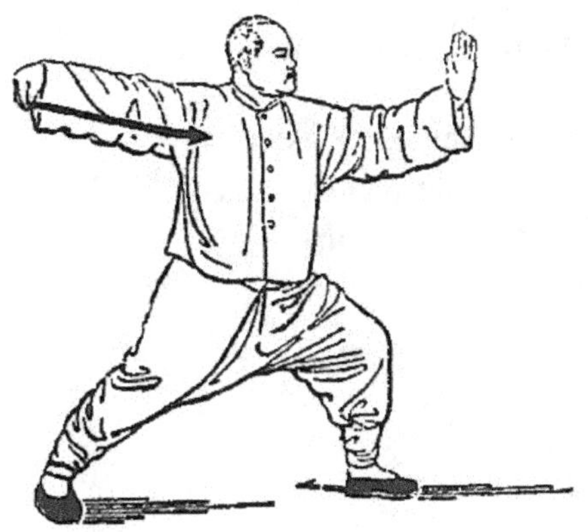

35.

高探馬

Gāo tàn mǎ

High Search of Horse.

Bending the right leg while straightening the left leg
to shift the weight westward to the right leg,
raise the left toes from the ground,
and *sōng* the right hand while quickly arcing it eastward
to southwest of the sternum while straightening its wrist
and turning its palm downward and northeastward
while straightening the left wrist
and turning its palm to the south.
The gaze is over the left hand.
Then, turning the torso eastward
while arcing the right hand upward and eastward
and then toward the north
for its palm to face downward from east of the chin,
lift the left knee eastward,
and draw the left hand downward and westward
to the east of the abdomen
for the palms to face one another as if holding a sphere.

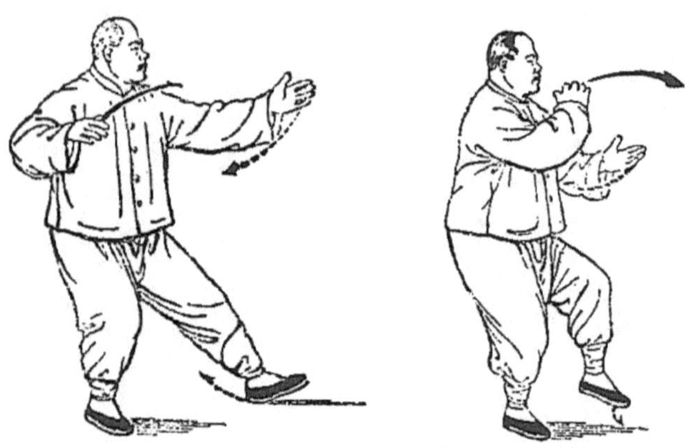

And then, setting the left foot on the ground *xū*
a half step east of the right heel,
extend the right hand upward and eastward
for its palm to face downward from east of the face,
and draw the left hand downward and northwestward
to northeast of the abdomen while turning its palm upward.
The gaze is toward the right hand extending.

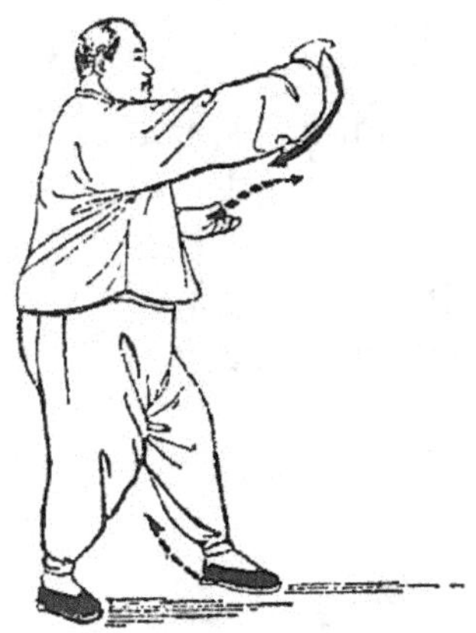

36.
右分脚
Yòu fēn jiǎo
Right Separating Foot.

Turning the torso southeastward
while lifting the left knee eastward,
shift the left hand upward and southeastward
while shifting the right hand downward and westward
for the palms again to face one another as if holding a sphere.
And then, shifting the right hand westward and upward
while shifting the left hand eastward
while turning its palm westward, step the left foot eastward
to begin to shift the weight eastward into a left bow stance.
The gaze shifts from the withdrawing right hand
to levelly eastward.

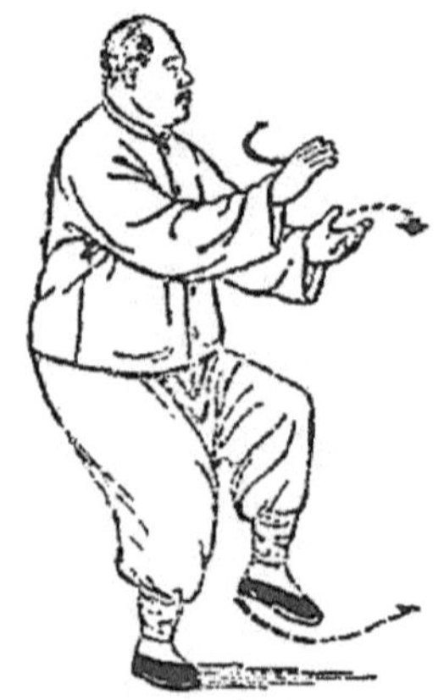
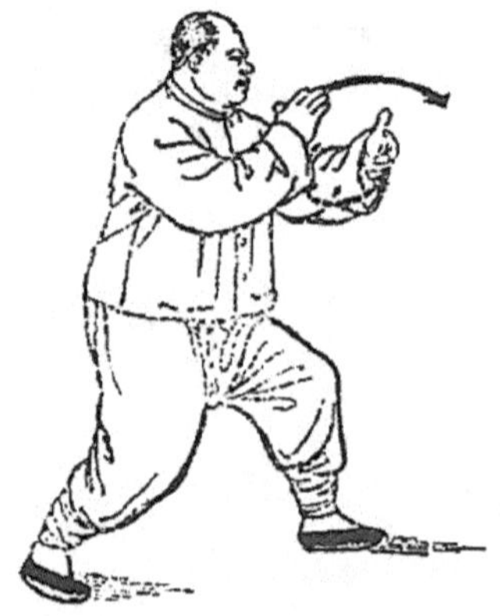

Then, turning the torso eastward
to complete the eastward shift into a left bow stance,
shift the left hand upward and northwestward,
and promptly arc the right hand eastward past the left hand
while settling its wrist for its palm to face downward and eastward.
The gaze is toward the arc of the right hand eastward.
And then shift the left foot on its ball southwestward,
and, lifting the right knee eastward
while circling the right hand downward
and then toward the north and then upward,
shift the left hand toward the south
while turning the right palm westward
to cross the hands with the right hand on the outside.
The gaze is over the crossing of the hands.

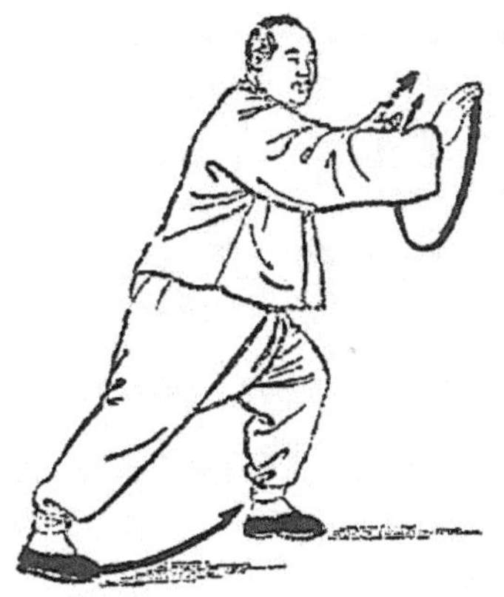 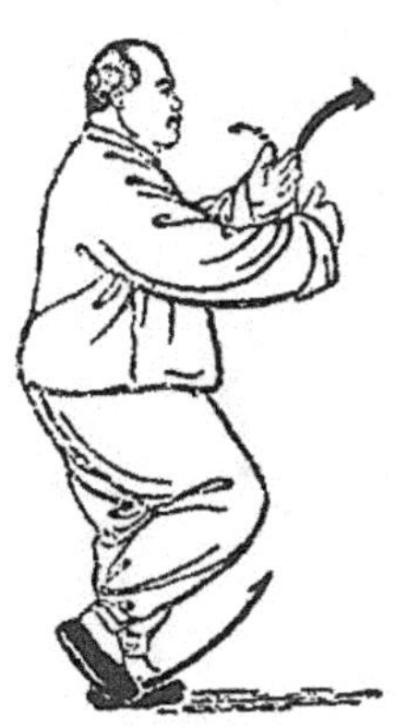

Then, continuing to lift the right knee upward
while shifting it southeastward,
shift the left hand upward and northwestward
while shifting the right hand upward and southeastward
to turn its palm toward the north.
And then straighten the left leg
to kick the right foot southeastward and upward
to the level of the *yāo*
while extending the left hand northwestward
and turning its palm toward the north
while extending the right hand southeastward
and turning its palm eastward.
The gaze shifts levelly in the direction of the right foot and hand.

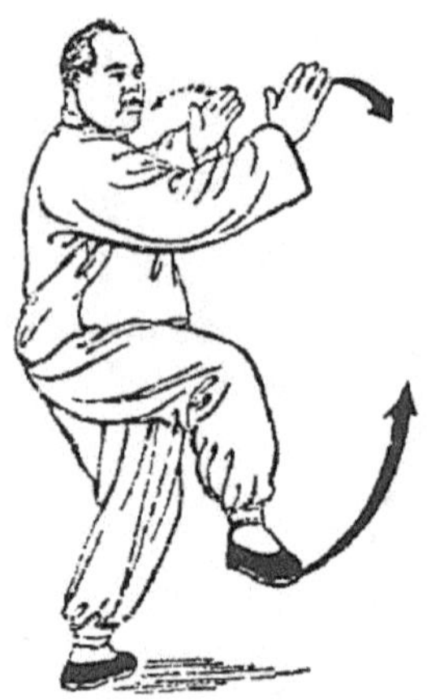 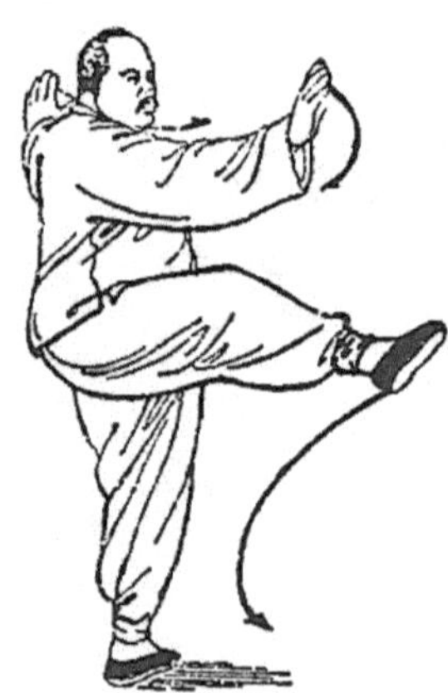

37.

左分脚

Zuǒ fēn jiǎo

Left Separating Foot.

Settling again onto the left leg
while lowering the right knee and letting the right foot drop *sōng*,
sink the elbows to draw the left hand southeastward
to east of the left shoulder
while turning its palm downward and southeastward
and shifting the right hand down to southeast of the right shoulder
while turning its palm northeastward.
And then, stepping the right foot southeastward
to begin to shift the weight southeastward into a right bow stance,
shift the right hand eastward
while turning its palm upward and toward the north
and shifting the left hand toward the right elbow
while turning its palm to face the elbow
with its fingers upward and southwestward.

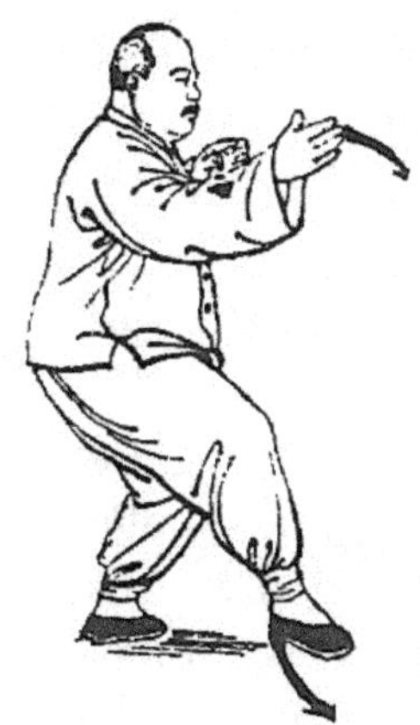
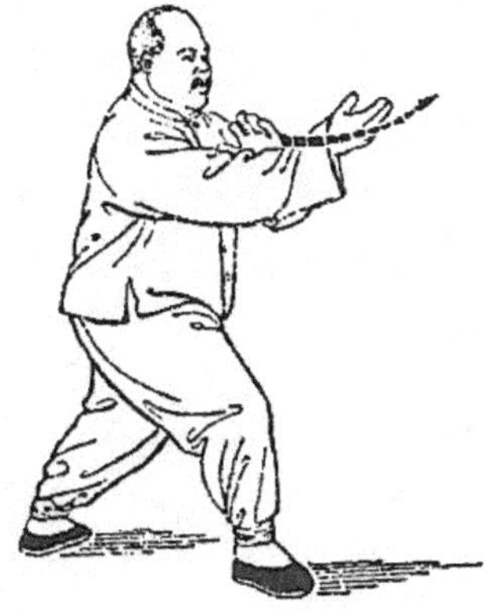

Then, completing the southeastward shift
into a right bow stance, extend the left hand eastward
while turning its palm upward and westward
and shifting the right hand northwestward
for its palm to face northwestward
with its fingers pointing toward the left wrist.
The gaze is toward the arc of the left hand eastward.
And then, lifting the left knee eastward
while shifting the right hand further westward,
circle the left hand
downward and southwestward and then upward
to cross the hands with the left hand on the outside.
The gaze is over the crossing of the hands.

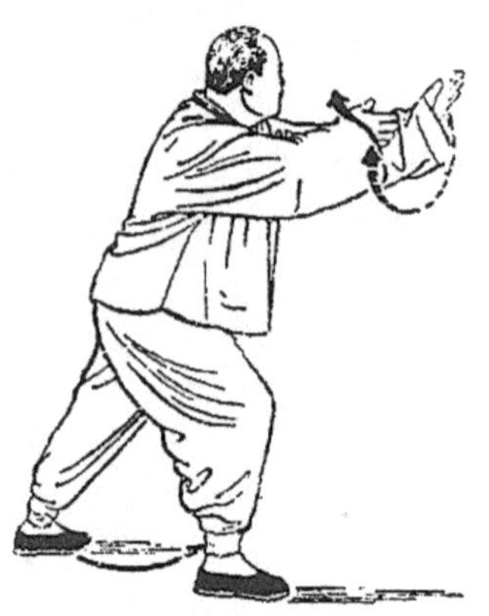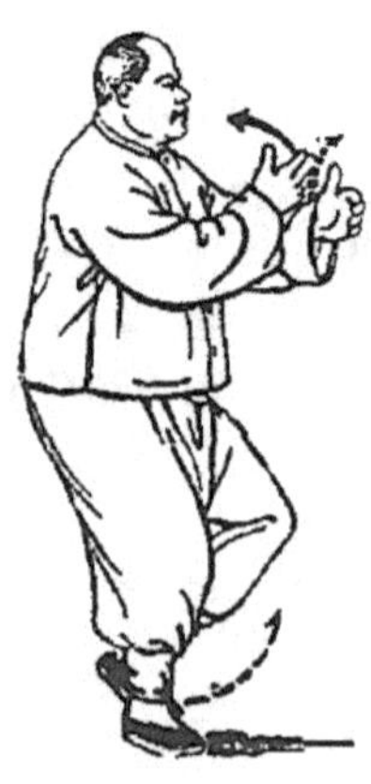

Fu Zhongwen doesn't say why the right foot in the first of these
two drawings is pointing more directly eastward than it is in the
drawing preceding it, or why no arrow indicates either the shift
eastward or the shift again southeastward that the second of these
two drawings indicates, but other such discrepancies suggest that
the reason is that Fu Zhongwen used some illustrations to illustrate
more than one form.

Then, continuing to lift the left knee eastward,
shift the left hand upward and eastward
while shifting the right hand upward and southwestward.
And then, kicking the left foot eastward and upward,
extend the left hand upward and northeastward
to turn its palm downward and southeastward,
and arc the right hand upward and southwestward
to turn its palm toward the south.
The gaze shifts levelly in the direction of the left hand.

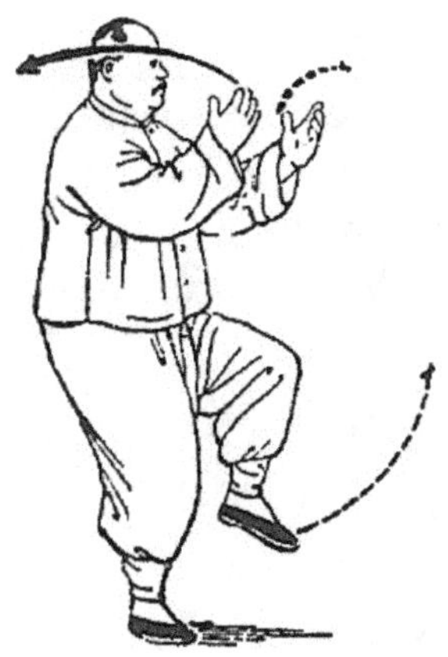 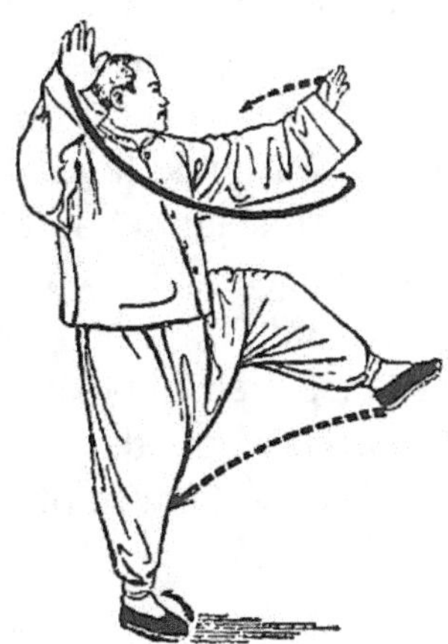

38.

左轉身蹬脚
Zuǒ zhuǎn shēn dēng jiǎo
Left Turning Body to Tread Foot.

Sōng the left knee, and lift the right toes
to pivot the right foot on its heel northeastward
while drawing the hands toward one another
to turn the palms to face one another
while beginning to swing the left knee northwestward
to begin to turn the torso northeastward.
And then, continuing the pivot of the right foot northwestward,
turn the torso to the north and then northwestward
while swinging the arms and the left knee with the turn
to settle the right foot flat and *shí* pointing northwestward
while crossing the hands
for their palms to face their opposite shoulders
with the left hand on the outside.
The gaze levelly follows the turn of the body.

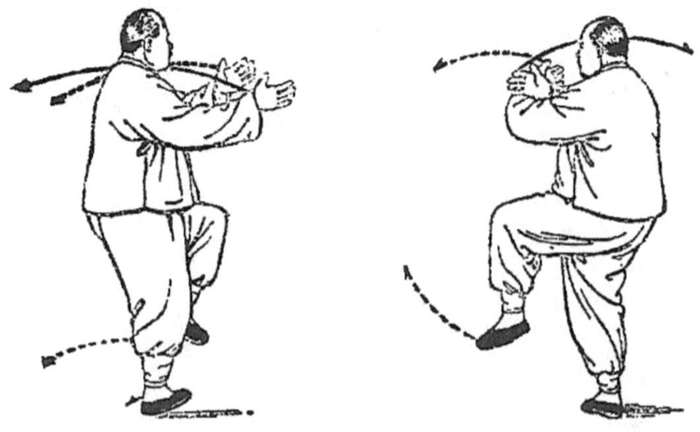

Then, kicking the left foot westward and upward
for its toes to point upward,
separate the hands to extend the left hand westward
to turn its palm northwestward,
while arcing the right hand northeastward
to turn its palm toward the north.
The gaze follows the left hand.

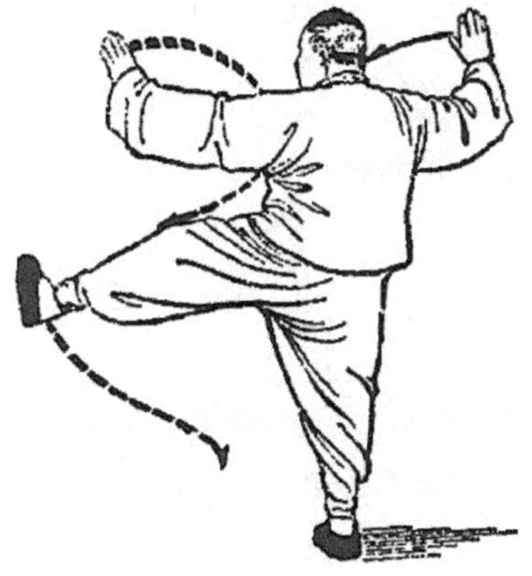

The *zì* separately literally meaning "tread" and "foot" together in
that order idiomatically mean "kick".

39.

左摟膝

Zuǒ lǒu xī
Left Drawing Knee.

Dropping the left foot *sōng*,
bend the right knee to settle onto the right leg,
and arc the left hand northeastward and downward past the chest
and then southwestward past the abdomen to above the left knee
for its palm to face downward from west of the *yāo*,
and sink the right elbow to draw the right hand
southwestward toward the right ear
while turning its palm westward.
The gaze follows the left hand and then shifts westward.
And then, turning the torso westward,
step the left foot westward into a left bow stance,
and brush the left hand to above and to the south of the left knee
while pushing the right palm westward
while settling its wrist to keep its palm facing westward.
The gaze is toward the right hand pushing forward.

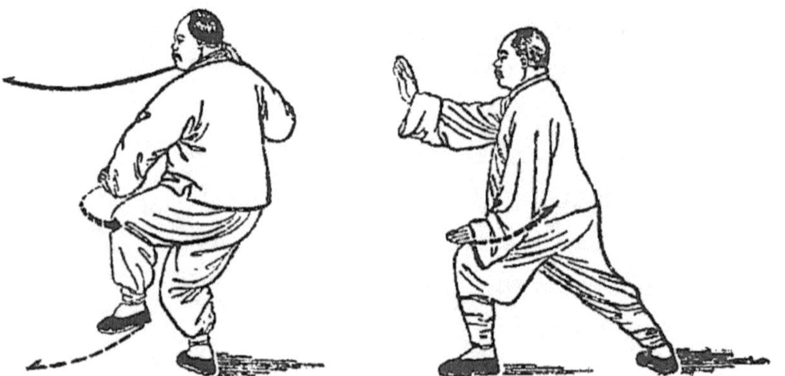

40.

右摟膝

Yòu lǒu xī

Right Drawing Knee.

Turning the left foot on its heel southwestward,
turn the torso southwestward
while swinging the arms with the turn,
sinking the right elbow until its forearm is horizontal,
turning the right palm southeastward
for its fingers to point upward and southwestward,
and shifting the left hand up to south of the left side of the *yāo*
while turning its palm toward the *yāo*.
And then, lifting the right knee westward,
arc the left hand eastward and upward
while turning its palm southwestward and upward
and shifting the right hand eastward and downward
to south of the abdomen
while turning its palm downward.
The gaze shifts from the right hand to the left hand.

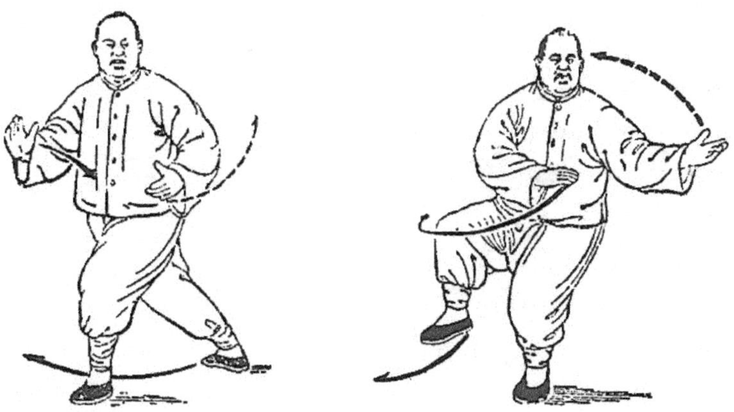

Then, stepping the right foot westward
to set its heel on the ground *xū*,
arc the right hand downward and westward
and then northeastward to southwest of the *yāo*
while arcing the left hand upward and westward
to southeast of the left ear
for its palm to face downward and northwestward.
And then, shifting the weight westward into a right bow stance,
turn the torso westward while pushing the left palm westward
while settling its wrist
and circling the right hand westward and downward
and then northeastward to north of the *yāo*
while keeping its palm facing downward.
The gaze shifts toward the right palm brushing past the knee
and then levels again past the left palm's forward push.

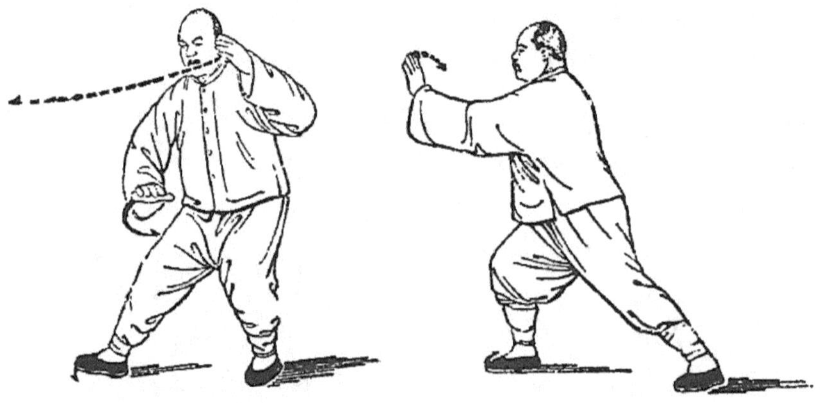

41.

進步栽錘

Jìn bù zāi chuí

Advance Step Imposing Hammer.

Turning the right foot on its heel northwestward
and lifting the left heel to shift into the tray stance,
begin to arc the left hand northeastward and downward.
Then, lifting the left knee westward past the right knee
to turn the torso northwestward,
circle the right hand upward and northeastward
and then downward and then southwestward to northeast of the *yāo*
while closing it into a fist with its heart toward the south
and continuing the arc of the left hand
northeastward and downward and then promptly southwestward
for its palm to face the left knee from above it.
The gaze is toward the left palm brushing downward.

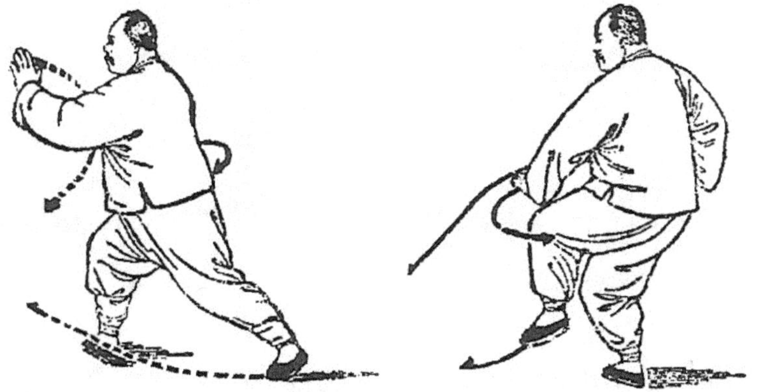

And then step the left foot westward into a left bow stance,
and lean the torso westward and downward
while brushing the left hand to south of the left knee
while keeping its palm facing downward
and hammering the right fist westward and downward
to below and to the northwest of the left knee.
The gaze is toward the right fist striking.

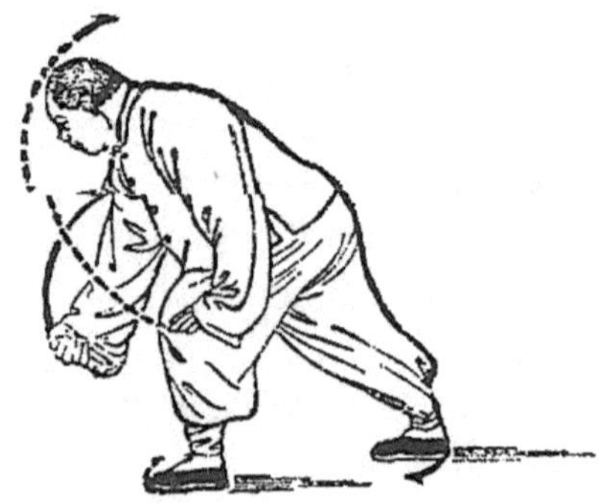

42.

翻身撇身錘

Fān shēn piē shēn chuí
Turning Body to Cast Body to Hammer.

Returning the torso to *xū líng dǐng jìn*
and promptly turning it to the north
while swinging the arms with the turn,
turn the left foot on its heel to the north,
and turn the right foot on its heel northeastward
while arcing the right fist upward and northeastward
to north of the sternum
and arcing the left hand upward and northeastward
to northwest of the left temple
while turning its palm toward the north.
The gaze follows the movement of the hands.
Then, pivoting the left foot on its heel northeastward,
promptly lift the right knee eastward
to turn the torso eastward
while shifting the right forearm upward with the turn
to the level of the sternum
and arcing the left hand downward with the turn
for its palm to face downward and northeastward
from east of the upper abdomen.
The gaze includes the motion of the hands.

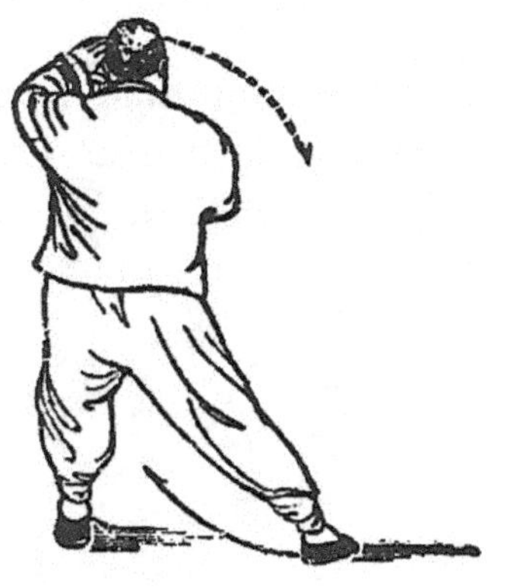 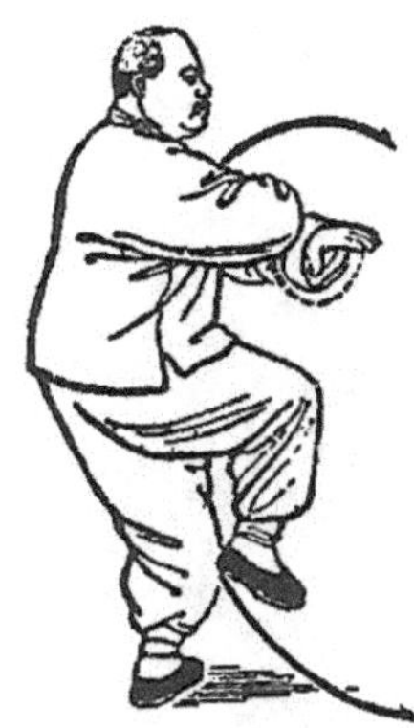

153

Then, stepping the right foot eastward
to touch its heel to the ground *xū*, press the back of the right fist
upward and eastward over the left hand.
And then, shifting the weight eastward into a right bow stance,
arc the right fist downward and southwestward
to southeast of right side of the *yāo*
while turning its heart upward
and extending the left hand eastward and upward
while turning its palm toward the south
for its fingers to point upward and eastward.

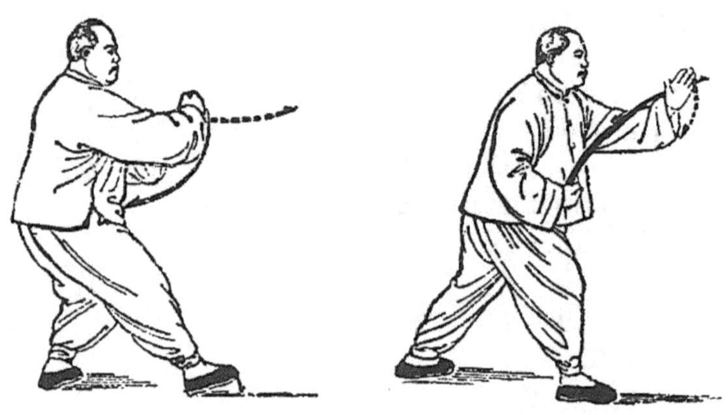

43.

進步搬攔錘

Jìn bù bān lán chuí

Advance Step Shift Block Hammer.

Turning the torso northeastward
while straightening the right knee and bending the left knee
to shift the weight westward onto the left leg,
arc the right fist upward and eastward to the level of the chin
while turning its heart downward and toward the north
and sinking the left elbow
to draw its hand downward and westward
to north of the right elbow while keeping its palm facing south.
The gaze is across the top of the right fist.
Then, shifting the right fist downward and northwestward
to east of the sternum,
draw the left hand northwestward to northeast of the abdomen.
The gaze shifts levelly toward the southwest.

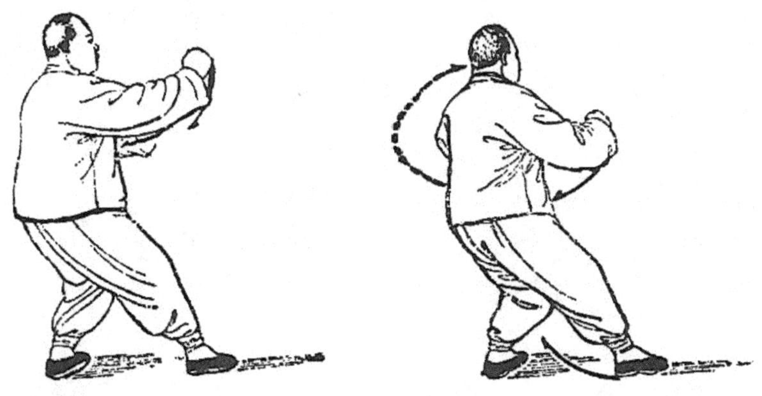

Chuí is the name of both the *zì* meaning "cudgel" and the *zì*
meaning "hammer" in the designations for the *bān lán chuí* forms.
And what Yang Chengfu calls shift block hammer is the same as
what he calls shift block cudgel. So, because the pronunciation is
identical and the meaning similar, that may be a dictation error.

And then, straightening the left leg somewhat
to lift the right knee eastward,
coil the right fist downward and westward to northeast of the *yāo*
while arcing the left hand downward and westward
and then upward and eastward to northwest of the left ear
while turning its palm eastward.
The gaze shifts with the motion of the hands
before returning levelly southwestward.
Then, turning the torso eastward, step the right foot southeastward
to set its heel on the ground *xū* to turn its toes southeastward
while arcing the right fist upward and eastward
and shifting the left hand southeastward and downward
to cross the hands with the left palm facing north
and the heart of the right fist facing northwestward.

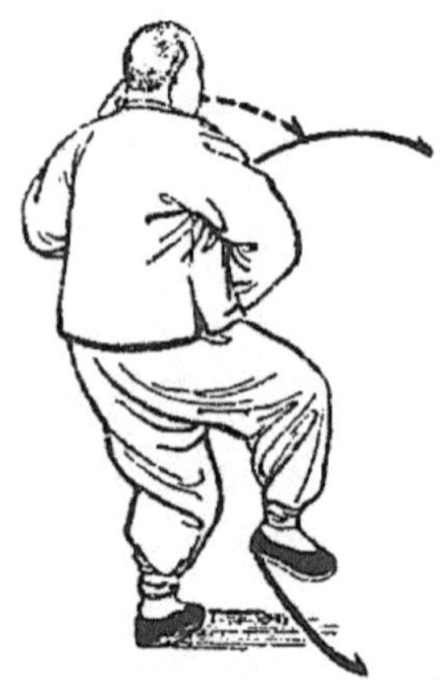 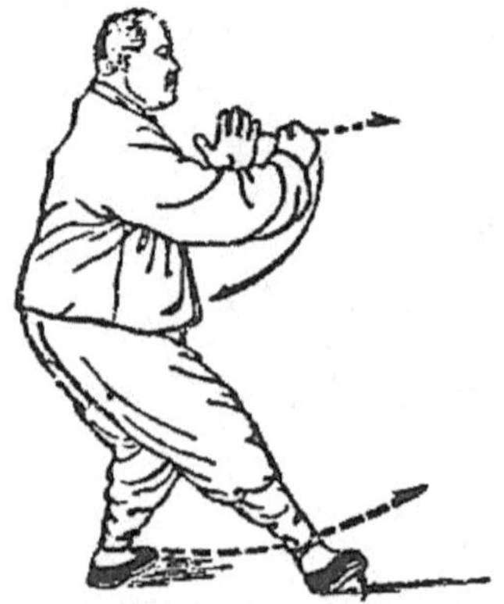

Then, settling the right foot flat and *shí*
and turning the torso southeastward,
bend the right knee to shift the weight to it
to lift the left knee eastward
while shifting the left hand eastward
and arcing the right fist downward and westward
for its heart to face upward and toward the north
from south of the abdomen.
And then, turning the torso further southeastward
to step the left foot eastward to touch its heel to the ground *xū*,
shift the right fist further westward
while shifting the left hand downward and further eastward.

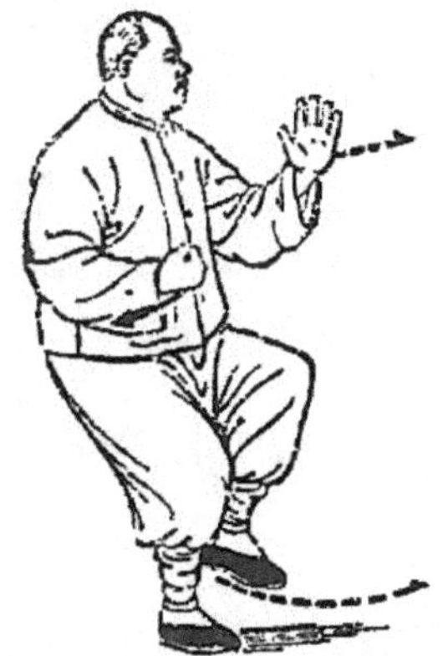 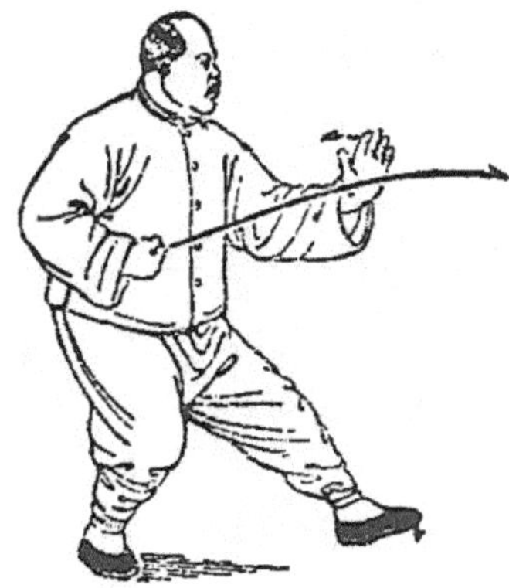

Then, turning the torso eastward
while shifting the weight eastward into a left bow stance,
hammer the right fist upward and eastward
while shifting the left hand southwestward
toward the right shoulder
as the right forearm glides eastward past it
until the right arm is nearly straight
with the left palm facing the right forearm
with its thumb nearly touching the right elbow.
The gaze follows the left palm before shifting to the right fist.

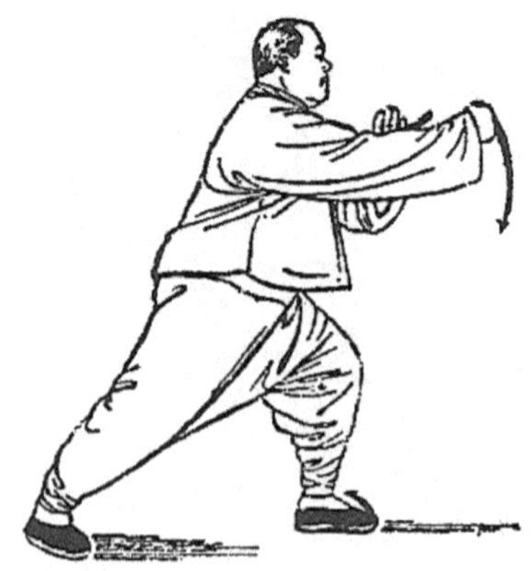

44.

右蹬脚

Yòu dēng jiǎo
Right treading Foot.

Turning the left foot on its heel northeastward,
lift the right heel to shift into the tray stance
while shifting the left hand downward and toward the north
for its fingers to point upward and eastward
from northeast of the sternum
and shifting the right hand downward to east of the abdomen
while opening it and turning its palm
downward and northwestward.
Then, lifting the right knee eastward,
shift the left hand upward and toward the south
while shifting the right hand northwestward and upward
to cross the hands in front of the clavicle
with the left palm facing southwestward
with its fingers upward and southeastward
and the right hand on the outside
with its palm facing inward.
The gaze is over the hands crossing.

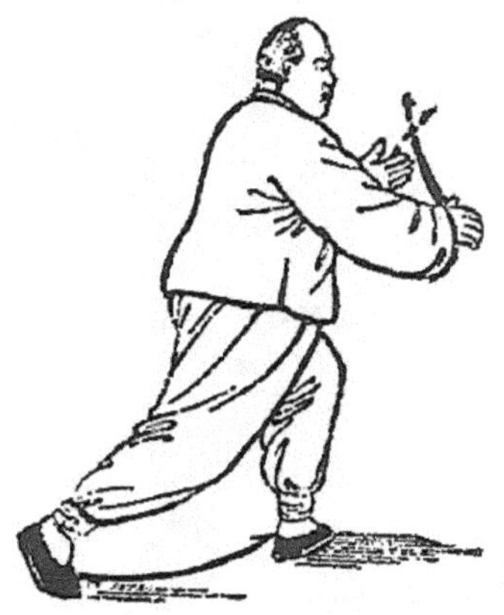 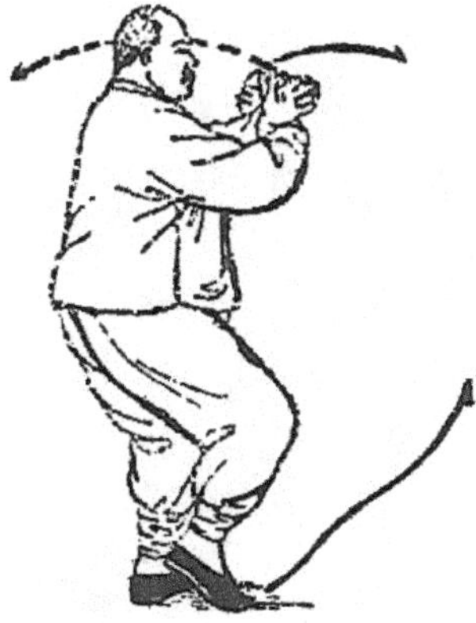

And then, continuing to lift the right knee
while turning the torso northeastward,
straighten the left knee to kick the right foot eastward
for its toes to point upward at the level of the *yāo*,
and spread the hands
upward and northwestward and southeastward
for the right palm to face northeastward and downward
while the left palm faces toward the north.
The gaze is level in the direction of the kick.

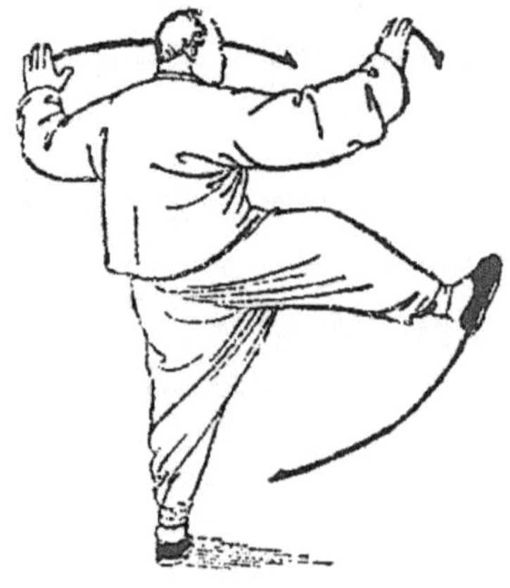

45.

左打虎式用法

Zuǒ dǎ hǔ shì yòng fǎ

Left Striking Tiger Form Use Method.

Settling again onto the left leg,
lower the right knee to drop its foot *sōng*,
and arc the left hand eastward to northeast of the left shoulder
while turning its palm toward the south
for its fingers to point upward and eastward
and shifting the right hand down to shoulder-level
while turning its palm downward and eastward.
The gaze shifts toward the right hand.
Then set the right foot on the ground
parallel to the left foot to settle into the horse stance
before lifting the left knee northeastward
while shifting the right hand down to the level of the sternum
while turning its palm further downward
and shifting the left hand down to the level of the right hand
while turning its palm upward.
The gaze shifts levelly northeastward.

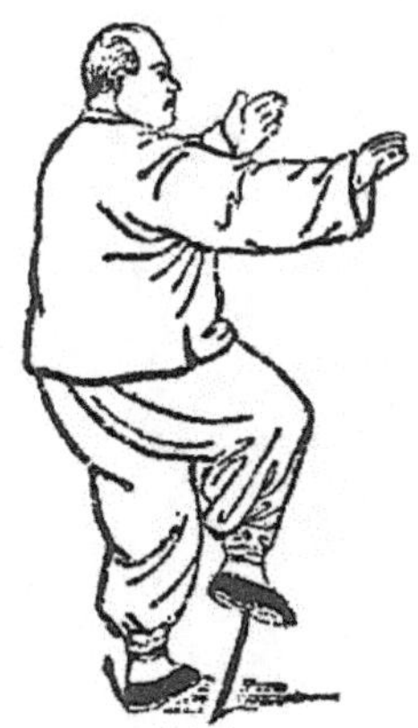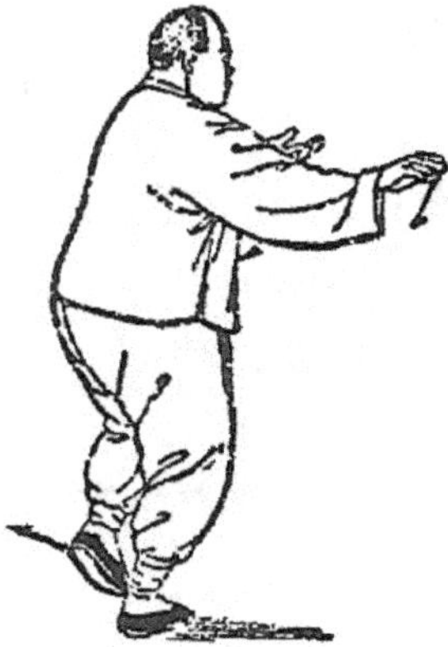

Then, turning the torso toward the north
while keeping the arms eastward
but shifting them down to the level of the abdomen,
swing the left knee northwestward.
And then step the left foot northwestward
to settle it flat and *shi* pointing toward the north,
and bend the left knee while straightening the right leg
to shift the weight to the left leg
while sweeping the left hand downward and westward
and then upward and eastward to northeast of the forehead
while closing it into a fist and turning its heart toward the north
and drawing the right hand downward and northwestward
to north of the abdomen and below the right fist
while closing it into a fist with its heart toward the abdomen.
The gaze follows the left hand until it's higher than the eyes
and then shifts levelly northeastward.

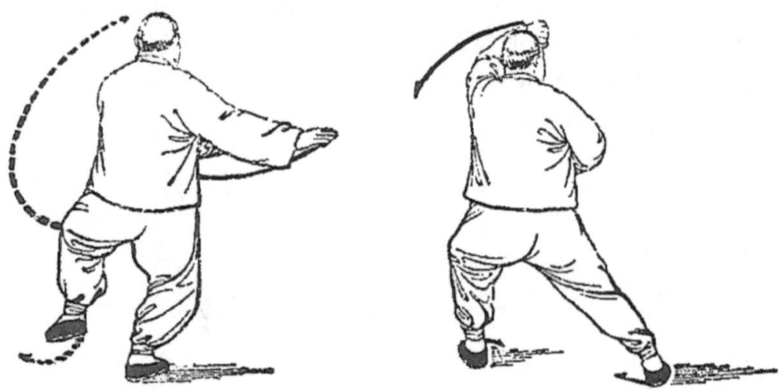

46.

右打虎式用法

Yòu dǎ hǔ shì yòng fǎ
Right Striking Tiger Form Use Method

Arcing the left hand northwestward
and downward to shoulder-level
while opening it and turning its palm downward,
turn the torso northeastward
while swinging the right arm with the turn
to shift its forearm up to the level of the sternum
while turning the left foot on its heel northeastward
to turn the right foot on its ball westward.
The gaze is briefly toward the left palm
before returning levelly northeastward.
Then, promptly lifting the right knee southeastward
to turn the torso southeastward,
arc the right hand southeastward and downward
and then southwestward to above and to the west of the right knee
while opening it and turning its palm northeastward
and arcing the left hand downward and southeastward
to above and to the northeast of the right knee
while settling its wrist to keep its palm facing downward.

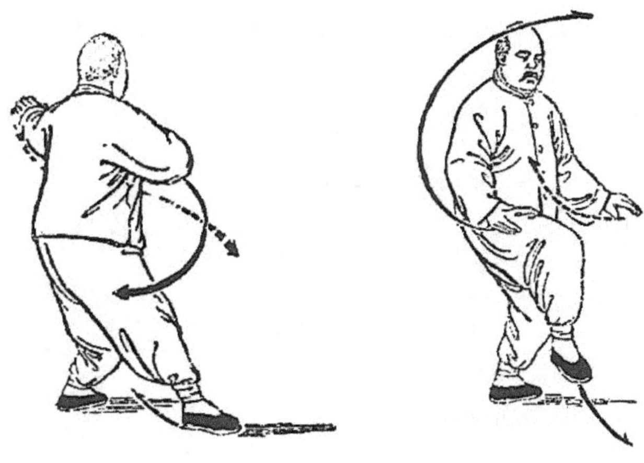

And then step the right foot southeastward into a right bow stance
while sweeping the right hand westward and upward
and then eastward to above and to the southeast of the forehead
while closing it into a fist with its heart toward the south
and arcing the left hand southwestward and upward
to southeast of the upper abdomen
while closing it into a fist with its heart toward the abdomen.
The gaze shifts levelly with the turn of the torso
but shifts briefly toward the right fist's upward arc
before returning levelly southeastward.

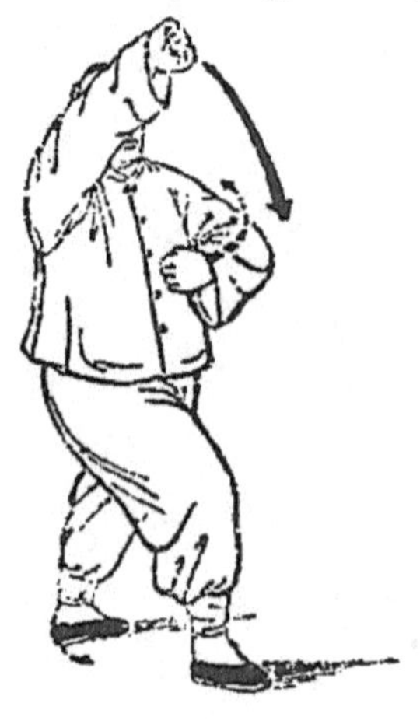

47.
回身右蹬脚同前
Huí shēn yòu dēng jiǎo tóng qián
Revert Body to Tread Right Foot Same as Before

Shifting the left foot on its ball further southwestward,
bend the left knee to shift the weight toward it
to turn the torso eastward
while arcing the right fist eastward and downward
while turning its heart northeastward
and shifting the left fist northeastward and upward
and then westward to east of the left shoulder.
The gaze follows the turn of the body.
Then, completing the shift of weight to the left leg,
lift the right knee eastward
to draw its foot northwestward toward the left foot,
and arc the left fist downward and southeastward and then upward
while arcing the right fist
downward and northwestward and then upward
while opening both hands and turning their palms inward
to cross them in front of the clavicle
with the right hand on the outside.
The gaze follows the left hand before leveling eastward.

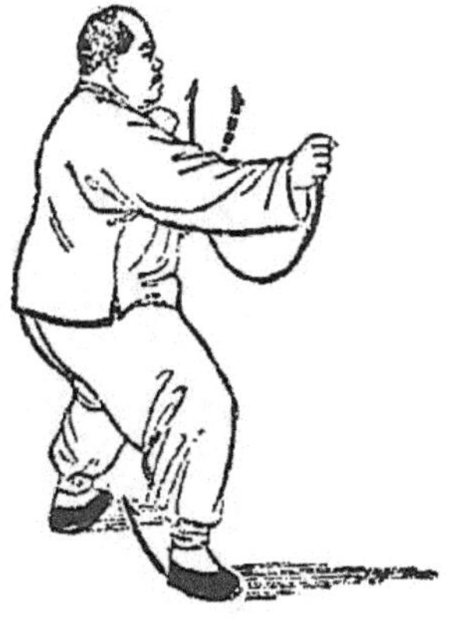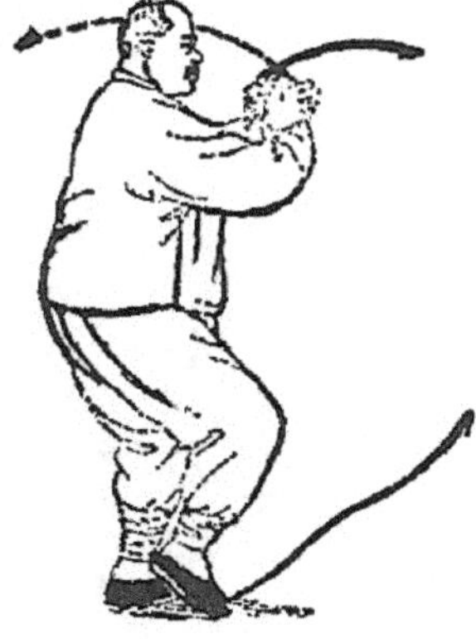

Then, separating the hands
while turning the torso northeastward
to kick the right heel eastward and upward
for its toes to point upward at the level of the *yāo*,
arc the left hand upward and northwestward
while turning its palm toward the north
and extending the right hand upward and eastward
while turning its palm northeastward.
The gaze follows the left hand before following the right hand.

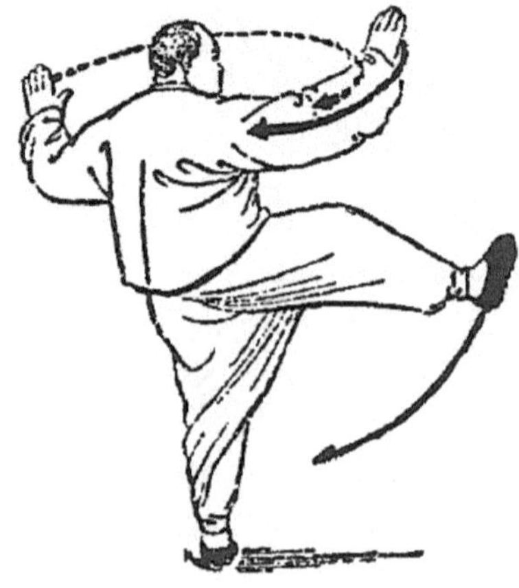

48.

雙風貫耳

Shuāng fēng guàn ěr
Double Winds Through Ears.

Sōng the right knee, and,
quickly pivoting the left foot on its ball westward,
swing the right knee southeastward to turn the torso southeastward
while swinging the hands with the turn
and quickly drawing them toward one another,
each to above and southeast of its shoulder,
while turning the palms toward the face.
The gaze levelly follows the turn.
And then, lowering the right knee
while extending its foot southeastward,
arc the left hand downward and then northeastward
while arcing the right hand downward and then southwestward
while turning the palms toward one another.

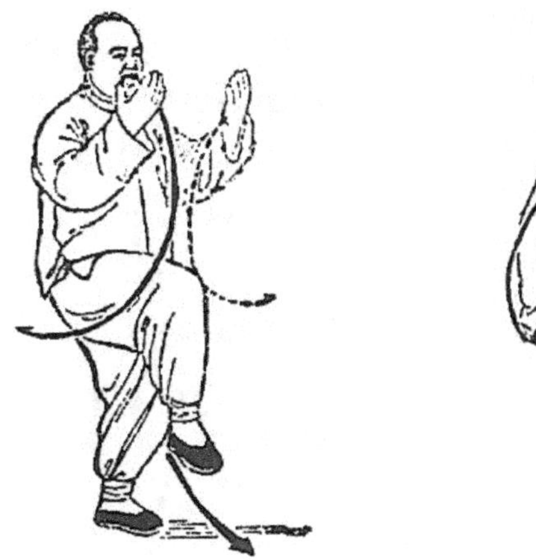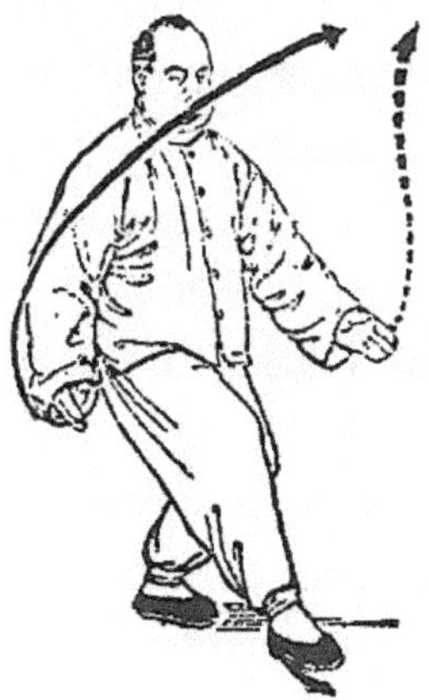

And then, completing the extension of the right foot southeastward
to shift the weight southeastward into a right bow stance,
swiftly arc the right hand westward and upward
and then northeastward to southeast of the forehead
while swiftly arcing the left hand eastward and upward
to east of the forehead while closing each hand into a fist
and turning the heart of the left fist southeastward
while turning the heart of the right fist toward the south.
The gaze is level toward the southeast.

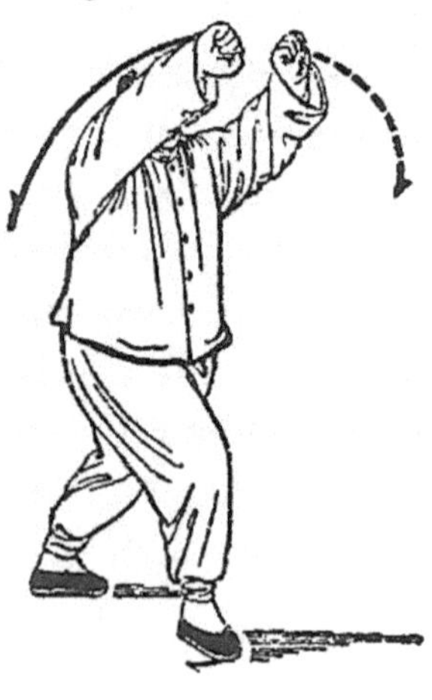

49.

左蹬脚用法

Zuǒ dēng jiǎo yòng fǎ

Left treading Foot Use Method.

Turning the right foot on its heel toward the south,
open the hands while quickly arcing them away from one another
and down to shoulder-level
while turning the left palm southwestward
for its fingers to point southeastward and upward
and turning the right palm southeastward and downward.
And then, shifting the weight to the right leg
to lift the left knee eastward,
continue the arc of the hands downward
and then toward one another
and then past one another and upward
to cross them in front of the sternum
with the palms facing inward with the left hand on the outside.
The gaze is between the arcing of the hands
before leveling eastward.

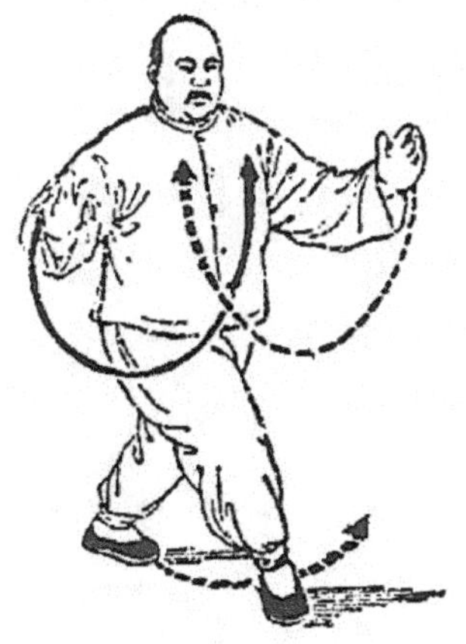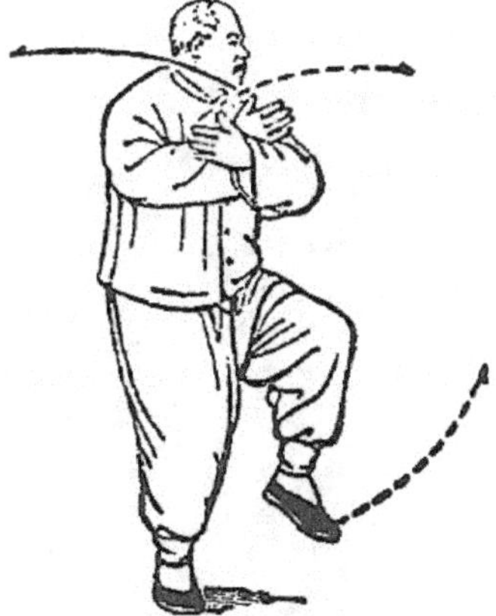

And then, quickly arcing the right hand upward and westward
while turning its palm southwestward
and quickly arcing the left hand upward and eastward
while turning its palm southeastward,
kick the left foot eastward and upward
for its toes to point upward at the level of the *yāo*.
The gaze shifts toward the separating of the hands
before returning eastward with the extending of the left hand.

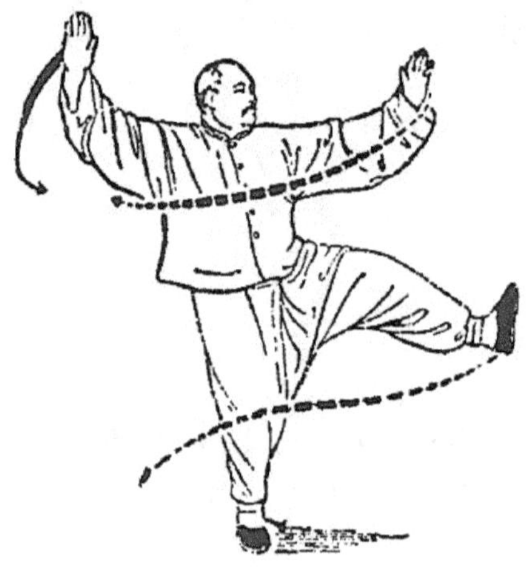

50.

轉身蹬脚用法

Zhuǎn shēn dēng jiǎo yòng fǎ

Turning Body to Tread Foot Use Method.

Lowering the left leg,
quickly pivot the right foot on its ball northeastward
to swing the left leg downward and southwestward
to turn the torso to the south and then southwestward
while arcing the right hand down to the level of the abdomen
while turning its palm downward and southwestward
and arcing the left hand downward and southwestward
while turning its palm northwestward toward the right hand.
And then, swinging the arms with the turn,
continue the pivot of the right foot on its ball
eastward and then toward the south and then westward
to continue the swing of the left leg northwestward
and then northeastward to turn the torso eastward,
and then settle the left foot on the ground *shi* north of the right foot
with its toes pointing northeastward
while crossing the hands in front of the clavicle
with the palms facing inward and the right hand on the outside
to begin to lift the right knee eastward.
The gaze levelly follows the pivot.

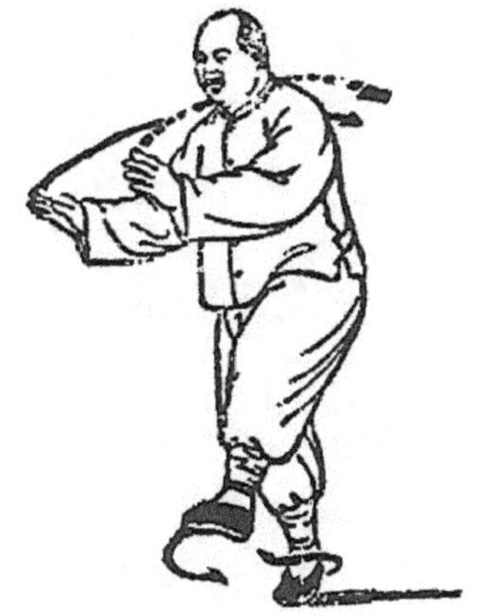
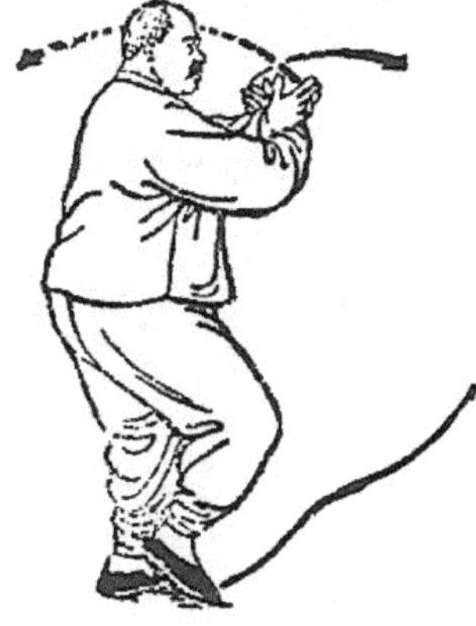

And then lift the right knee
while turning the torso northeastward,
and straighten the left knee to kick the right foot eastward
for its toes to point upward at the level of the *yāo*,
and arc the left hand upward and northwestward
while turning its palm toward the north
and arcing the right hand upward and eastward
while turning its palm northeastward.
The gaze is toward the right hand.

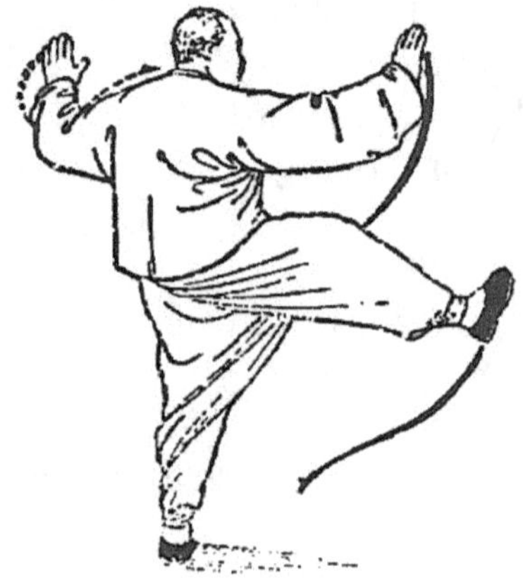

51.

進步搬攔錘

Jìn bù bān lán chuí
Advance Step Shift Block Hammer.

Sōng the right knee to settle again onto the left leg
while closing the right hand into a fist
and coiling it downward and northwestward
to northeast of the abdomen while turning its heart downward
and circling the left hand westward and downward
and then eastward and upward to northwest of the left ear
while turning its palm eastward.
The gaze shifts from the right hand to levelly forward.
Then, turning the torso again eastward,
step the right foot southeastward to touch its heel to the ground *xū*
to turn it southeastward with its toes upward
while arcing the right fist upward and eastward
and arcing the left hand southeastward and downward
to cross the hands in front of the sternum
with the left palm facing south with its fingers upward
and the right fist on the outside with its heart northwestward.

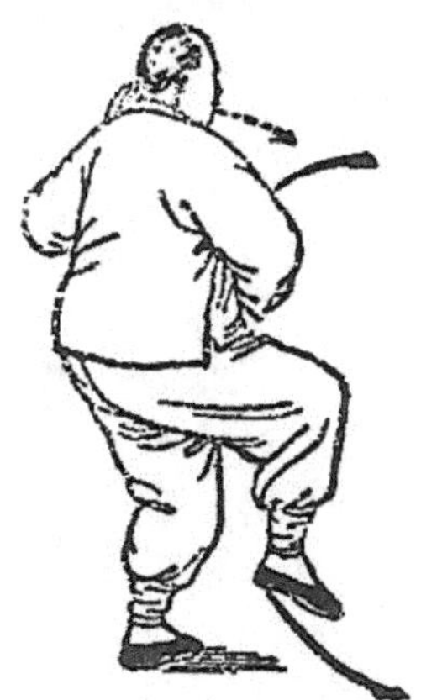 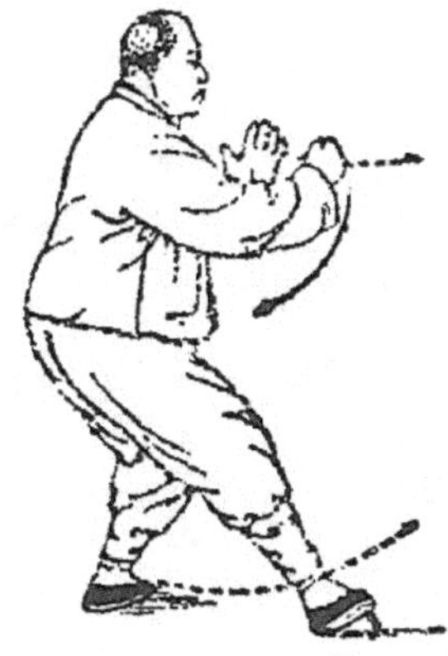

Then, turning the torso southeastward
while settling the right foot flat and *shí* pointing southeastward,
bend the right knee to shift the weight to it
to lift the left knee eastward
while arcing the right fist downward and southwestward
to south of the abdomen
and beginning to shift the left hand eastward.
The gaze is over the left hand.
And then, turning the torso further southeastward,
step the left foot eastward to touch its heel to the ground *xū*
while continuing the shift of the left hand eastward
and shifting the right fist downward and further westward.

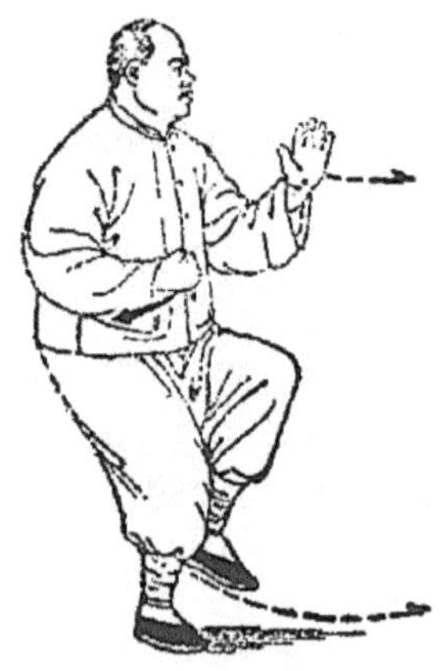
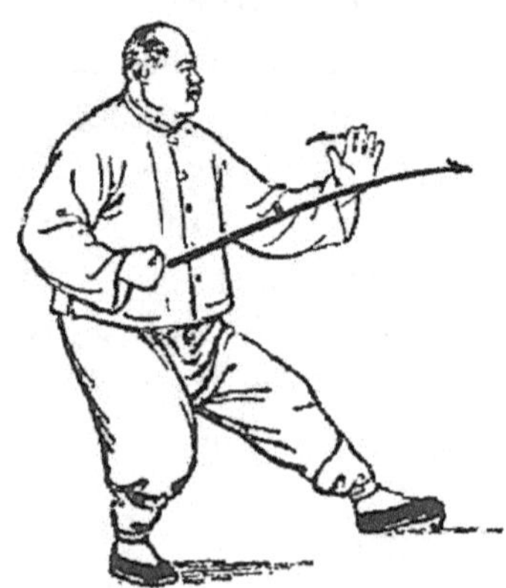

And then, turning the torso eastward
and shifting the weight eastward into a left bow stance,
hammer the right fist upward and eastward
while drawing the left hand southwestward
toward the right shoulder
as the right forearm glides eastward past it
until the right arm is nearly straight
with the left palm facing the right forearm
with its thumb nearly touching the right elbow.
The gaze follows the left palm before shifting to the right fist.

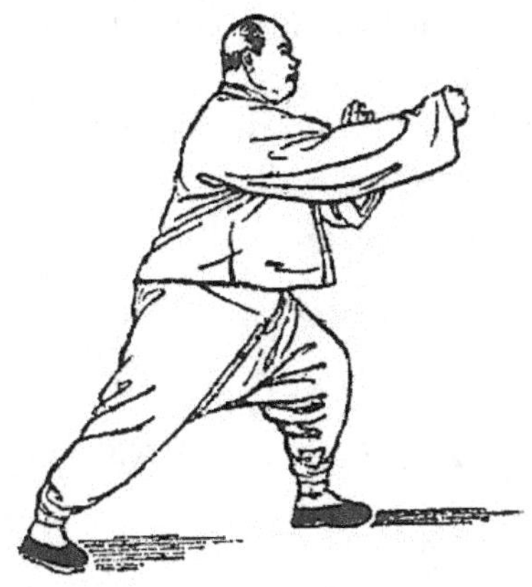

52.
如封似閉
Rú fēng shì bì
As Sealing Like Closing.

Thread the left hand beneath the right elbow
and to the southeast of it to turn the left palm southwestward
while opening the right hand
to turn its palm upward and northwestward.
Then, bending the right knee to shift the weight westward onto it,
sink the right elbow to draw its hand westward toward the clavicle
while shifting the left hand upward to cross the hands
for both palms to face the clavicle with the left hand on the outside
with its fingers pointing upward and toward the south
while the right fingers point upward and toward the north.
The gaze includes the palms.

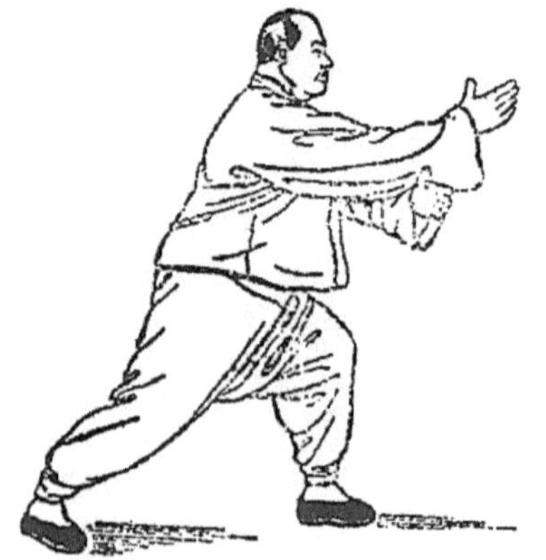 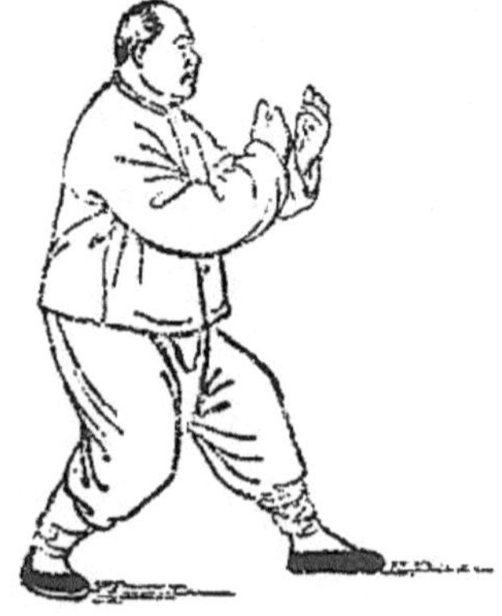

Then, shifting the left hand downward and northwestward while shifting the right hand downward and southeastward, turn the palms to face one another at the level of the sternum. And then, shifting the weight eastward into a left bow stance, push both hands upward and eastward to east of the clavicle while settling their wrists and turning their palms eastward. The gaze is levelly eastward.

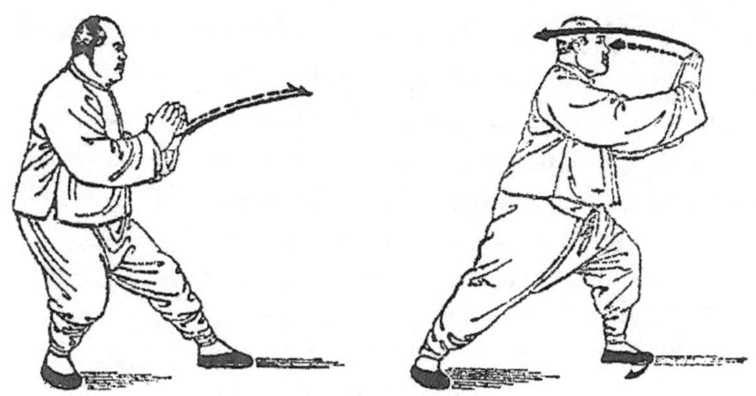

53.

十字手

Shí zì shǒu
Ten *Zì* Hands.

Keeping the weight on the left leg
while turning its foot on its heel to the south,
quickly turn the torso to the south
while swinging the hands with turn
and turning the right foot on its heel southwestward
while spreading the elbows apart
for the right fingers to point upward and eastward
while the left fingers point upward and westward.
The gaze is through the space between the palms.
Then arc the hands upward and away from one another
and then downward to shoulder-level
for the right fingers to point upward and westward
while the left fingers point upward and eastward

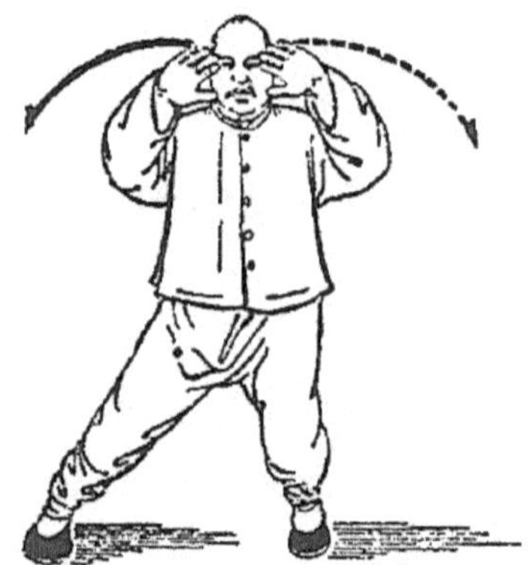 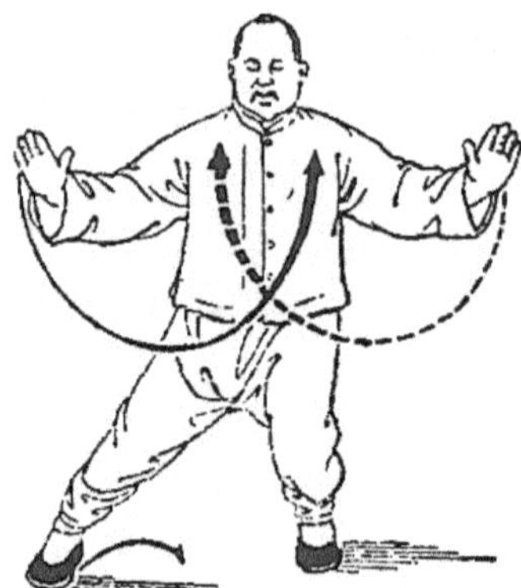

And then, stepping the right foot toward the left foot
into the horse stance,
arc the hands downward and toward one another and then upward
to cross them in front of the clavicle
with the palms facing inward with the right hand on the outside.
The gaze is over the intersection of the wrists.

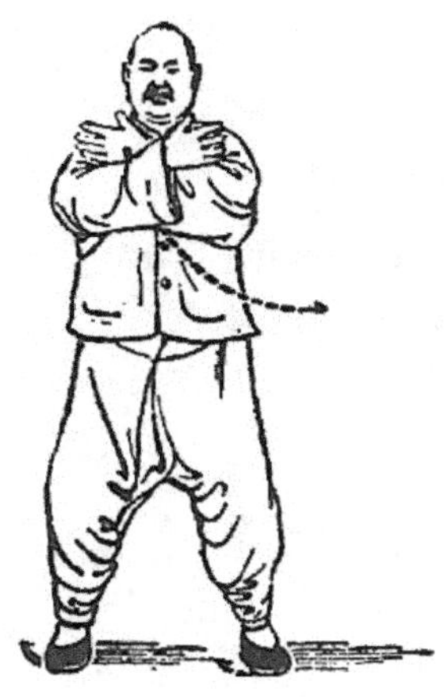

54.

抱虎歸山

Bào hǔ guī shān

Embrace Tiger and Return to Mountain.

Right drawing knee.

Turning the right foot on its heel westward,
promptly turn the torso southwestward
while turning the left foot on its heel southwestward
and arcing the left hand downward and southeastward
to southeast of the *yāo* while turning its palm northwestward.
And then, continuing the southwestward turn of the torso,
lift the right knee westward
while shifting the right hand downward and westward
to southwest of the abdomen while turning its palm downward
and arcing the left hand eastward and upward to shoulder-level
while turning its palm upward and westward.
The gaze follows the left hand.

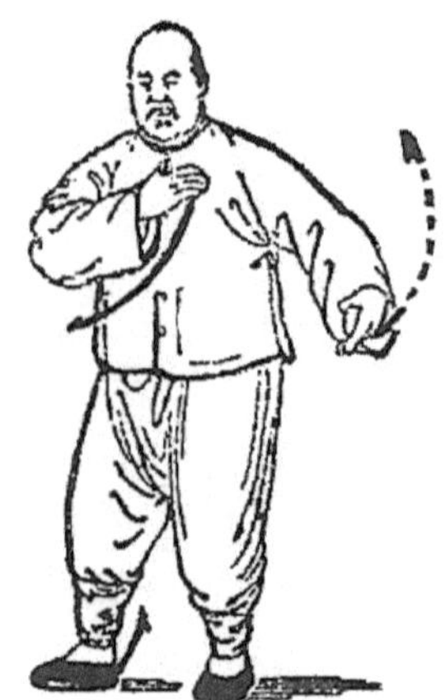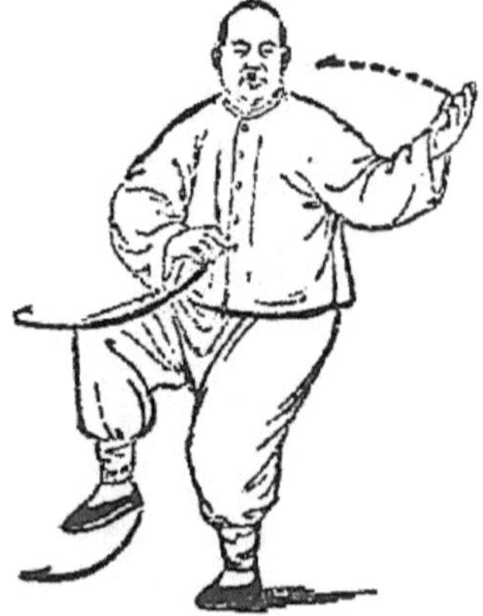

Then, continuing to turn the torso southwestward
while extending the right leg northwestward
to touch its heel to the ground *xū*,
arc the left hand upward and westward to southeast of the left ear
for its palm to face downward and northwestward,
and shift the right hand downward and northwestward
to west of the *yāo*.
And then push the left hand northwestward while settling its wrist
and shifting the weight northwestward into a right bow stance
while turning the torso northwestward
and swinging the right hand to north of the *yāo*
while keeping its palm facing downward.
The gaze shifts levelly with the turn
and follows the left hand pushing forward.

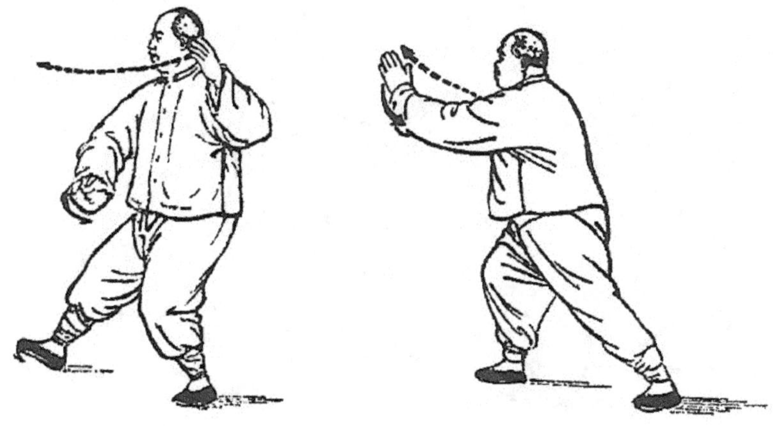

The remainder of this segment is a repetition of the eighteenth
segment with neither separate naming nor separate numbering.

Stroke (Rollback).

Sinking the left elbow
to shift its hand down to the level of the sternum,
arc the right hand westward and upward
for its palm to face downward and westward
from west of the right shoulder.
And then, turning the torso southwestward,
straighten the right leg to bend the left knee
to shift the weight southeastward onto the left leg
to roll the right hand downward and eastward
to the level of the sternum
while sinking the left elbow to roll the left hand southeastward
while turning its palm toward the north.

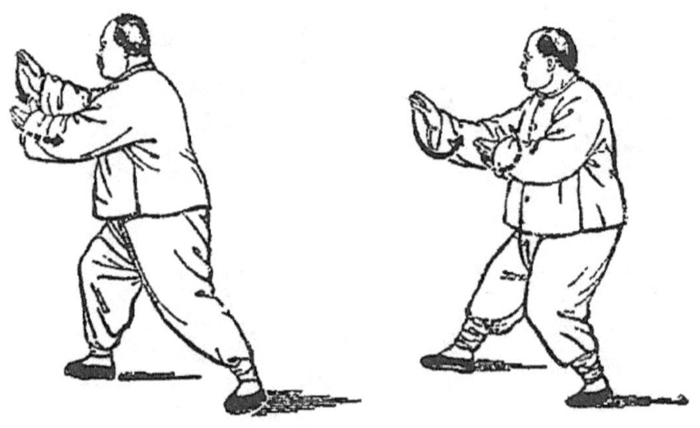

Press.

Then, turning the torso westward,
circle both hands downward and southeastward and then upward
for the left palm to face downward and northwestward
at shoulder-level with the right palm facing the left wrist
from northwest of the left forearm.
And then, turning the torso northwestward
while shifting the weight again northwestward
into a right bow stance,
press the back of the right hand northwestward and upward,
while pushing the left hand northwestward while settling its wrist
to press the right forearm further northwestward.
The gaze is toward the right forearm.

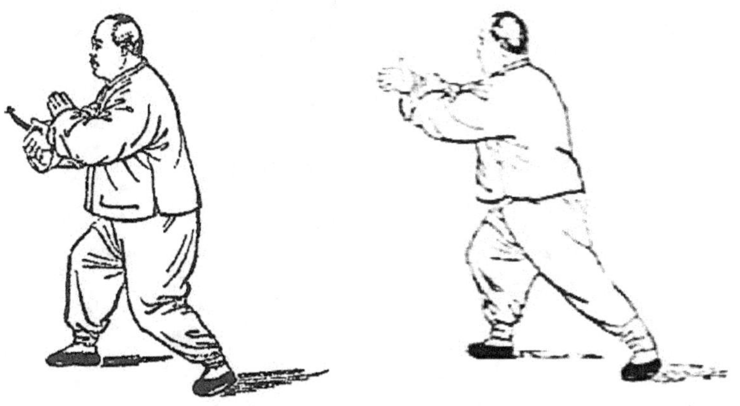

Push.

Then pass the left hand over the right wrist
while turning both palms to face downward at shoulder-level,
and then spread the hands shoulder-width apart.
And then, bending the left knee while straightening the right leg
to shift the weight southeastward onto the left leg,
sink the elbows to draw the hands toward their shoulders
for the left palm to face northwestward
while the right palm faces westward.
The gaze is level and northwestward.

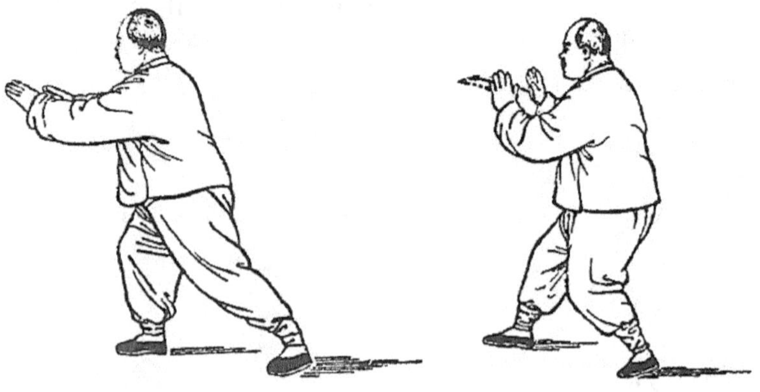

And then, quickly pushing the palms
upward and northwestward while settling their wrists,
again shift the weight northwestward into a right bow stance.
The gaze remains level and forward.

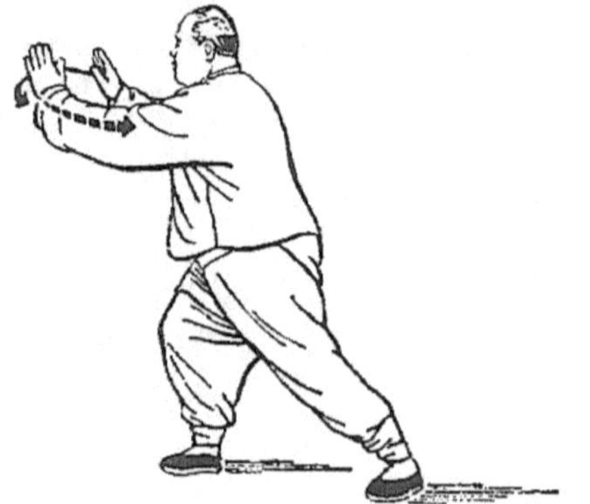

55.

斜單鞭
Xié dān biān
Oblique Solitary Whip.

Bending the left knee and straightening the right leg
to shift the weight to the left leg, turn the torso southwestward
while swinging the hands with the turn
and shifting them down to shoulder-level
while turning the left palm downward
and turning the right palm southwestward.
Then, turning the right foot on its heel southwestward,
bend the right knee while straightening the left knee
to return the weight to the right leg
while turning the torso toward the south
and swinging the arms with the turn
while turning the right palm downward and southeastward
and sinking the elbows to draw the hands toward the sternum.

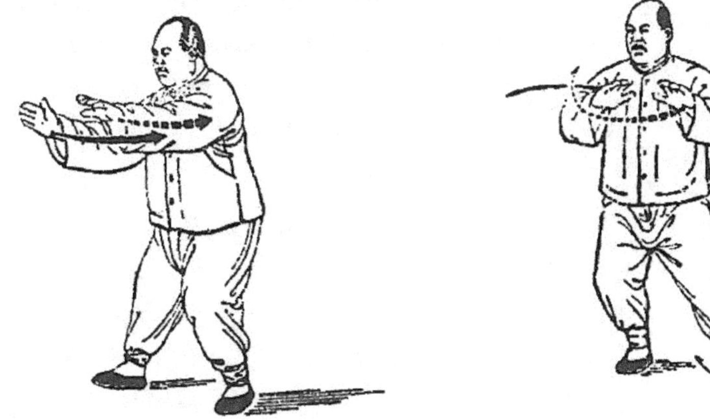

Then, keeping the weight on the right leg,
again turn the torso southwestward, and *sōng* the right wrist
while gathering its fingers and thumb to each other
and extending the right arm northwestward
while arcing the left hand northwestward and upward
to southwest of the face while turning its palm toward the face
and lifting the left knee to shift the left heel northwestward
to begin extending the left foot southeastward.
And then, completing the step of the left foot southeastward
to shift into a left bow stance,
shift the right hand upward until its fingertips are at shoulder-level,
and arc the left hand southeastward to southeast of the face
while turning its palm toward the south.
The gaze follows the left hand.

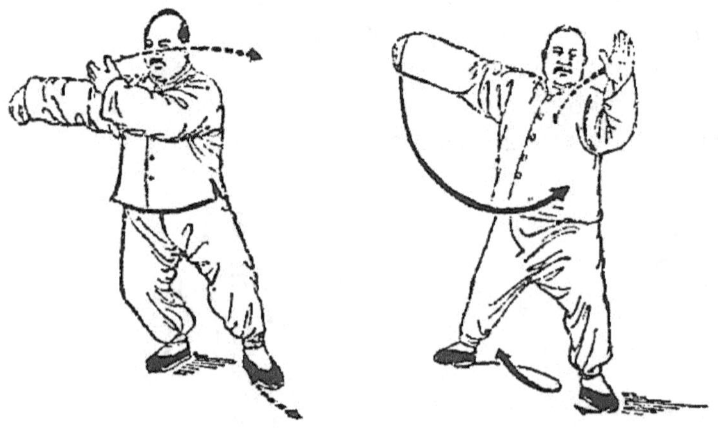

What makes this Solitary Whip form oblique is that its ending
orientation is southeastward while the ending orientation of the
other Solitary Whip forms is directly eastward.

56.

野馬分鬃右式

Yě mǎ fēn zōng yòu shì
Wild Horse Parts Mane, Right Form.

Turning the left foot on its heel southwestward
and lifting the right knee to circle the right foot
toward the left foot and then westward,
sōng the right hand, and arc it downward and southeastward
and then upward to south of the left side of the abdomen
while turning its palm upward
and arcing the left hand westward and downward
to above the right hand
while turning its palm to face the right palm as if to hold a sphere.
And then, quickly stepping the right foot westward
into a right bow stance,
quickly turn the torso further southwestward
while arcing the left hand downward and southeastward
to south of the *yāo*
while settling its wrist for its palm to remain facing downward
and arcing the right hand upward and northwestward
for its fingers to point upward and westward
with its palm facing upward and southeastward.
The gaze is toward the right palm.

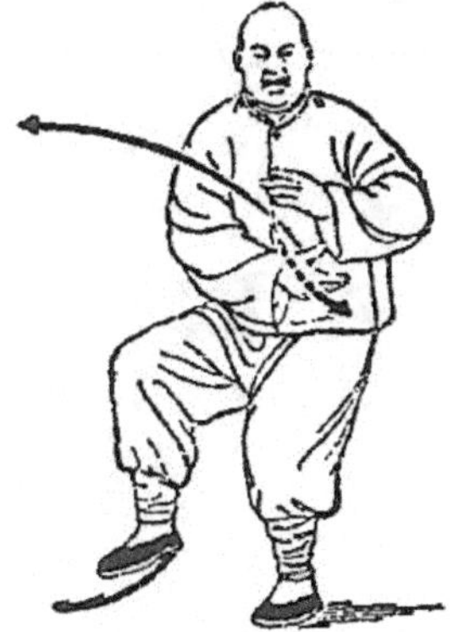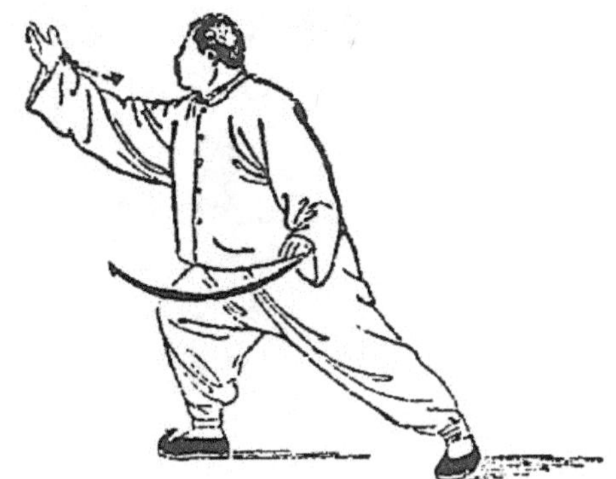

57.

野馬分鬃左式

Yě mǎ fēn zōng zuǒ shì
Wild Horse Parts Mane, Left Form.

Completing the turn of the torso westward
while shifting the right foot on its heel northwestward,
shift the right elbow toward the north
to draw the right hand toward the right shoulder
while turning its palm toward the south
and shifting the left hand westward to southwest of the *yāo*.
And then lift the left knee to swing it westward past the right knee
while turning the torso northwestward
and drawing the right hand toward the sternum
while turning its palm downward
and drawing the left hand northeastward to west of the *yāo*
while turning its palm upward
to face the right palm as if to hold a sphere.
The gaze follows the right palm before leveling northwestward.

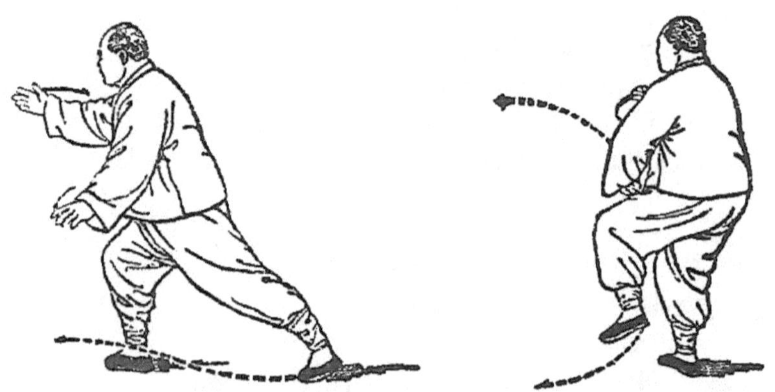

Then, quickly stepping the left foot westward
into a left bow stance,
arc the left hand upward and westward
while turning its palm northeastward,
and pluck the right hand downward and northeastward
to north of the *yāo* while turning its palm downward.
The gaze shifts toward the left palm extending westward.

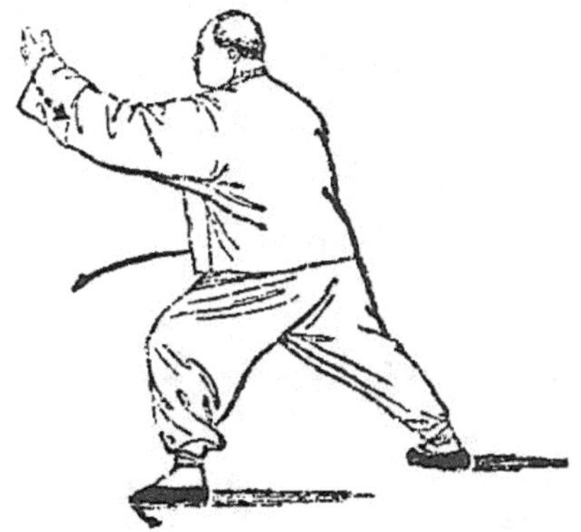

Right form.

Turn the torso again westward
while swinging the arms with the turn
and turning the left foot on its heel southwestward.
And then swing the right knee westward past the left knee
while turning the torso southwestward
and drawing the left hand
downward and northeastward toward the sternum
while turning its palm downward
and drawing the right hand
southeastward and upward to south of the abdomen
while turning its palm upward
to face the left palm as if to hold a sphere.
The gaze follows the left palm before leveling to the south.

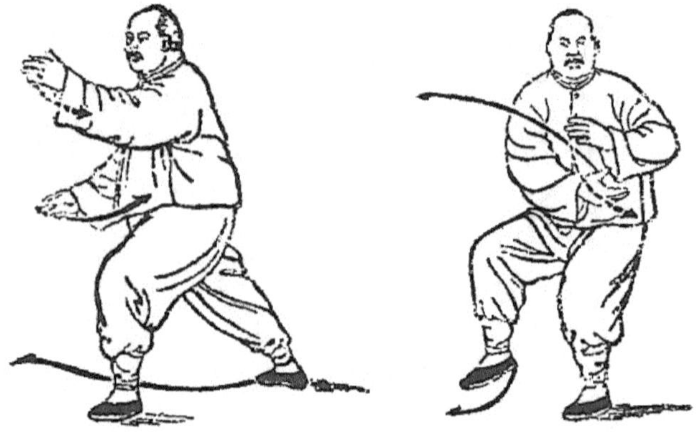

Then, quickly stepping the right foot westward
into a right bow stance,
arc the right hand upward and northwestward
for its palm to face upward and southeastward
from west of the eyes,
and pluck the left hand downward and southeastward
to south of the *yāo* while turning its palm downward.
The gaze shifts toward the right palm extending westward.

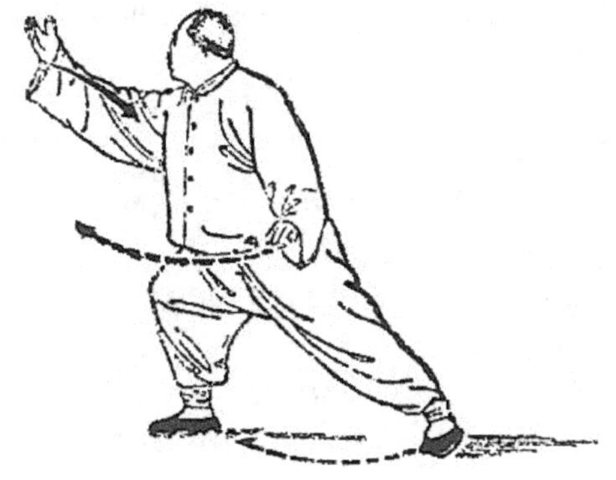

58.
攬雀尾
Lǎn què wěi
Grasp Sparrow Tail.

Arrow Quiver Cover (Ward-Off).

Turn the right foot on its heel southwestward,
and draw the left foot westward to southeast of the right ankle
to lift the left knee toward the south
while arcing the left hand westward to southwest of the *yāo*
while turning its palm northeastward
and arcing the right hand downward and southeastward
to southwest of the sternum
to turn the palms to face one another as if to hold a sphere.
The gaze follows the right hand.
Then, stepping the left foot to the south into a left bow stance,
arc the right hand upward and then westward and downward
to west of the *yāo* while turning its palm downward
and shifting the left hand up to shoulder-level
while turning its palm upward and northeastward.

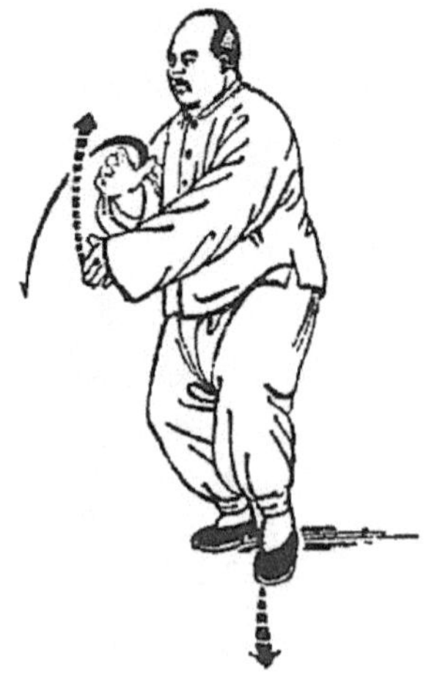
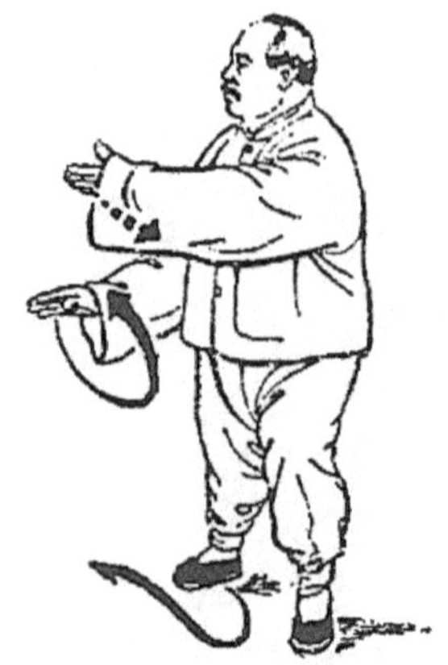

Then, shifting the left foot on its ball northeastward
and lifting the right knee
to circle the right foot toward the left foot and then westward,
circle the right hand downward and southeastward
and then upward to southwest of the abdomen
while turning its palm upward and southeastward
and sinking the left elbow to draw the left hand eastward
to turn its palm toward the right palm as if to hold a sphere
with the left hand at the level of the sternum
and the right hand at the level of the left wrist.
The gaze remains levelly southwestward.
And then, stepping the right foot westward
to touch its heel to the ground *xū*,
press the back of the right hand westward and upward,
while shifting the left hand westward to south of the right elbow
for its fingers to point toward the right wrist.

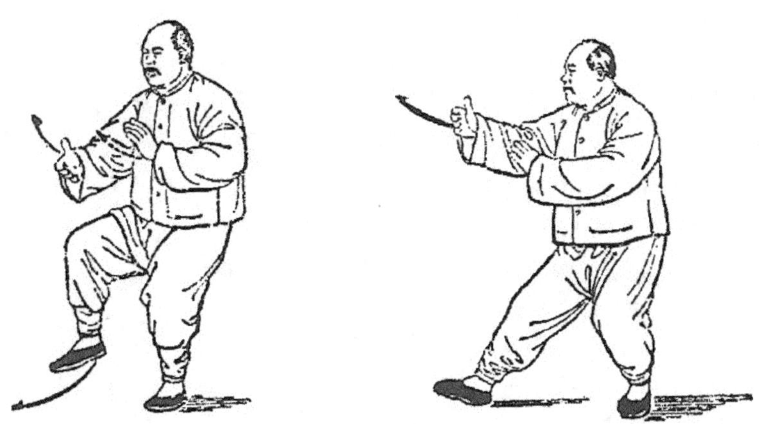

And then, shifting the weight westward into a right bow stance
while shifting the right hand further westward and upward
to west of the face for its palm to face the face,
shift the left hand with the right hand
while settling its wrist for its fingertips to point further upward.

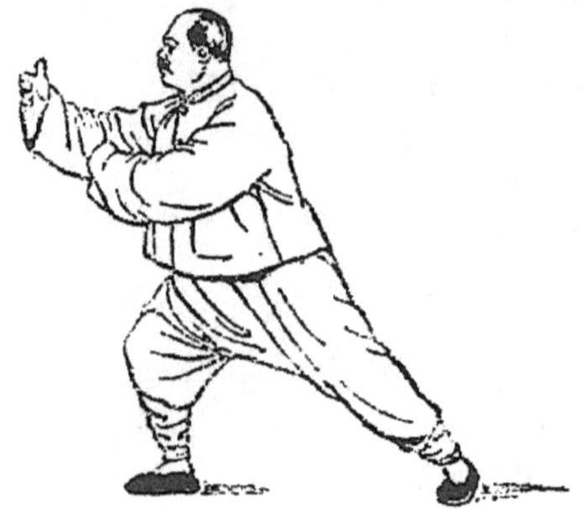

Stroke (Rollback).

Turning the right palm downward and westward
while turning the left palm upward and toward the north,
begin to roll the hands downward and eastward.
Then, to continue rolling the hands downward and eastward,
bend the left knee to straighten the right leg
to shift the weight eastward onto the left leg.

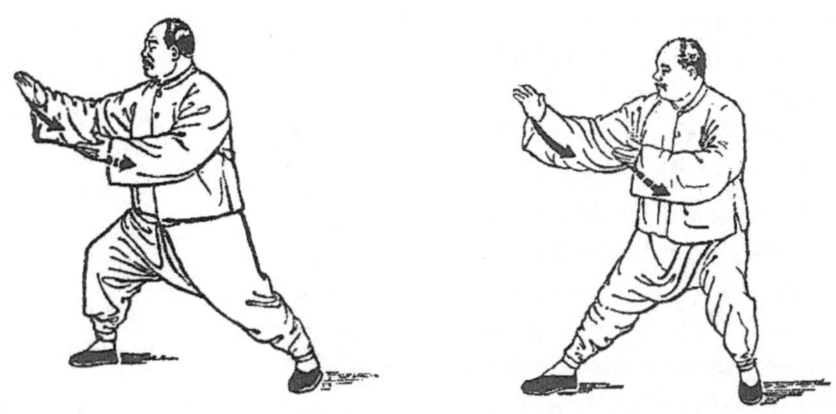

And then, keeping the elbows at least a fist's width from the torso,
continue rolling the hands downward and eastward
while turning the right palm southeastward.
The gaze attends to the left hand before following the right hand.

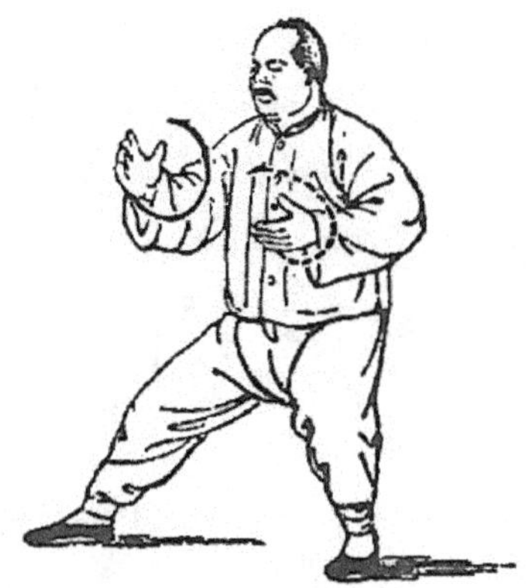

Press

Beginning to shift the weight westward,
circle both hands downward and southeastward
and then upward and westward
to turn the left palm downward and westward
while turning the right palm eastward.
And then, completing the shift of the weight
westward again into a right bow stance
press the back of the right hand westward and upward
for its palm to face the face,
and push the left hand westward and upward
while settling its wrist to press the right forearm further westward.
The gaze is toward the right wrist.

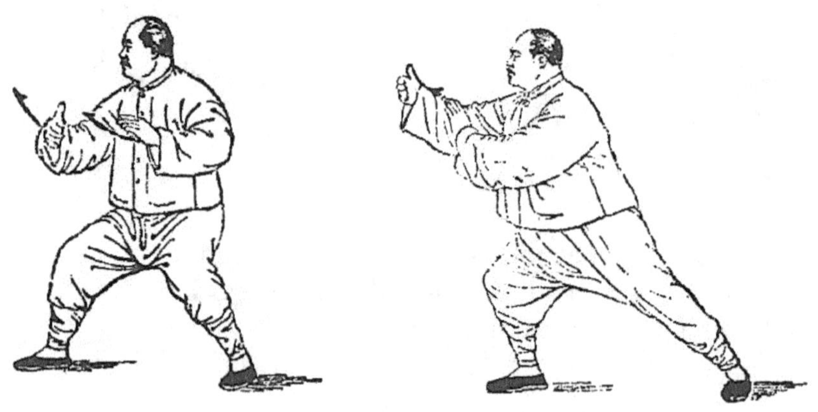

Push

Turning the torso westward,
shift the right hand down to shoulder-level,
and pass the left hand over the right wrist
while turning both palms downward
to spread them shoulder-width apart.
Then, turning the palms to face one another
for their fingers to point upward and westward,
sink the elbows to draw the hands toward the sternum
while bending the left knee to straighten the right leg
to shift the weight to the left leg.
The gaze is level and westward.

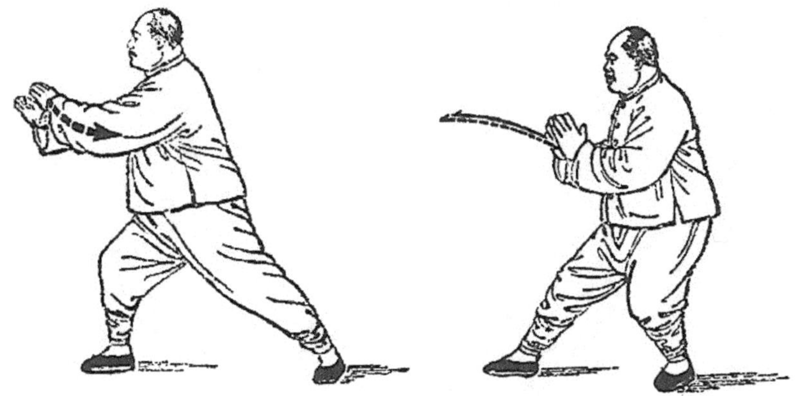

And then quickly straighten the wrists
to turn the palms downward
to push them upward and forward while settling their wrists
and shifting the weight westward again into a right bow stance.
The gaze remains levelly forward.

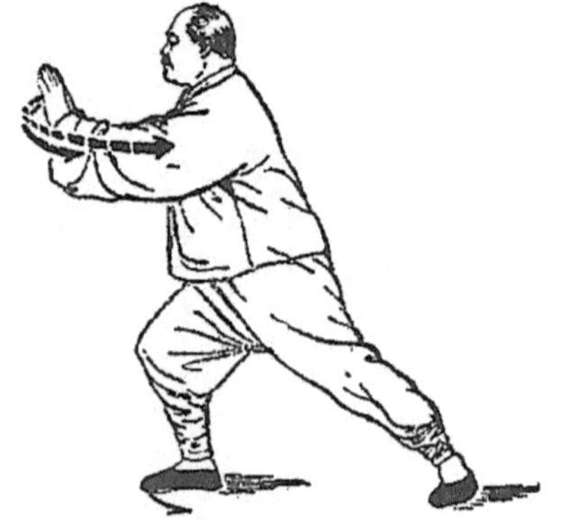

59.

單鞭

Dān biān
Solitary whip.

Bending the left knee and straightening the right leg
to shift the weight to the left leg, turn the torso southwestward,
and turn the right foot on its heel southwestward
while swinging the hands with the turn
and beginning to turn the palms downward.
And then, turning the torso southeastward
while swinging the arms with the turn
and continuing to turn the palms downward,
turn the left foot on its ball northwestward,
and turn the right foot on its ball also northwestward
while bending the right knee while straightening the left knee
to shift the weight to the right leg.
The gaze levelly shifts with the turn.

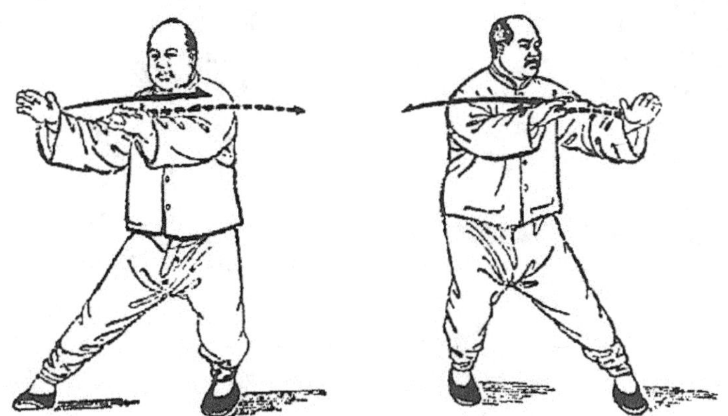

Then, keeping the weight on the right leg,
turn the torso again southwestward
while swinging the arms with the turn
and shifting the gaze with the turn.
And then, again turning the torso southeastward
while shifting the left hand
upward and eastward to southeast of the chin
to turn its palm toward the chin,
lift the left knee eastward,
and *sōng* the right wrist while extending its hand westward
and gathering its fingers and thumb to each other
for the hand to hang downward
to form a hook shape with its wrist.
The gaze shifts levelly with the turn.

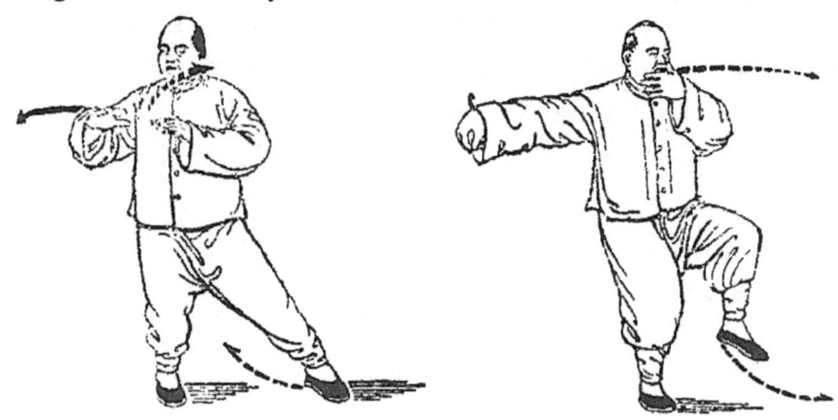

And then, shifting the right hand upward
until its fingertips are at shoulder-level,
step the left foot eastward into a left bow stance
while extending the left hand eastward
while turning its palm downward
before settling its wrist and turning its palm southeastward.
The gaze shifts levelly with the motion of the left hand.

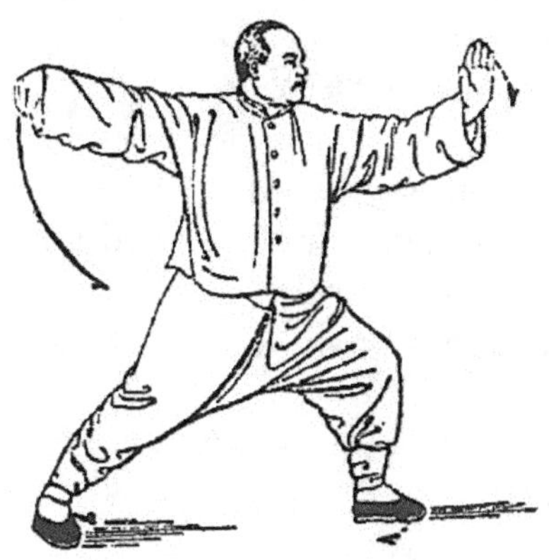

60.

玉女穿梭頭一手左式

Yù nǚ chuān suō tóu yī shǒu zuǒ shì

Jade Female Threads Shuttle Head, One Hand, Left Form.

Turning the left foot on its heel to the south
to turn its knee toward the south
while lifting the right heel northeastward,
sōng the right hand, and arc it downward and eastward
to southwest of the *yāo*
while settling its wrist for its palm to face downward
and sinking the left elbow to shift the left hand southwestward
while turning its palm toward the south.
And then, promptly turning the torso southwestward,
lift the right knee westward
while arcing the right hand downward and southeastward
and then upward and quickly westward
while turning its palm eastward
to point its fingers toward the south
while arcing the left hand downward and westward
to south of the left side of the *yāo*
while turning its palm downward.
The gaze shifts from the downward motion of the left hand
to the upward motion of the right hand.

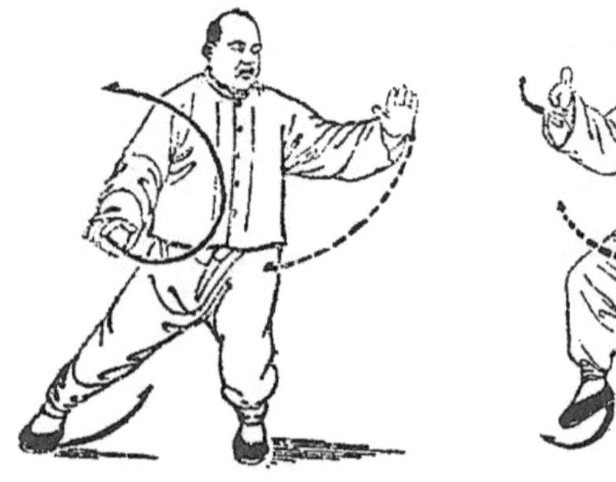
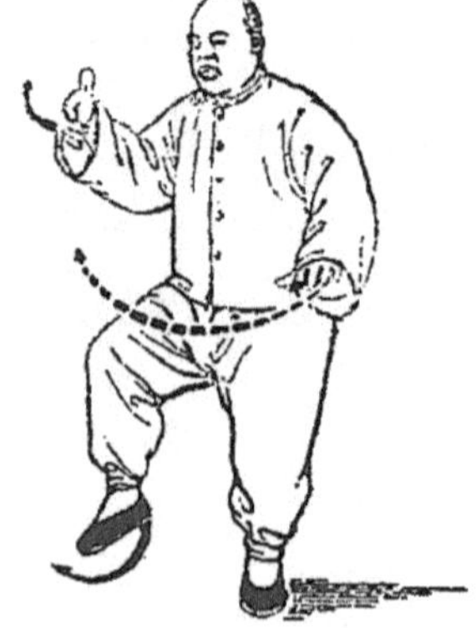

Then, continuing the turn of the torso westward,
swing the arms with the turn,
and shift the right foot downward and westward.
And then, setting the right foot on the ground
a half step west of the left heel
with its toes pointing northwestward,
lift the left knee southwestward
to swing the left foot past the right ankle
while shifting the right hand eastward toward the clavicle
for its palm to face the left shoulder
and shifting the left hand northeastward toward the abdomen
to beneath the right hand.
The gaze follows the right hand during the turn
and then shifts levelly westward.

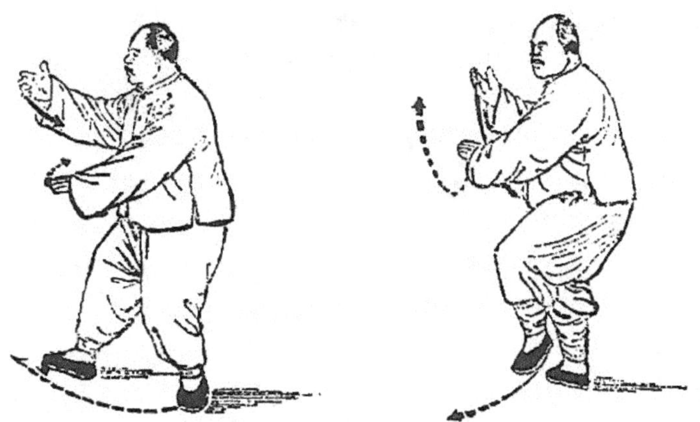

Then, extending the left foot southwestward
to set its heel on the ground *xū* with its toes pointing westward,
arc the left hand from beneath the right hand
downward and southwestward and then upward
to west of the left shoulder
while arcing the right hand downward and eastward
to west of the right side of the abdomen.
The gaze follows the left hand.
And then, shifting the weight southwestward
into a left bow stance,
arc the left hand upward and eastward
to above and to the southwest of the left temple
while turning its palm westward and extending the right hand
westward and upward to shoulder-level
while settling its wrist and turning its palm southwestward.
The gaze includes the right palm pushing forward.

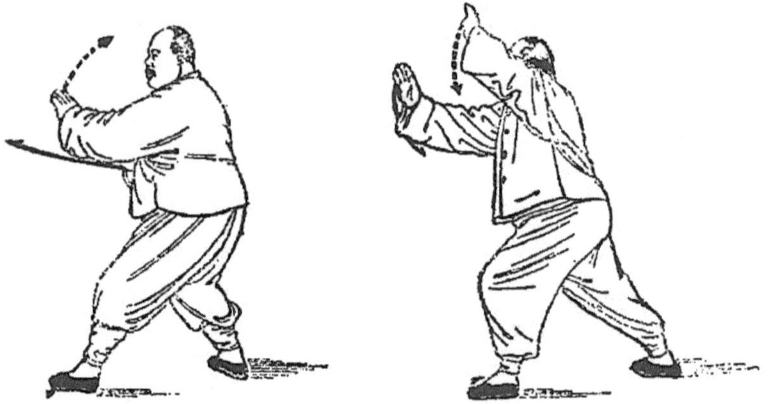

Yang Chengfu, while the drawings may not make it clear, directs
assuring that the directions of these four Jade Female Threads
Shuttle segments are to each of the four corners.

61.

玉女穿梭頭一手右式

Yù nǚ chuān suō tóu yī shǒu yòu shì

Jade Female Threads Shuttle Head, One Hand, Right Form.

Promptly turn the left foot on its heel toward the north
to turn the torso northwestward while sinking the left elbow
to arc the left hand downward to northwest of the face
while turning its palm toward the face
and sinking the right elbow to draw its hand downward
toward the left elbow while turning its palm toward the elbow.
The gaze is toward the left palm.
And then pivot the left foot on its heel northeastward
to lift the right knee
to circle the right foot southwestward
toward the left heel and then on to the north
and northeastward and then to the south and then eastward
and on southeastward to turn the torso northeastward
while swinging the arms with the turn and,
settling the weight onto the left leg,
shifting the left hand down to the level of the clavicle
while shifting the right hand up to the level of the clavicle
to turn both palms toward the face.
The gaze shifts from the left hand to the right hand.

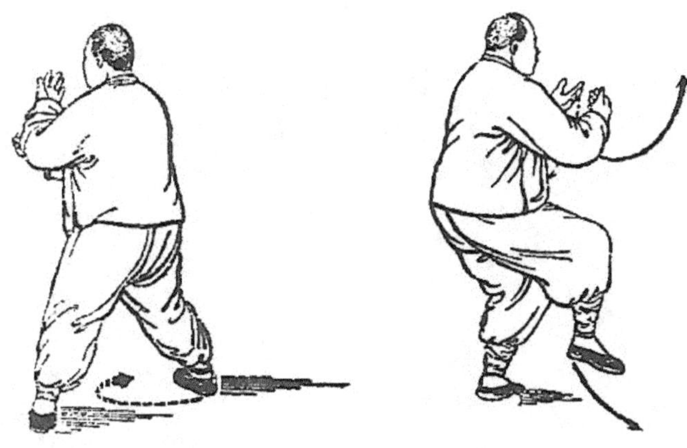

Then, turning the torso eastward
and stepping the right foot southeastward
to touch its heel to the ground *xū*,
shift the left hand down to the level of the sternum
while turning its palm downward and southeastward,
and circle the right hand downward and southeastward
and then upward to shoulder-level
to turn its palm downward and northeastward.
The gaze follows the left hand.
And then, shifting the weight southeastward
into a right bow stance,
arc the right hand upward to above and east of the right temple
for its palm to face upward and eastward
with its fingers pointing upward and toward the north,
and arc the left hand eastward and upward while settling its wrist
to keep its fingers at the level of the sternum.
The gaze includes the left palm pushing eastward.

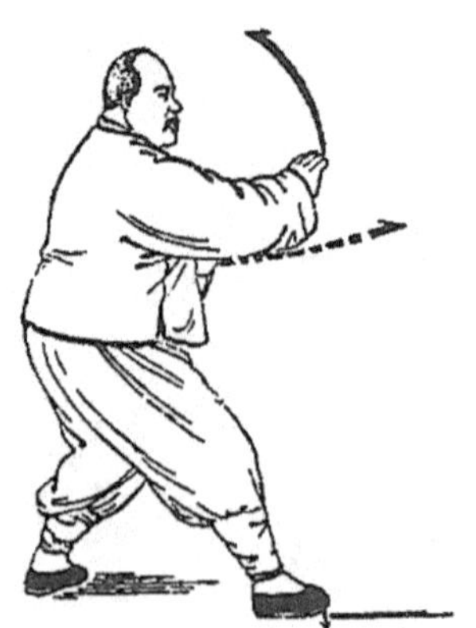 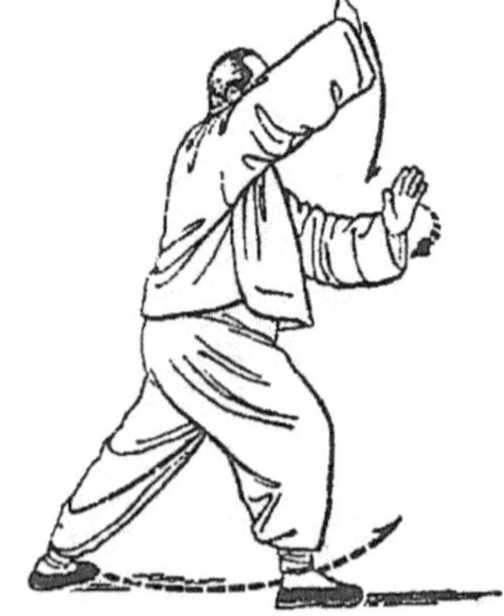

62.

玉女穿梭
Yù nǚ chuān suō
Jade Female Threads Shuttle.

Left Thread the Shuttle.

Turn the right foot on its heel southeastward,
and, lifting the left knee eastward
to swing its foot eastward past the right ankle and upward,
turn the left palm further downward,
and arc the right hand down to east of the sternum
while turning its palm toward the left shoulder.
The gaze follows the right palm past the left hand until it's level.
Then, turning the torso southeastward,
step the left foot northeastward to touch its heel to the ground *xū*,
and arc the left hand downward and eastward
and then upward to shoulder-level
for its palm to face downward and eastward,
and shift the right hand downward
to southeast of the upper abdomen
while turning its palm downward and northeastward.
The gaze follows the left hand.

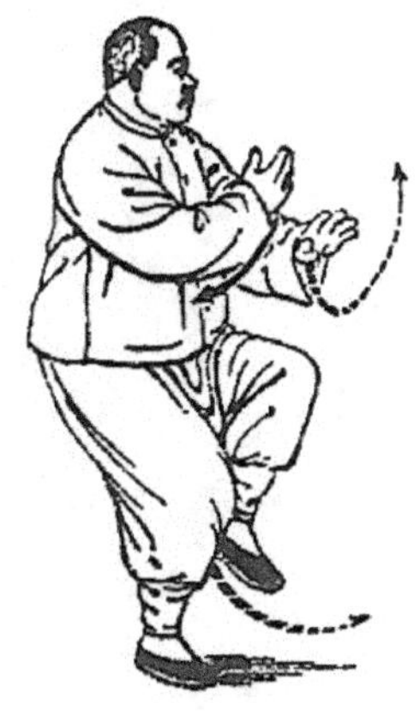
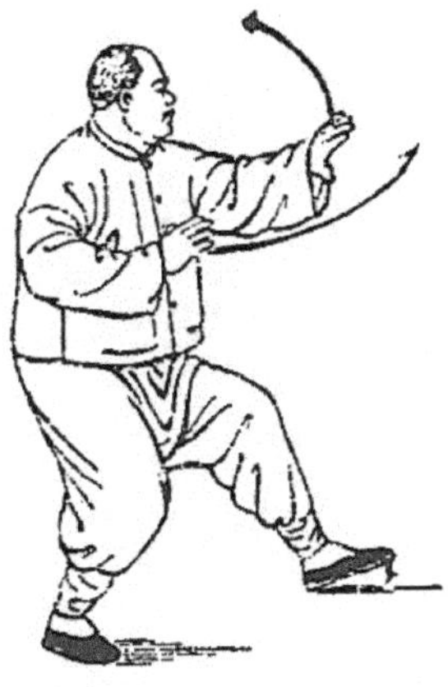

And then, shifting the weight northeastward into a left bow stance,
arc the left hand upward and westward
to above and to the northeast of the forehead
for its palm to face eastward
with its fingers upward and toward the south,
and arc the right hand eastward and upward
while settling its wrist to keep its palm facing northeastward.
The gaze includes the right palm pushing forward.

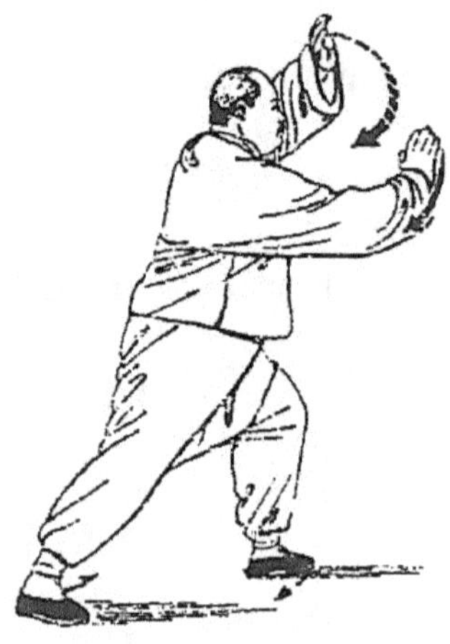

63.

玉女穿梭
Yù nǚ chuān suō
Jade Female Threads Shuttle.

Right Thread the Shuttle.

Promptly turning the left foot on its heel southwestward,
also turn the right foot on its heel southwestward
to turn the torso southeastward
while swinging the arms with the turn,
shifting the right hand down to the level of the abdomen
while straightening its wrist, turning its palm toward the north,
and sinking the left elbow to arc its hand eastward and downward
and then westward to southeast of the clavicle
while turning its palm toward the clavicle.
The gaze is toward the left palm.
And then, lifting the right knee westward
to turn the torso southwestward
while swinging the arms with the turn
and shifting the left hand down to the level of the sternum
for its palm to face the clavicle,
shift the right hand toward the upper abdomen
for its palm to face the sternum from beneath the left fingers.
The gaze shifts with the hands.

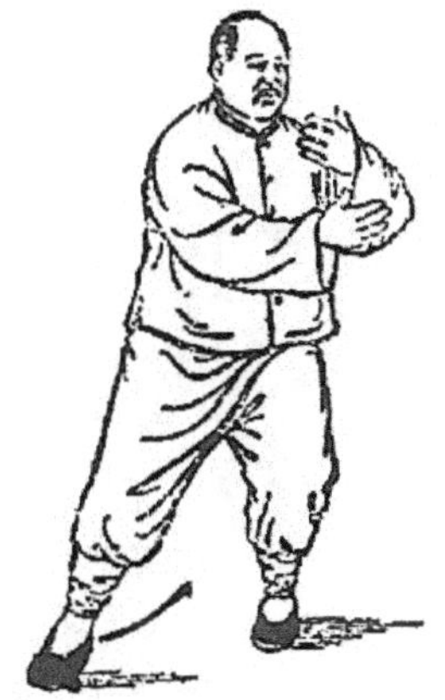
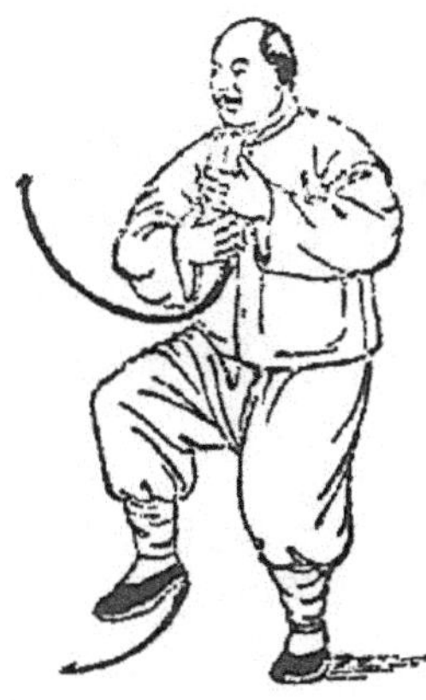

Then, shifting the left foot on its ball northeastward
to step the right foot northwestward
to touch its heel to the ground *xū*,
arc the right hand downward and westward
and then upward to shoulder-level
while turning its palm downward and westward
and shifting the left hand down to the level of the upper abdomen
while turning its palm downward and northwestward
The gaze follows the left hand.
And then, turning the torso northwestward,
shift the weight northwestward into a right bow stance
while arcing the right hand upward
to above and northwest of the forehead
for its palm to face northwestward
with its fingers pointing upward and southwestward
and arcing the left hand northwestward and upward
to shoulder-level while turning its palm northwestward.
The gaze follows the hands.

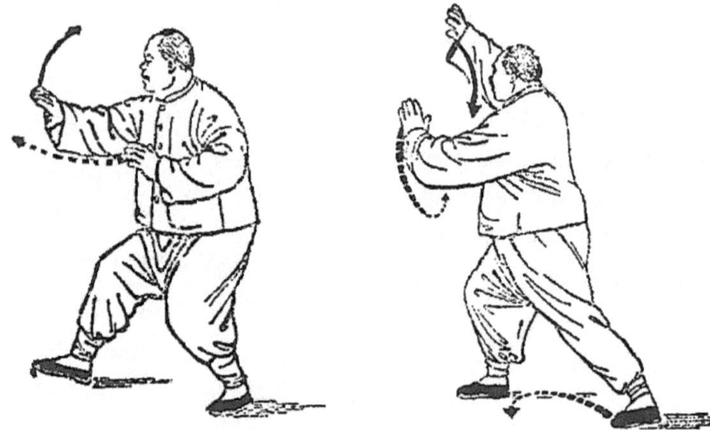

64.

攬雀尾
Lǎn què wěi
Grasp Sparrow Tail.

Arrow Quiver Cover (Ward-Off).

Lifting the left knee
and pivoting the right foot on its ball northeastward
to swing the left foot past the right ankle and then toward the south
while turning the torso southwestward,
arc the right hand downward to southwest of the sternum,
and circle the left hand downward and northeastward
to southwest the abdomen
while turning the palms to face one another as if to hold a sphere.
The gaze follows the right hand.
And then, stepping the left foot to the south into a left bow stance
arc the right hand upward and then westward and downward
to west of the *yāo*
for its palm to face downward and toward the south,
and shift the left hand up to west of the left shoulder
for its palm to face upward and toward the north.

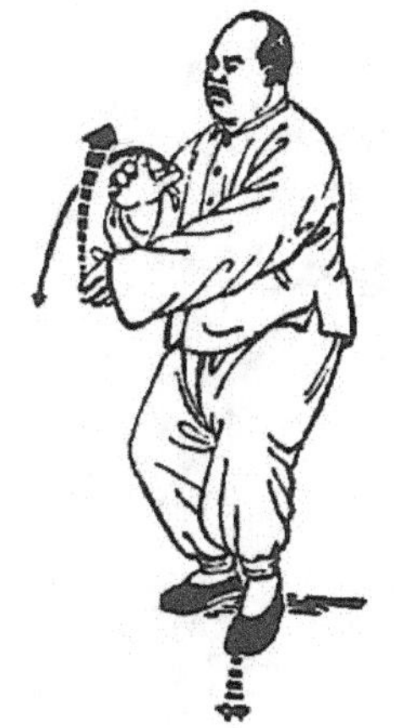 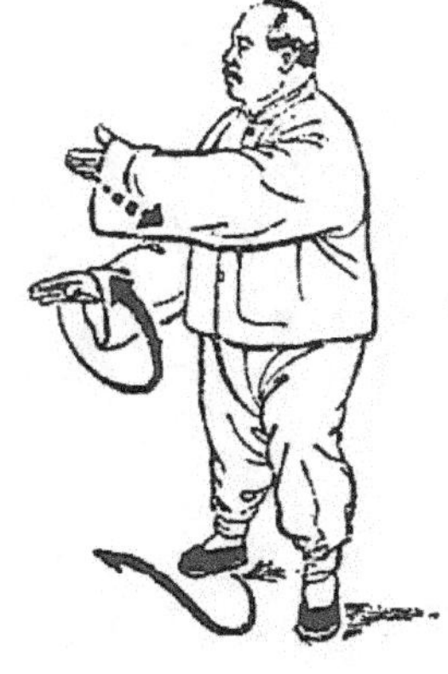

Then, shifting the left foot on its ball northeastward
and lifting the right knee
to circle the right foot toward the left foot and then westward,
circle the right hand downward and southeastward
and then upward and southwestward to southwest of the abdomen
while turning its palm upward and southeastward
and sinking the left elbow to draw the left hand eastward
while turning its palm toward the right palm as if to hold a sphere
with the left hand at the level of the sternum
and the right hand at the level of the left wrist.
The gaze remains levelly southwestward.
And then, stepping the right foot westward
to touch its heel to the ground *xū*,
press the back of the right hand westward and upward,
while shifting the left hand westward to south of the right elbow
for its fingers to point toward the right wrist.

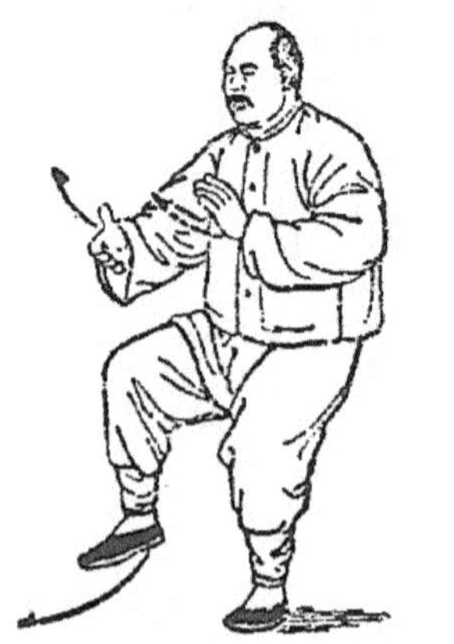
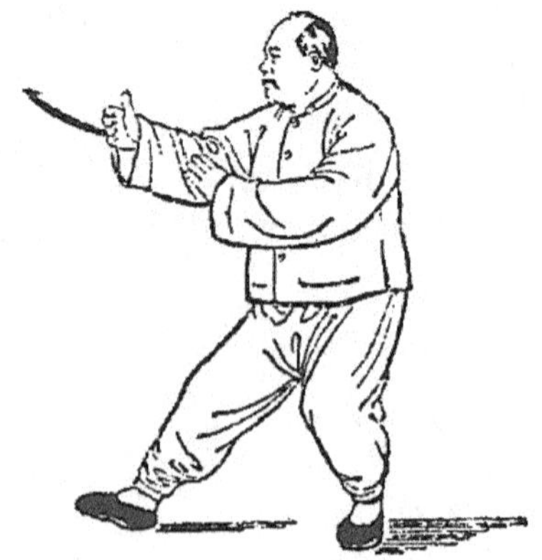

And then, shifting the weight westward into a right bow stance
while shifting the right hand further westward and upward
to west of the face for its palm to face the face,
shift the left hand with the right hand
while settling its wrist for its fingertips to point further upward

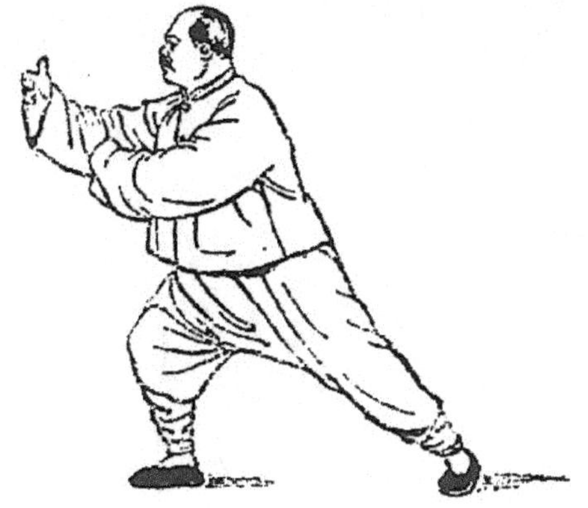

Stroke (Rollback).

Turning the right palm downward and westward
while turning the left palm upward and toward the north,
begin to roll the hands downward and eastward.
Then, to continue rolling the hands downward and eastward,
bend the left knee while straightening the right leg
to shift the weight eastward onto the left leg.

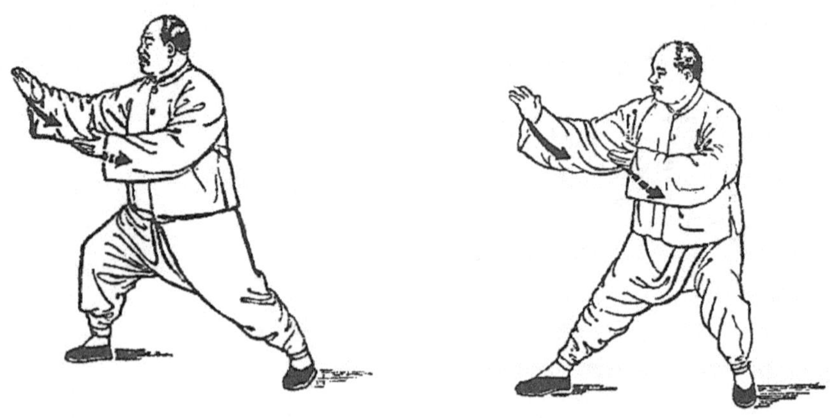

And then, keeping the elbows at least a fist's width from the torso,
continue rolling the hands downward and eastward
while turning the right palm southeastward.
The gaze attends to the left hand before following the right hand.

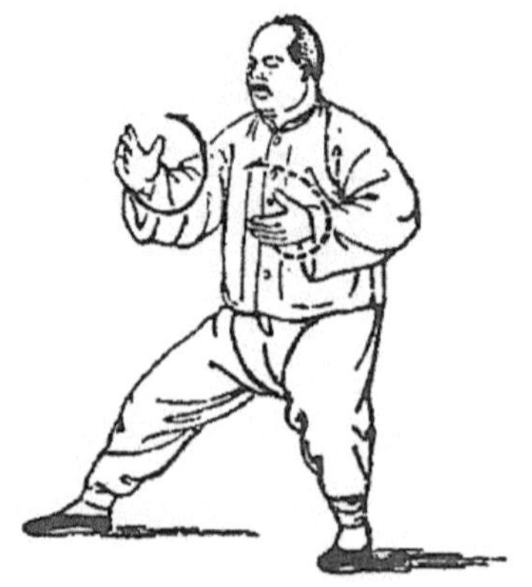

Press.

Beginning to shift the weight westward,
circle both hands downward and southeastward
and then upward and westward
to turn the left palm downward and westward
while turning the right palm eastward.
And then, completing the shift of the weight
westward again into a right bow stance
press the back of the right hand westward and upward
for its palm to face the face,
and push the left hand westward and upward
while settling its wrist to press the right forearm further westward.
The gaze is toward the right forearm.

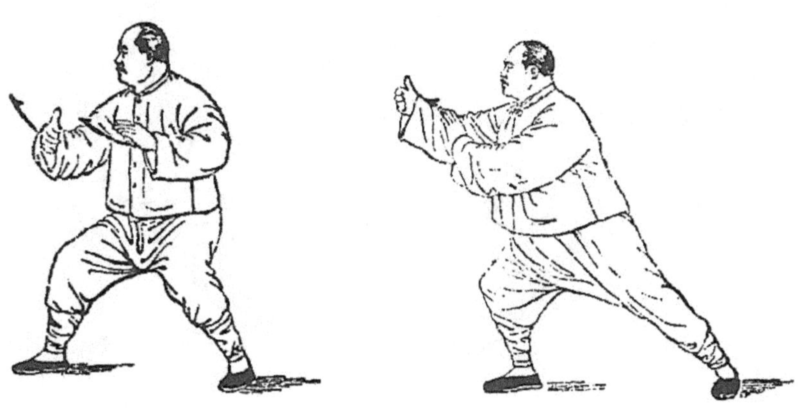

Push.

Turning the torso westward,
shift the right hand down to shoulder-level,
and pass the left hand over the right wrist
while turning both palms downward
to spread them shoulder-width apart.
Then, turning the palms to face one another
for their fingers to point upward and westward,
sink the elbows to draw the hands eastward toward the sternum
while bending the left knee to straighten the right leg
to shift the weight to the left leg.
The gaze is level and westward.

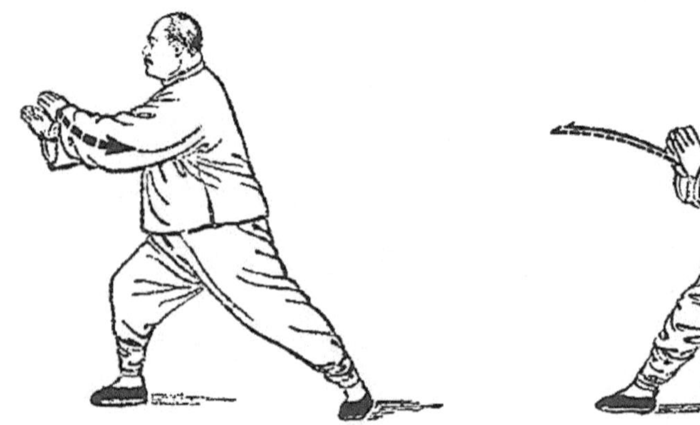

And then quickly straighten the wrists
to turn the palms downward
to push them upward and forward while settling their wrists
and shifting the weight westward again into a right bow stance.
The gaze remains level and forward.

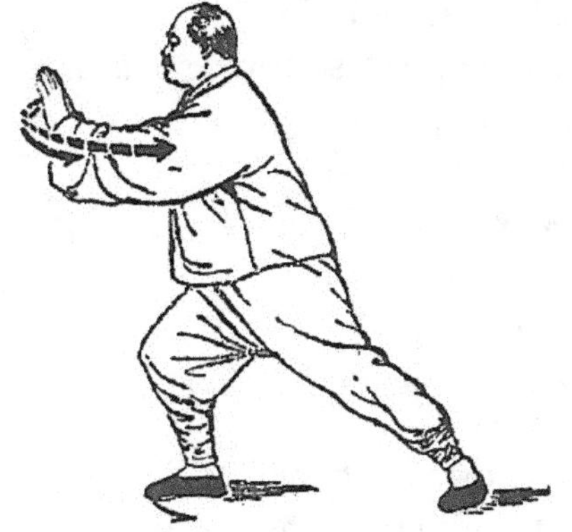

65.

單鞭

Dān biān

Solitary Whip.

Bending the left knee and straightening the right leg
to shift the weight to the left leg, turn the torso southwestward,
and turn the right foot on its heel southwestward
while swinging the hands with the turn
and beginning to turn the palms downward.
And then, turning the torso southeastward
while swinging the arms with the turn
and continuing to turn the palms downward,
turn the left foot on its ball northwestward,
and turn the right foot on its ball also northwestward
while bending the right knee while straightening the left knee
to shift the weight to the right leg.
The gaze levelly shifts with the turn.

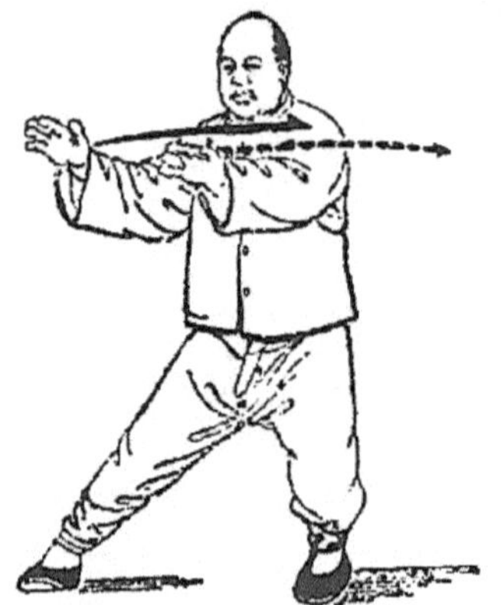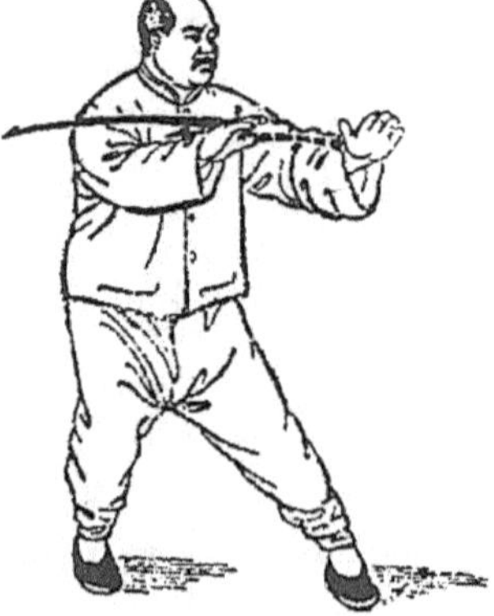

Then, keeping the weight on the right leg,
turn the torso again southwestward
while swinging the arms with the turn
and shifting the gaze with the turn.
And then, again turning the torso southeastward
while shifting the left hand
upward and eastward to southeast of the chin
to turn its palm toward the chin,
lift the left knee eastward,
and *sōng* the right wrist while extending its hand westward
and gathering its fingers and thumb to each other
for the hand to hang downward
to form a hook shape with its wrist.
The gaze shifts levelly with the turn.

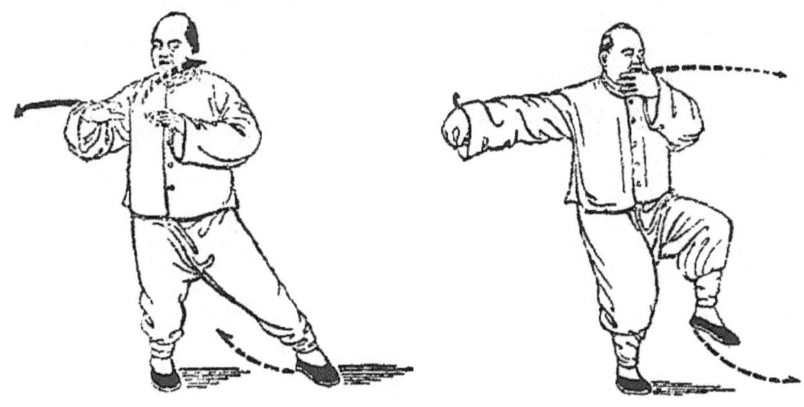

Then, shifting the right hand upward
until its fingertips are at shoulder-level,
step the left foot eastward into a left bow stance
while extending the left hand eastward
while turning its palm downward
before settling its wrist and turning its palm southeastward.
The gaze shifts levelly with the motion of the left hand.

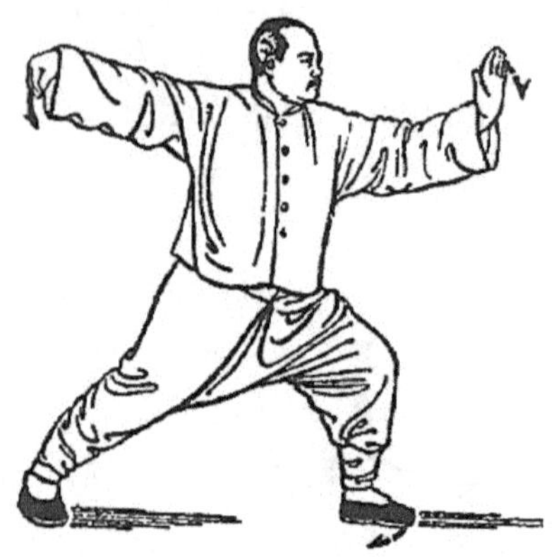

66.

扖手
Yǔn shǒu
Cloud Hands.

Right.

Lifting the left toes
to turn the left foot on its heel toward the south,
sōng the right hand while turning the left palm toward the south,
and begin to arc both hands downward.
Then, settling the left foot flat,
lift the right heel northeastward
to shift all the weight onto the left leg
while turning the torso to the south
and promptly arcing the right hand downward and eastward
while settling its wrist
for its palm to face downward and northeastward
from southwest of the *yāo*
and shifting the left hand down to southeast of the abdomen
while turning its palm downward for its fingers to point south
and beginning to lift the right heel eastward.
The gaze shifts levelly to the southwest.

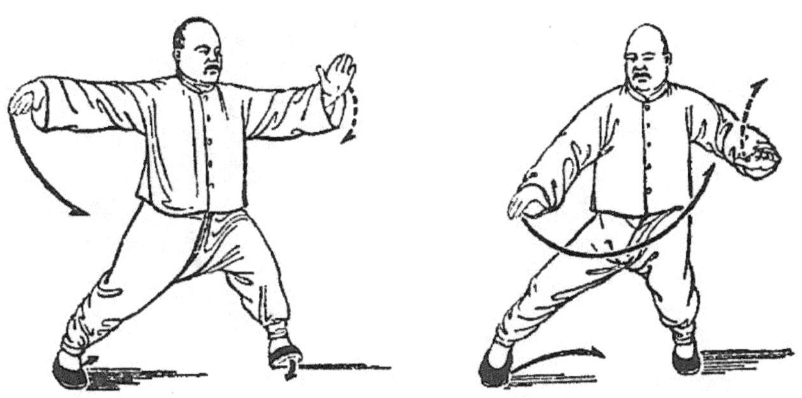

Then, lifting the right knee toward the south
while turning the torso southeastward,
continue the arc of the right hand downward and eastward
and then upward for its palm to face north
with its fingers eastward,
and shift the left hand upward for its palm to face south
with its fingers upward and eastward
and the right thumb south of the left elbow.
The gaze follows the right hand.
And then, turning the torso again to the south,
set the right foot on the ground flat to settle into the horse stance
while arcing the right hand upward and westward
for its palm to face the face from southwest of the face
and arcing the left hand downward and westward
for its palm to face the abdomen from south of the abdomen.
The gaze continues to follow the right hand.

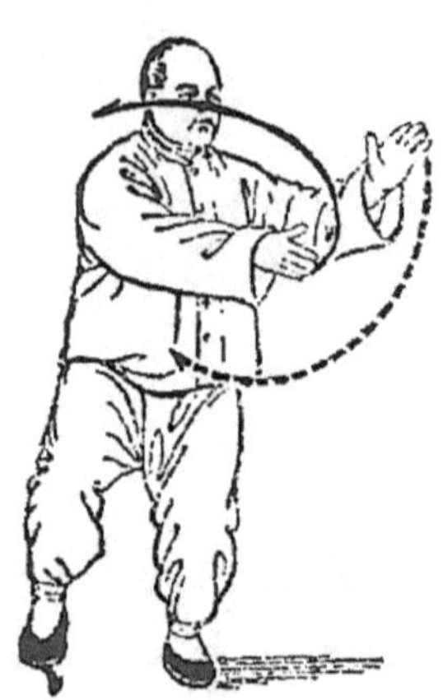
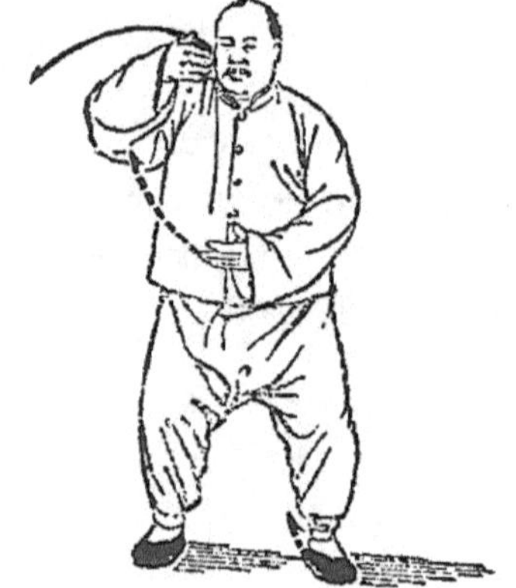

Left

Lifting the left knee to the south
while turning the torso southwestward,
arc the right hand westward for its palm to face south
with its fingers pointing upward and westward,
and arc the left hand westward and upward
while turning its palm downward and northwestward.
The gaze continues to follow the right hand.
And then, turning the torso again to the south,
step the left foot eastward into a wide horse stance,
and, arcing the left hand upward and eastward
for its palm to face the face from southeast of the face,
arc the right hand downward and eastward and upward
for its palm to face the abdomen from south of the abdomen.
The gaze shifts to the left palm.

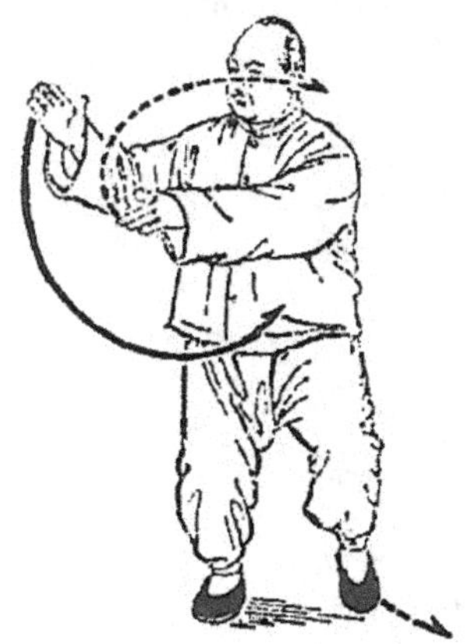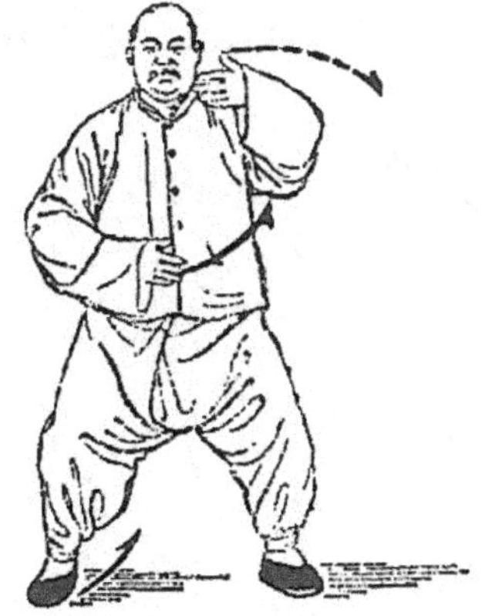

Right.

Lifting the right knee toward the south
while turning the torso southeastward,
arc the left hand eastward
while turning its palm toward the south
to point its fingers upward and eastward
and arcing the right hand eastward and upward
for its fingers to point eastward
with its thumb south of the left elbow.
The gaze continues to follow the left hand.
And then, turning the torso again to the south,
set the right foot on the ground flat to settle into the horse stance
while arcing the right hand upward and westward
for its palm to face the face from southwest of the face
and arcing the left hand downward and westward
for its palm to face the abdomen from south of the abdomen.
The gaze shifts to the right palm.

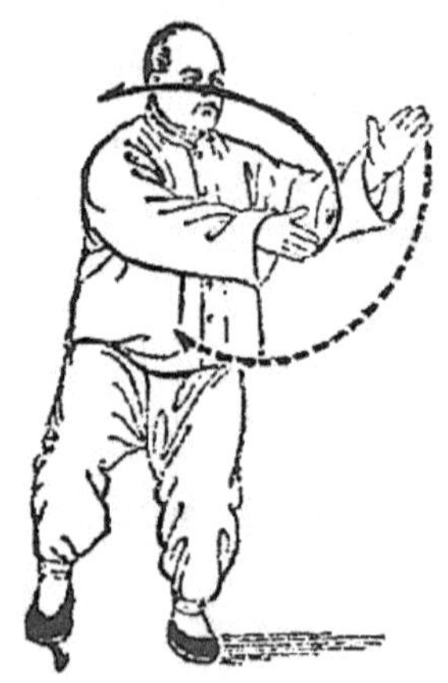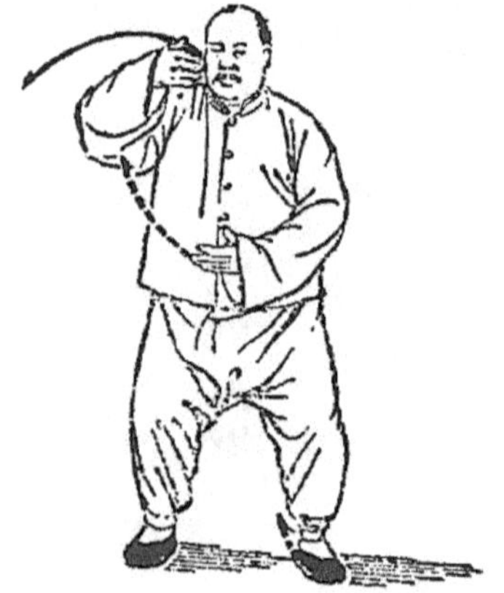

Left

Lifting the left knee to the south
while turning the torso southwestward,
arc the right hand westward for its palm to face south
with its fingers pointing upward and westward,
and arc the left hand westward and upward
while turning its palm downward and northwestward.
The gaze continues to follow the right hand.
And then, turning the torso again to the south,
step the left foot eastward into a wide horse stance,
and, arcing the left hand upward and eastward
for its palm to face the face from southeast of the face,
arc the right hand downward and eastward and upward
for its palm to face the abdomen from south of the abdomen.
The gaze shifts to the left palm.

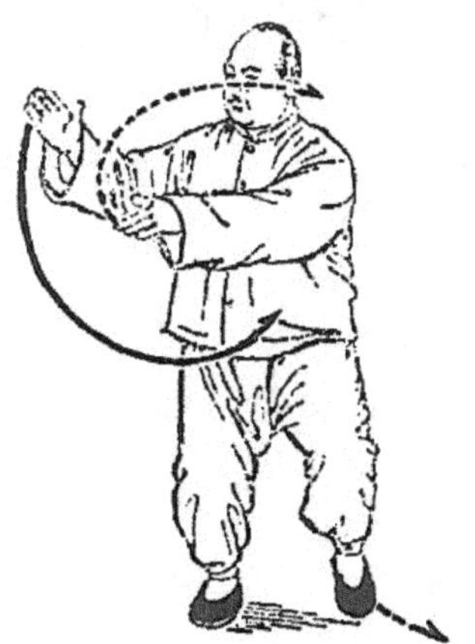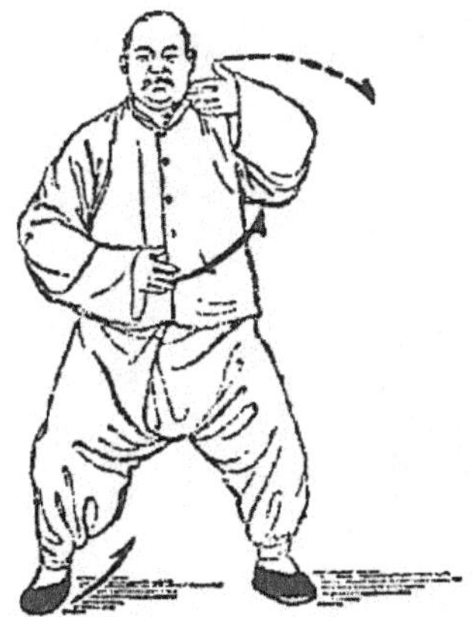

Right.

Lifting the right knee toward the south
while turning the torso southeastward,
arc the left hand eastward
while turning its palm toward the south
to point its fingers upward and eastward,
and arc the right hand eastward and upward
for its fingers to point eastward
with its thumb south of the left elbow.
The gaze continues to follow the left hand.
And then, turning the torso again to the south,
set the right foot on the ground flat to settle into the horse stance
while arcing the right hand upward and westward
for its palm to face the face from southwest of the face
and arcing the left hand downward and westward
for its palm to face the abdomen from south of the abdomen.
The gaze shifts to the right palm.

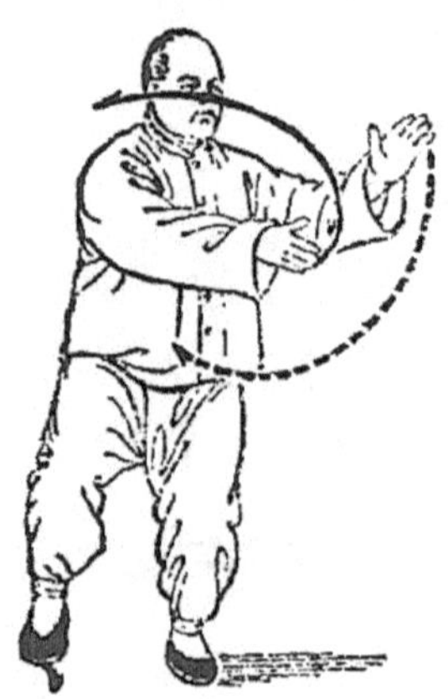
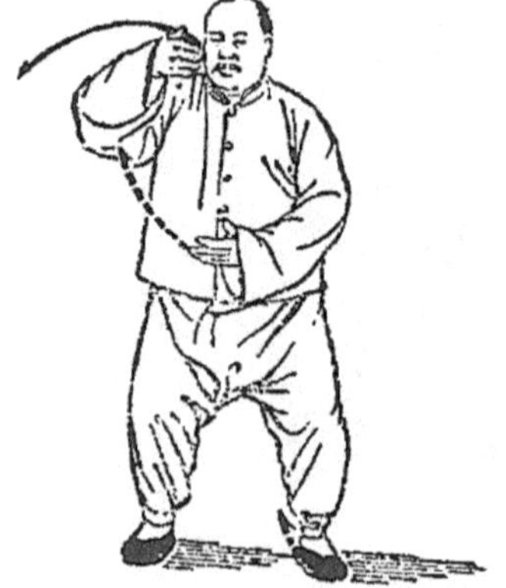

Left

Lifting the left knee to the south
while turning the torso southwestward,
arc the right hand westward for its palm to face south
with its fingers pointing upward and westward,
and arc the left hand westward and upward
while turning its palm downward and northwestward.
The gaze continues to follow the right hand.
And then, turning the torso again to the south,
step the left foot eastward into a wide horse stance,
and, arcing the left hand upward and eastward
for its palm to face the face from southeast of the face,
arc the right hand downward and eastward and upward
for its palm to face the abdomen from south of the abdomen.
The gaze shifts to the left palm.

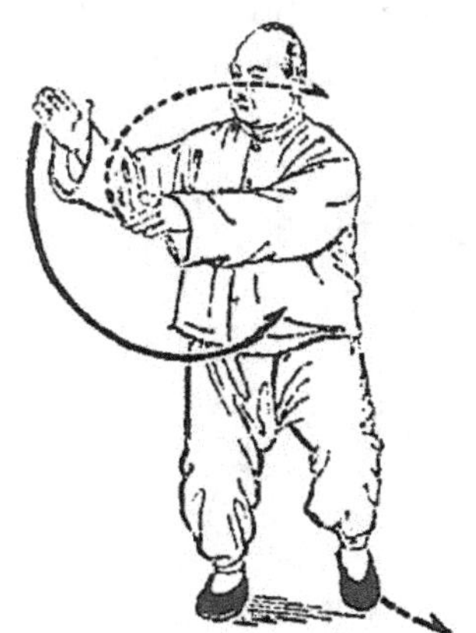 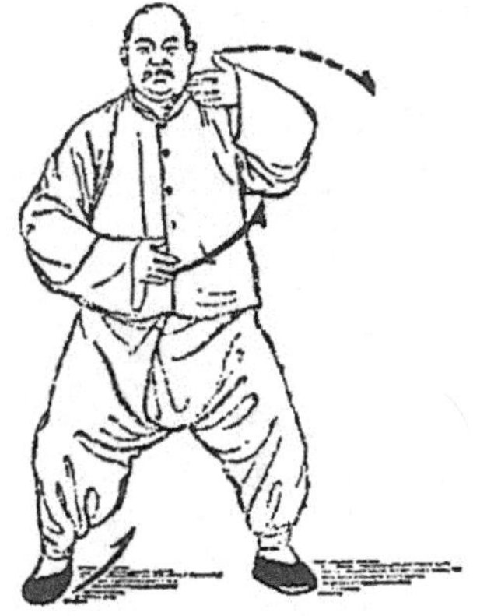

Right.

Lifting the right knee toward the south
while turning the torso southeastward,
arc the left hand eastward
while turning its palm toward the south
to point its fingers upward and eastward,
and arc the right hand eastward and upward
for its fingers to point eastward
with its thumb south of the left elbow.
The gaze continues to follow the left hand.
And then, turning the torso again to the south,
set the right foot on the ground flat to settle into the horse stance
while arcing the right hand upward and westward
for its palm to face the face from southwest of the face
and arcing the left hand downward and westward
for its palm to face the abdomen from south of the abdomen.
The gaze shifts to the right palm.

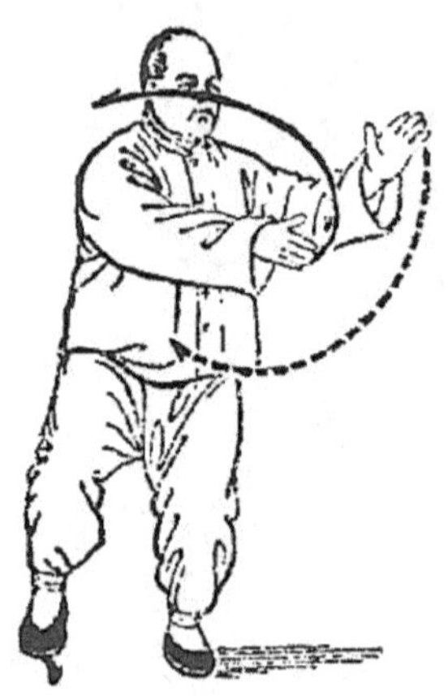
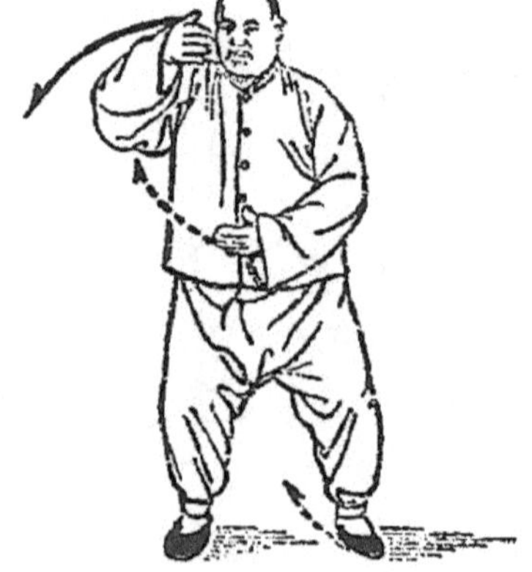

67.

單鞭下式
Dān biān xià shì
Solitary Whip Low Form.

Shifting the right foot on its ball northwestward
and shifting the weight to the right leg
to lift the left knee southeastward
while turning the torso southwestward,
sōng the right wrist while arcing its hand westward and downward
to the level of the sternum
and arcing the left hand westward and upward
while turning its palm downward and toward the north.
And then, turning the torso southeastward,
extend the right arm fully westward
while gathering its fingers and thumb to each other
for the hand to form a hook shape with its wrist
and arcing the left hand upward and eastward
to southeast of the chin while turning its palm toward the chin.
The gaze, after following the movement of the right hand,
shifts to the southeast over the left hand.

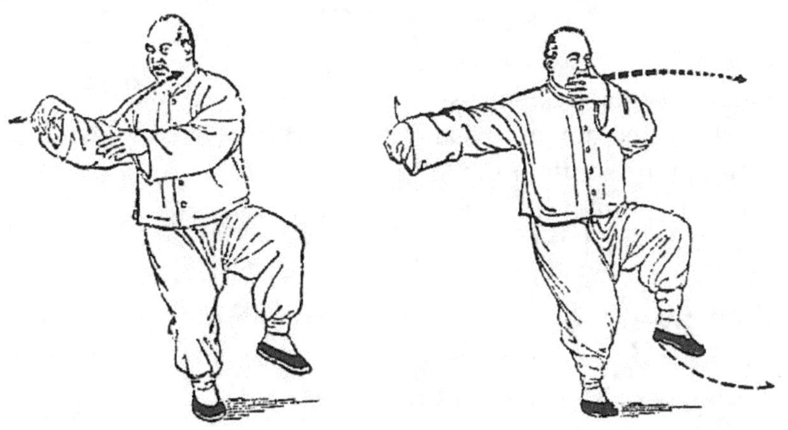

And then, stepping the left foot eastward
into a left bow stance, shift the right hand upward
until its fingertips are at shoulder-level,
and extend the left hand eastward while turning its palm downward
before settling its wrist and turning its palm southeastward.
The gaze shifts levelly with the motion of the left hand.
Then, turning the right foot on its heel southwestward,
bend the right knee while straightening the left leg
to shift the weight westward to the right leg,
and promptly settle low onto the right foot
while arcing the left hand southwestward and downward
and turning its palm to the south.

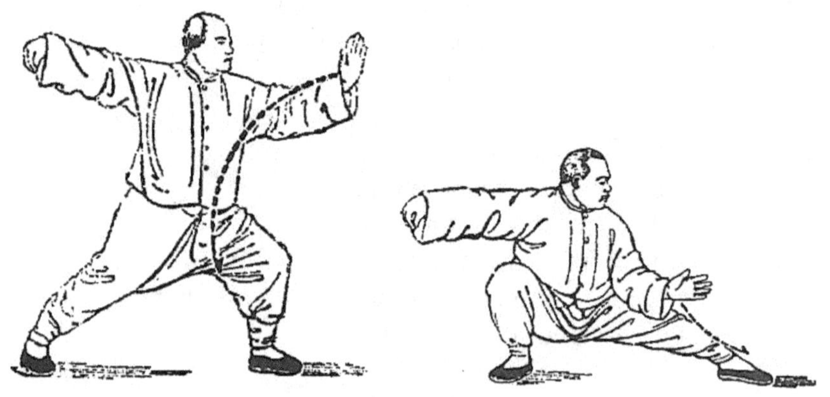

And then lean the torso southeastward
to shift the left hand downward and eastward
to above and to the south of the left ankle
for its fingers to point downward and eastward.
The gaze follows the left hand.

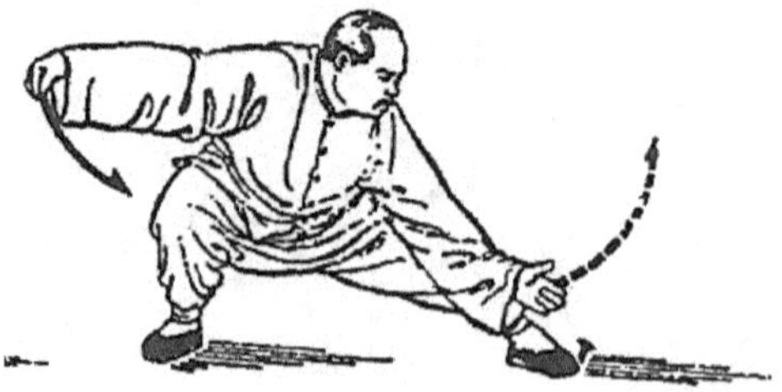

68.

金雞獨立右式

Jīn jī dú lì yòu shì
Golden Bird Single Stance, Right Form.

Turning the left foot on its heel northeastward,
bend the left knee while straightening the right leg
to shift into a low and wide left bow stance
while shifting the right hand downward and eastward
and arcing the left hand eastward and upward
while returning the torso to *xū líng dǐng jìn.*
The gaze shifts levelly eastward.
Then, promptly shifting all of the weight to the left leg,
begin to straighten it
while beginning to draw the right foot eastward
and beginning to draw the left hand northwestward
toward the left side of the *yāo*
while settling its wrist to turn its palm downward
and opening the right hand while beginning to arc it eastward.

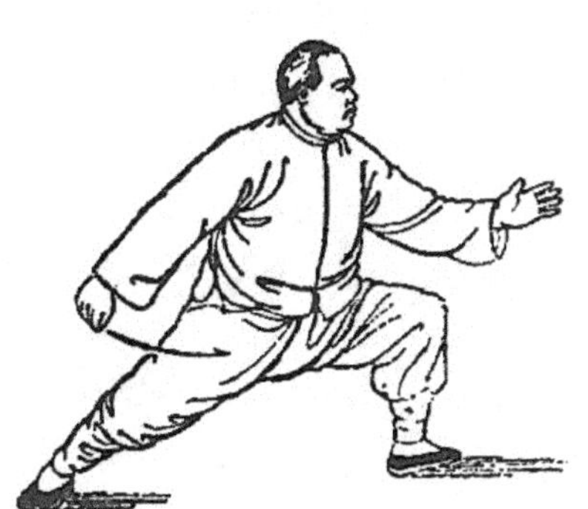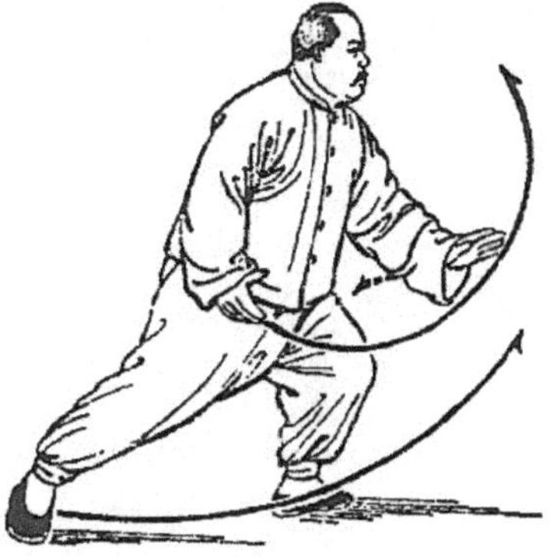

And then, continuing to straighten the left leg,
promptly lift the right knee eastward
to the level of the top of the *yāo*
while continuing the arc of the right hand eastward
and then upward to east of the face
to point its fingers upward while turning its palm to the north
and completing the draw of the left hand to north of the *yāo*
while completing the turn of its palm downward.
The gaze shifts toward the right hand to follow its rise.

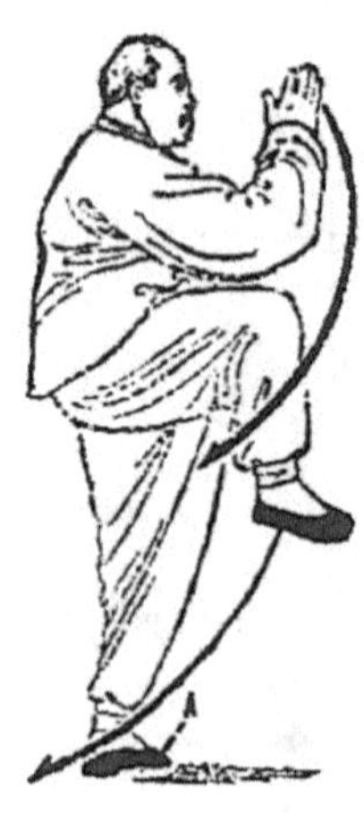

69.
金雞獨立左式
Jīn jī dú lì zuǒ shì
Golden Bird Single Stance, Left Form.

Settling a little lower onto the left leg,
set the right foot on the ground flat and *shí* south of the left foot
with its toes pointing southeastward,
and then, bending the right knee to settle onto it,
begin to lift the left knee eastward
while beginning to arc the left hand eastward
while turning its palm to the south
and arcing the right hand downward and southwestward
to southeast of the *yāo* while settling its wrist
and beginning to turn its palm downward.
And then, promptly straightening the right leg
to continue lifting the left knee eastward
until it's at the level of the top of the *yāo*,
continue the arc of the left hand upward
to east of the face for its fingers to point upward and eastward,
and continue the arc of the right hand downward and westward
for its palm to face downward and westward
from below and to the south of the *yāo*.
The gaze is toward the right hand arcing downward
before shifting toward the left hand arcing upward.

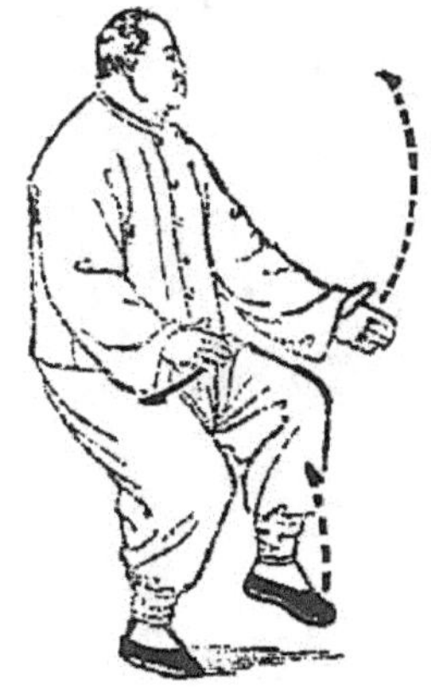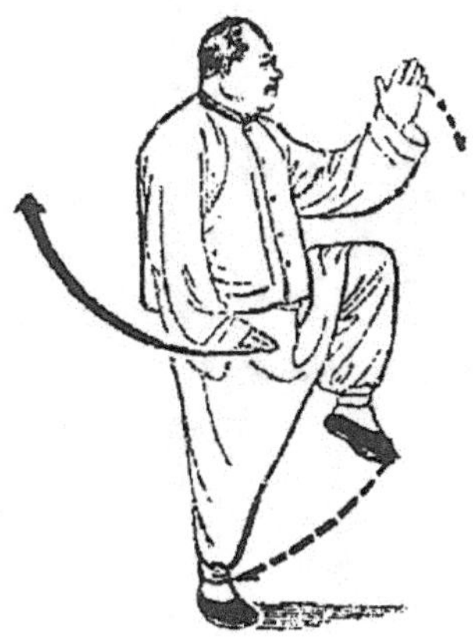

70.

倒輦猴

Dào niǎn hóu
Invert Monkey Carriage

Left.

Lowering the left knee
to begin to swing the left foot westward past the right ankle,
arc the right hand southwestward and upward to shoulder-level
while turning its palm southeastward
and extending the left hand eastward and downward
to the level of the sternum.
The gaze follows the right hand.
Then, turning the right foot on its heel eastward
to begin to turn the torso eastward,
complete the swing of the left foot westward
to set its toes on the ground to shift into the tray stance
while pushing the right palm eastward to south of the right ear
while turning its palm eastward and turning the left palm upward
while shifting it northwestward.

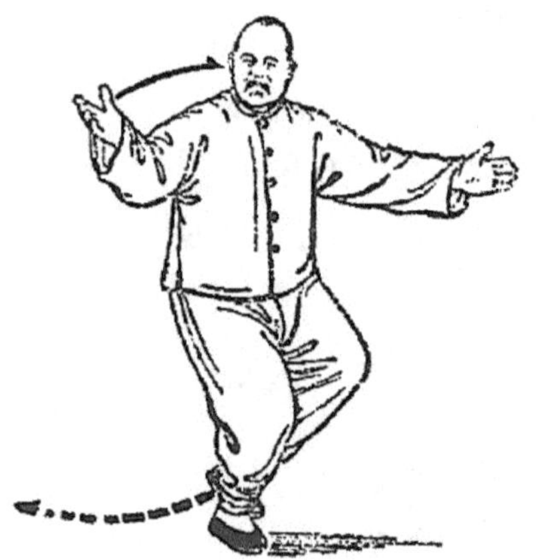
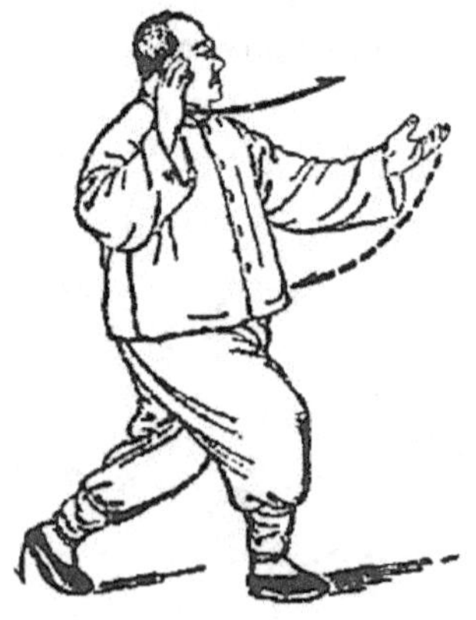

And then, completing the turn of the torso eastward
while pushing the right hand eastward
and settling its wrist while turning its palm northeastward,
arc the left hand downward and westward to north of the *yāo*
while bending the left knee and straightening the right leg
to turn the left foot on its ball southwestward to settle it flat
to shift the weight from the right foot to the left foot.
The gaze is toward the right hand pushing forward.

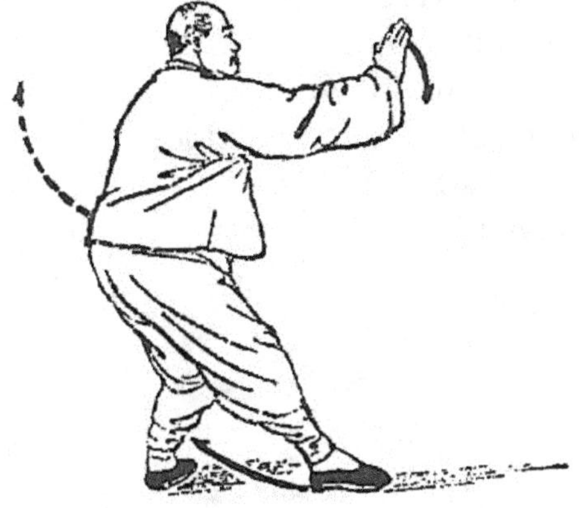

Right

Arcing the left hand northwestward and upward
while turning its palm northeastward,
shift the right hand down to east of the sternum
while turning its palm northwestward and lifting the right knee
to swing the right foot westward past the left ankle.
The gaze shifts toward the arcing right hand.
Then, swinging the right foot southwestward
to set its toes on the ground into the tray stance,
push the left hand southeastward to north of the left ear
while turning its palm eastward and sinking the right elbow
to begin to arc its hand downward and southwestward
while beginning to turn its palm upward

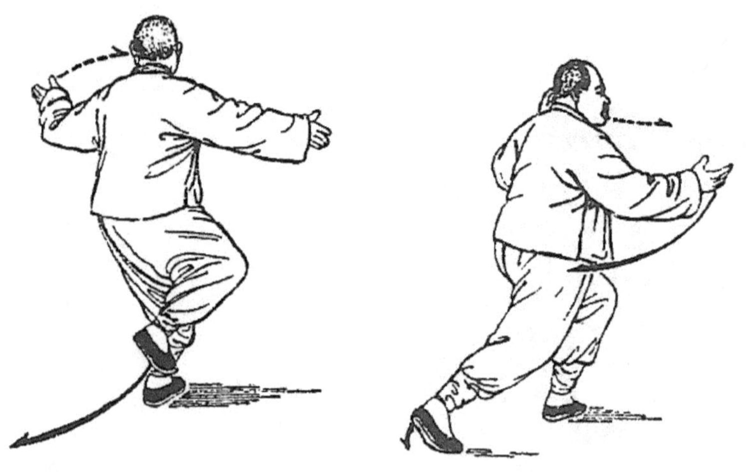

And then, turning the torso toward the south
while pushing the left hand eastward and settling its wrist
while turning its palm southeastward,
turn the left foot on its heel eastward,
and turn the right foot on its ball to the north to settle it flat
while arcing the right hand downward and westward
to south of the right side of the *yāo* while turning its palm upward
and bending the right knee while straightening the left leg
to shift the weight to the right leg.
The gaze is toward the left hand pushing forward.

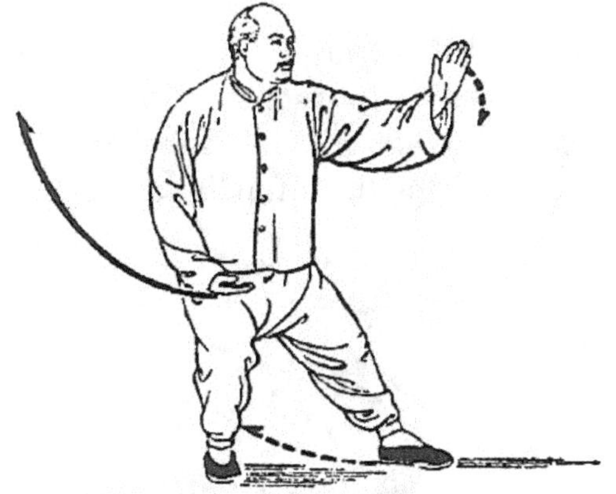

Left.

And then, turning the torso southeastward
while shifting the right foot on its ball northwestward,
arc the right hand southwestward and upward
while turning its palm upward and eastward
and shifting the left hand down to the level of the sternum
while turning its palm toward the south and lifting the left knee
to begin to swing the left foot westward past the right ankle.
The gaze shifts toward the arcing right hand.
Then, turning the right foot on its heel eastward,
begin to turn the torso eastward,
and complete the swing of the left foot westward
to set its toes on the ground to shift into the tray stance
while pushing the right palm eastward to south of the right ear
while turning its palm eastward and turning the left palm upward
while shifting it northwestward.

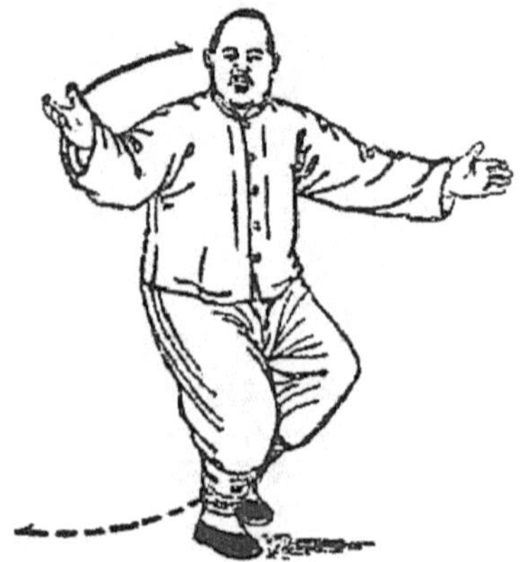 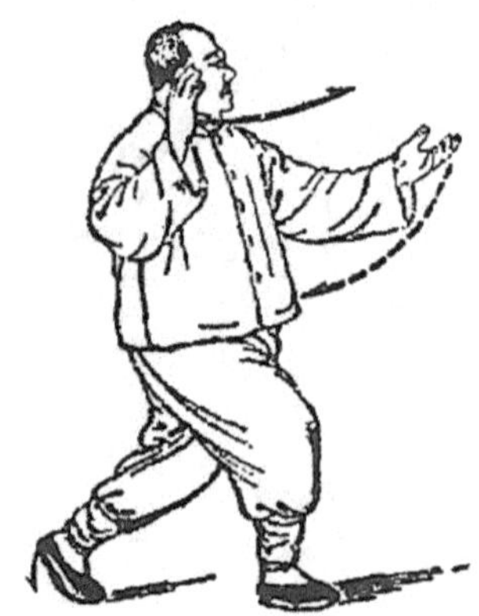

And then, completing the turn of the torso eastward
while pushing the right hand eastward
and settling its wrist while turning its palm northeastward,
arc the left hand downward and westward to north of the *yāo*
while bending the left knee and straightening the right leg
to turn the left foot on its ball southwestward to settle it flat
to shift the weight from the right foot to the left foot.
The gaze is toward the right hand pushing forward.

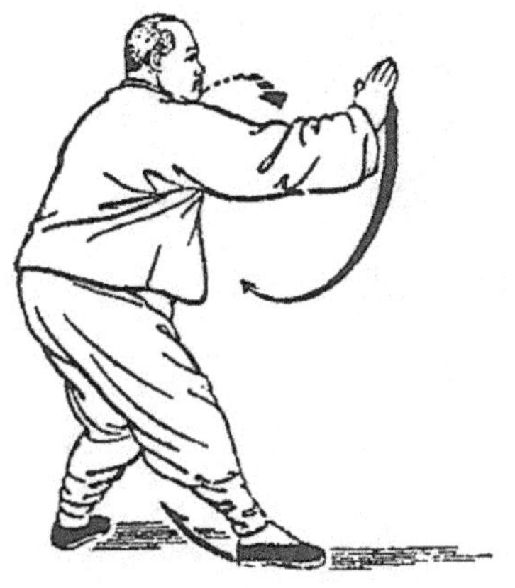

71.

斜飛式

Xié fēi shì

Oblique Flying Form.

Continuing the arc of the left hand northwestward and upward
and then promptly southeastward and downward
to east of the sternum
while turning its palm downward and toward the south,
arc the right hand downward and then quickly northwestward
to east of the *yāo* while turning its palm upward
and beginning to lift the right knee.
The gaze is over the left hand.
Then, pivoting the left foot on its heel eastward
while turning the torso southeastward
and swinging the arms with the turn,
lift the right knee southeastward
to swing the right foot southwestward
to set its heel on the ground *xū*
with its toes upward and southwestward
while drawing the hands toward one another
to turn their palms toward one another as if to hold a sphere.

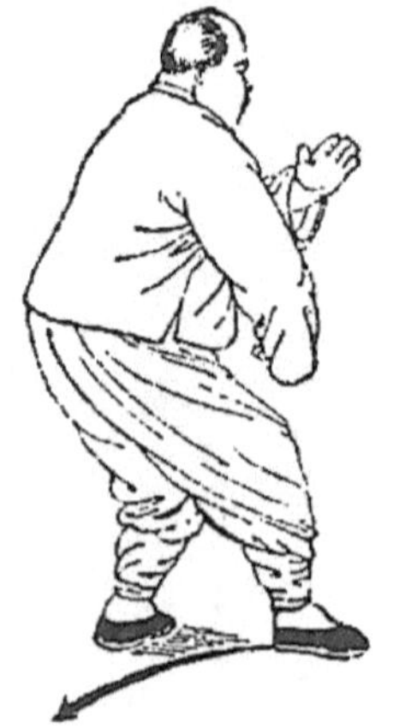
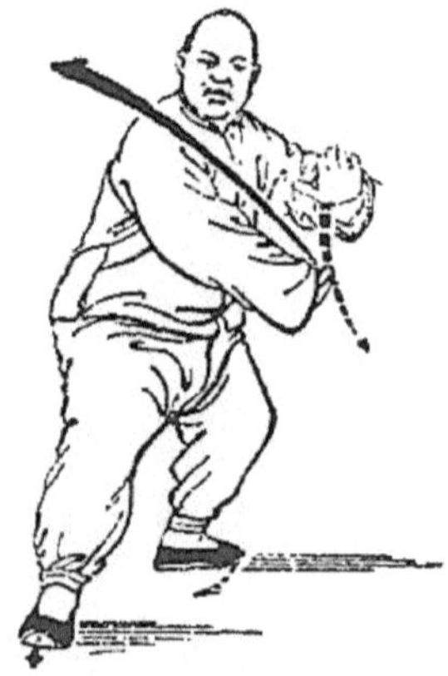

And then, turning the torso to the south
while shifting the left foot on its heel southeastward,
shift the weight southwestward into a right bow stance
while arcing the right hand upward and southwestward
for its palm to face eastward
with its fingers pointing upward and toward the south
from southwest of the face
and arcing the left hand downward to southeast of the *yāo*
for its palm to face downward with its fingers toward the south.
The gaze follows the motion of the right hand.

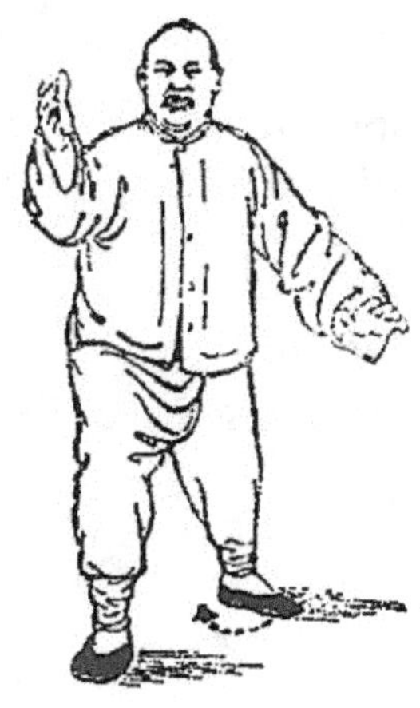

72.
提手上式
Tí shǒu shàng shì
Raise Hands Up Form.

Turn the left foot on its heel toward the south,
and lift its heel to shift the weight fully to the right leg
while shifting the right fingers downward and southwestward.
And then turn the left foot on its ball northwestward
to settle it flat to bend the left knee
to straighten the right leg to lift its toes
to shift the weight to the left leg
while arcing the left hand southwestward and upward
for it fingers to point upward and southwestward
from south of the sternum
and shifting the right hand eastward and upward
to above and directly east of the right shoulder
for its fingers again to point upward
and more directly toward the south.
The gaze continues to follow the right palm.

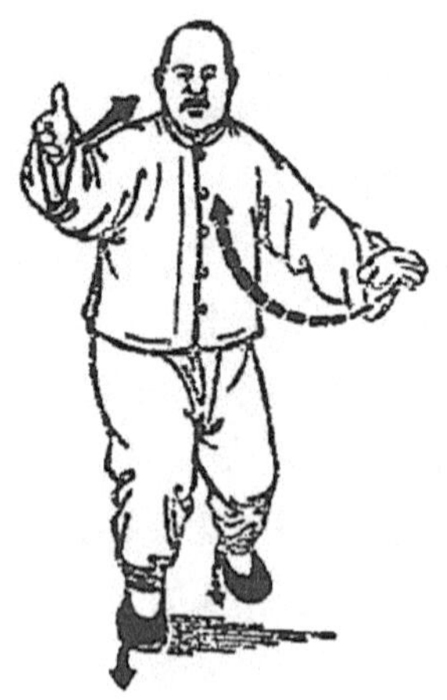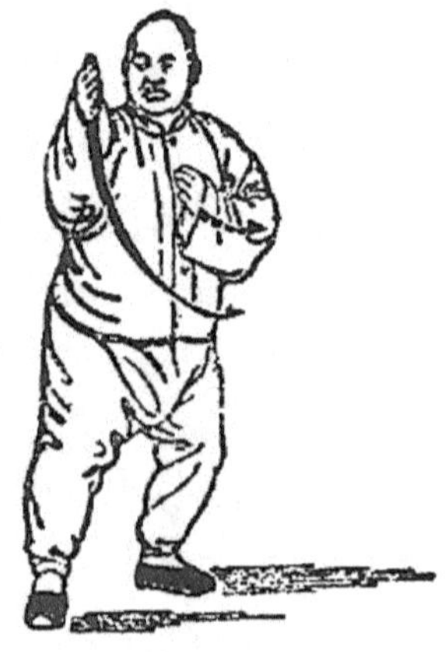

73.
白鶴亮翅
Bái hè liàng chì
White Crane Shines Wings.

Turning the torso southeastward,
arc the right hand downward and eastward
to southeast of the abdomen
while turning its palm downward and northeastward
and shifting the left hand southeastward
to turn its palm downward and northwestward.
And then turn the palms toward one another
as if to hold a sphere
while beginning to lift the right knee to the south
to shift the right hand eastward and upward
while turning its palm northeastward.
The gaze follows the right hand before shifting upward
before leveling toward the south.

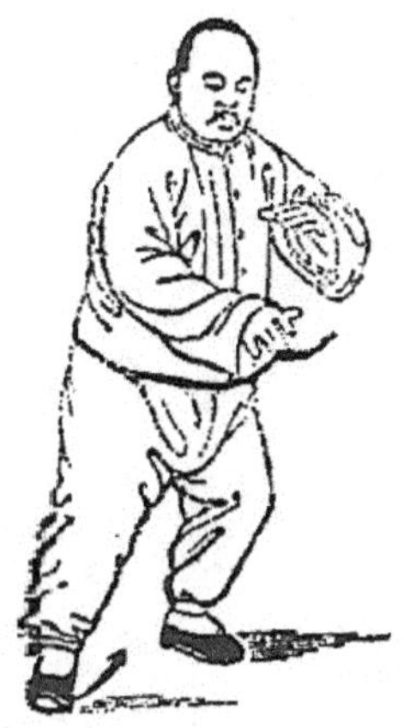
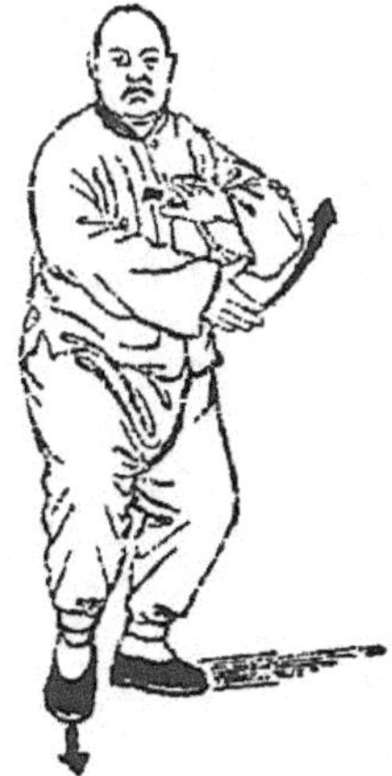

Then, stepping the right foot to the south
into a right bow stance with the right toes pointing southeastward,
turn the torso further southeastward
while continuing the arc of the right hand eastward and upward
to east of the right shoulder
and swinging the left hand with the turn
for its fingers to point upward and over the right elbow.
The gaze follows the motion of the right forearm and hand.
And then, turning the torso eastward,
step the left foot southeastward to east of the right heel
to set it on the ground *xū,*
and arc the left hand downward and toward the north
to above and to the north of the left knee
while settling its wrist to keep its palm downward
and arcing the right hand southwestward and upward
to above and to the southeast of the forehead
while turning its palm eastward.
The gaze levelly shifts to the east with the turn.

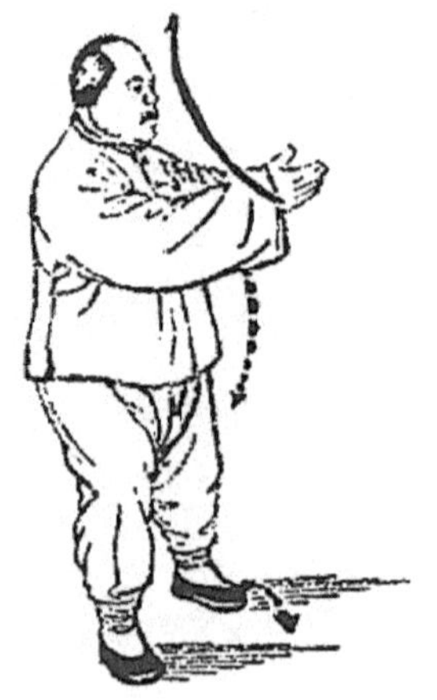

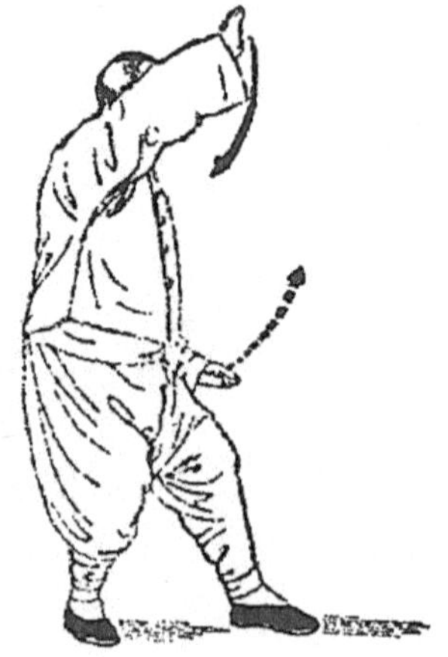

74.

搂膝拗步用法

Lǒu xī ǎo bù yòng fǎ
Draw and Bend Knee to Step Use Method.

Turning the torso southeastward, sink the right elbow
to draw the right hand down to southeast of the face
while turning its palm toward the face
and arcing the left hand southeastward and upward
for its fingers to point upward and toward the south
from east of the sternum.
And then arc the right hand downward and westward
to south of the right side of the *yāo*
while turning its palm toward the abdomen
and drawing the left hand westward toward the sternum.
The gaze follows the right palm.

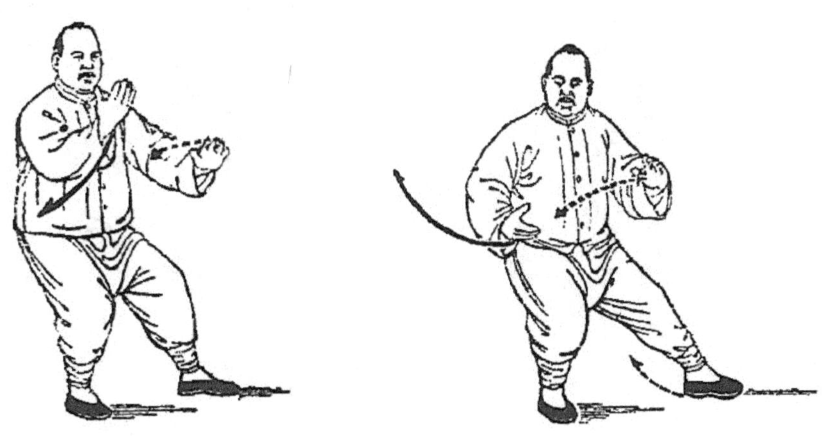

Then, lifting the left knee eastward,
arc the right hand westward and upward
while turning its palm upward and southeastward,
and arc the left hand southwestward and downward
to south of the abdomen.
The gaze continues to follow the right palm.
And then, arcing the right hand upward and eastward
to southwest of the right ear
while turning its palm downward and northeastward,
step the left foot eastward to touch its heel to the ground *xū*,
and arc the left hand downward and eastward
to southeast of the *yāo*,
while turning its palm downward.

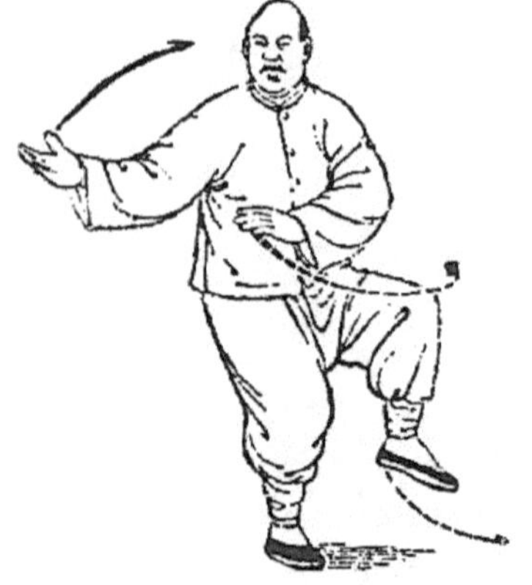
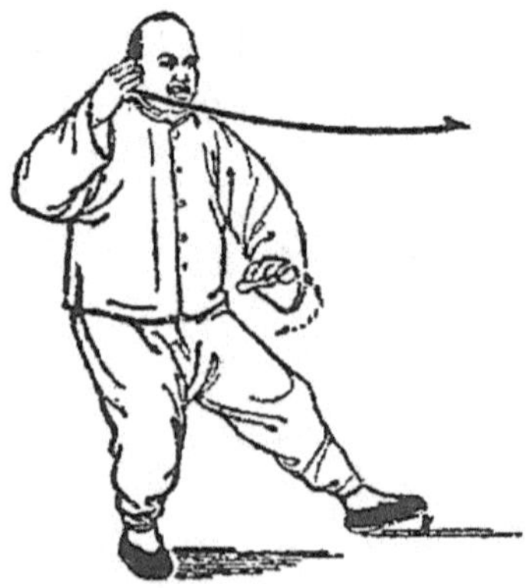

And then, turning the torso eastward,
shift the weight eastward into a left bow stance
while pushing the right hand eastward
while settling its wrist and brushing the left hand
eastward and downward toward the north
and then westward to above and to the north of the left knee
while keeping its palm facing downward.
The gaze follows the right hand.

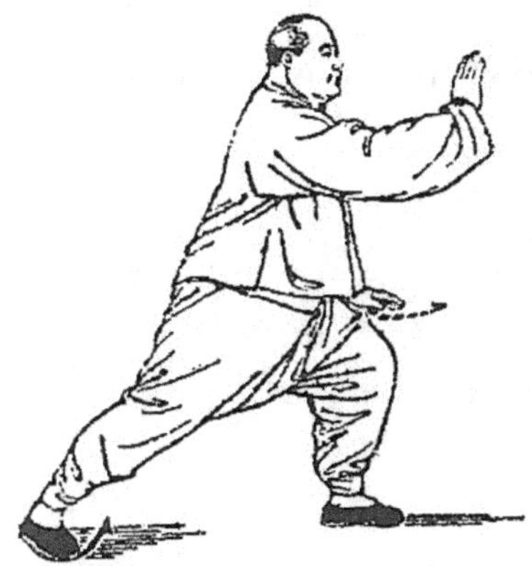

75.
海底針
Hăi dĭ zhēn
Sea Bottom Needle.

Lifting the right heel to shift into the tray stance
while shifting the left hand eastward,
extend the right hand further eastward while straightening its wrist
and turning its palm toward the north.
And then step the right foot eastward to south of the left foot
to settle it *shí* pointing southeastward,
and lift the left knee eastward
while promptly sinking the right elbow
to draw the right hand toward the right shoulder
while shifting the right fingers more levelly eastward
and shifting the left hand upward and toward the south
to above and to the west of the left knee
for its palm to face the left knee.

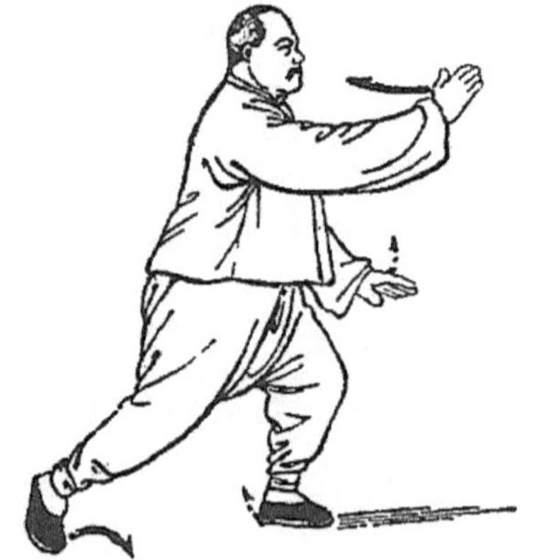
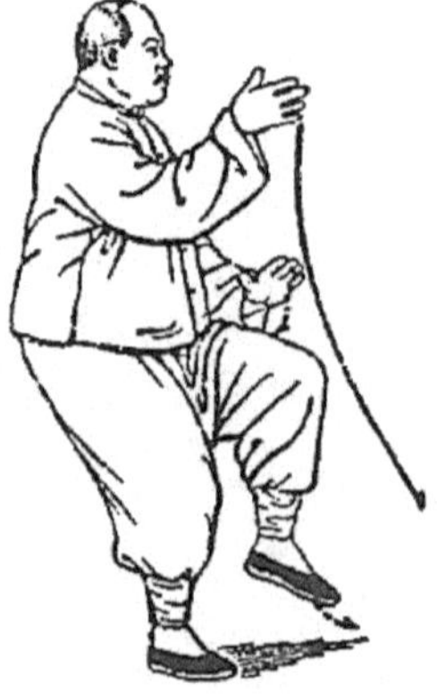

And then set the ball of the left foot on the ground
a half step east of the right heel,
and, bending the torso eastward and downward
while brushing the left hand northwestward
to above and to the northwest of the left knee, *sōng* the right wrist,
and promptly arc the right hand downward and southeastward
to scoop it toward the north.
The gaze is toward the right hand as it arcs toward the ground.

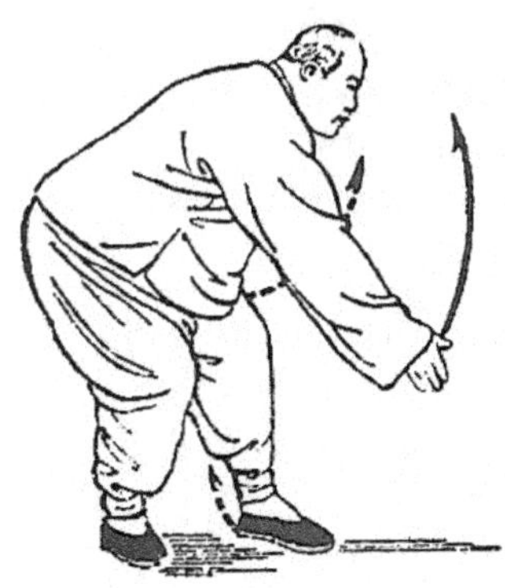

76.
扇通臂
Shàn tōng bì
Fan Through Arms.

Returning the torso to *xū líng dǐng jìn*,
lift the left knee eastward,
and quickly arc the right hand upward to east of the right shoulder
while turning its palm downward and southeastward
and arcing the left hand southeastward and upward
to north of the right forearm and east of the sternum
for its fingers to point upward and southeastward
toward the right forearm.
The gaze continues to follow the right hand.
Then, turning the torso toward the south,
step the left foot eastward into a left bow stance,
and extend the left hand eastward and upward
to east of the clavicle while settling its wrist
for its palm to face downward and southeastward
and arcing the right hand upward and westward
to south of the top of the head
while turning its palm toward the south.
The gaze is toward the left hand.

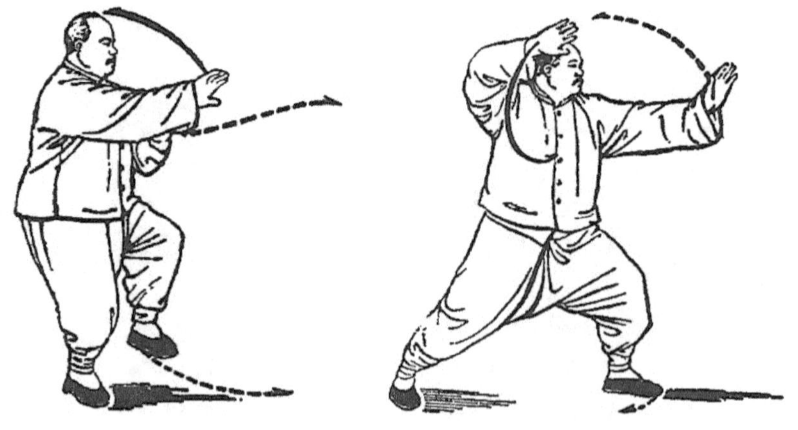

77.

轉身白蛇吐信
Zhuǎn shēn bái shé tǔ xìn
Turning Body White Snake Spits Truth.

Turning the left foot on its heel toward the south
and turning the right foot on its heel southwestward,
circle the right hand southwestward and downward
and then northeastward to south of the sternum
while closing it into a fist with its heart downward
and arcing the left hand upward and southwestward
to south of the top of the head while turning its palm to the south.
The gaze shifts with the turn to follow the arc of the left hand
before following the arc of the right hand
before shifting levelly to the south.
And then, pivoting the left foot on its ball northeastward
to turn the left knee southwestward
to turn the torso southwestward,
promptly lift the right knee westward
while shifting the right fist upward with the turn
to turn its heart toward the sternum
and arcing the left hand downward with the turn
for its palm to face downward and northwestward
from below and southwest of the right fist.
The gaze includes the motion of the hands.

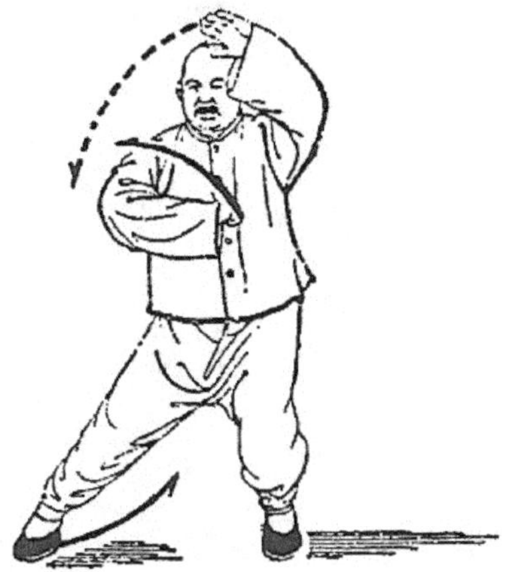 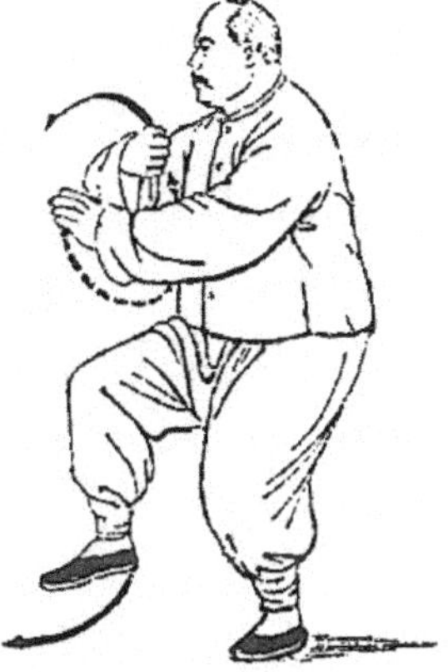

Then, stepping the right foot westward
to touch its heel to the ground *xū,*
circle the left hand downward and northeastward
and upward and southwestward to southwest of the sternum
while arcing the right hand upward and westward
and then downward to the level of the sternum
while opening it for its palm to face south.
And then, turning the torso westward,
shift the weight westward into a right bow stance
while arcing the left hand upward and westward
for its palm to face northwestward with its fingers upward
and arcing the right hand downward and eastward
to west of the right side of the *yāo*
while turning its palm upward.
The gaze is toward the left palm pushing forward.

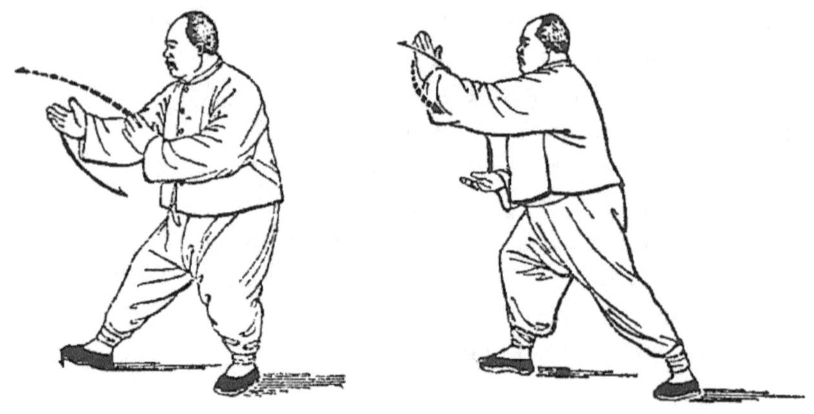

78.

搬攔捶

Bān lán chuí

Shift Block Cudgel.

Bending the left knee while straightening the right leg
to shift the weight eastward onto the left leg
while turning the torso southwestward,
sink the left elbow to draw the left hand downward and eastward
while turning its palm to the north
and closing the right hand into a fist
while arcing it upward and southwestward
for its heart to face downward toward the left hand.
The gaze is toward the right fist.
Then, turning the torso further southwestward,
shift the right fist down to the level of the sternum
while sinking the left elbow
to draw the left hand eastward to the south of the abdomen.
The gaze shifts levelly southwestward.

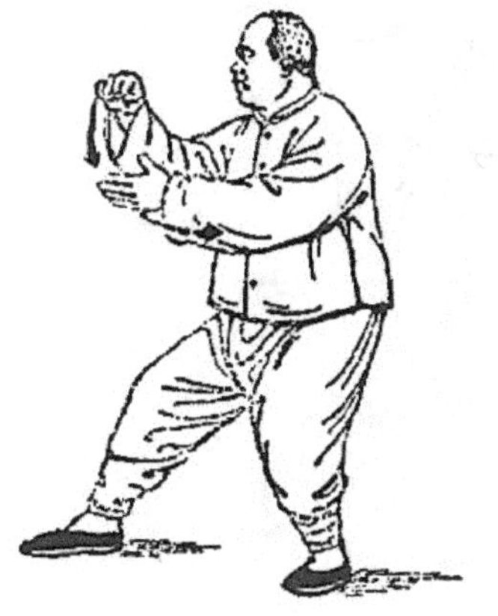
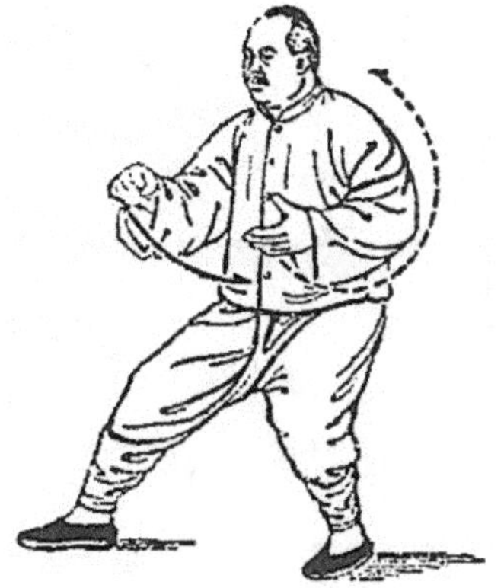

And then, lifting the right knee westward,
coil the right fist downward and eastward
to the south of the abdomen
while arcing the left hand downward and eastward
and then upward and westward to southeast of the face
while turning its palm downward and westward.
The gaze follows the hands
before returning levelly southwestward.
Then, turning the torso westward, step the right foot westward
to touch its heel to the ground *xū*
while arcing the right fist upward and westward
and shifting the left hand northwestward and downward
to cross the hands with the left palm facing north
and the heart of the right fist facing southeastward.

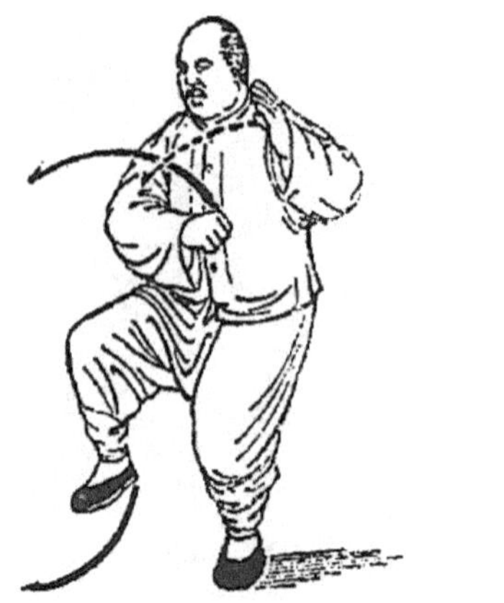 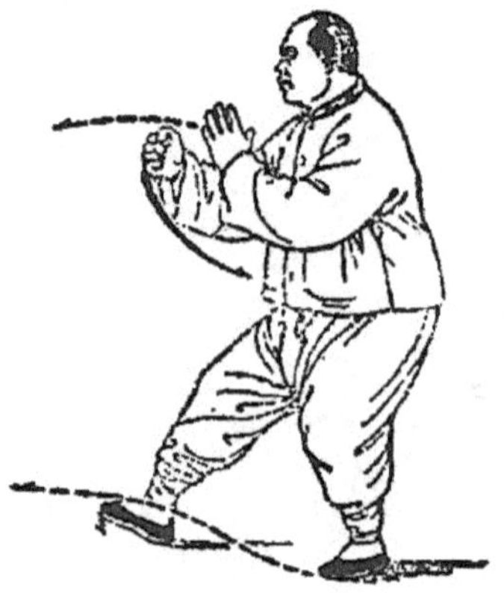

And then, turning the right foot on its heel northwestward,
shift the weight to it to lift the left knee westward
while turning the torso northwestward
and extending the left hand further westward
while arcing the right fist downward and eastward
to north of the *yāo*.
Then, bending the right knee further
to settle lower onto the right leg,
step the left foot westward to touch its heel to the ground *xū*
while continuing to extend the left hand westward
and continuing to draw the right fist eastward.

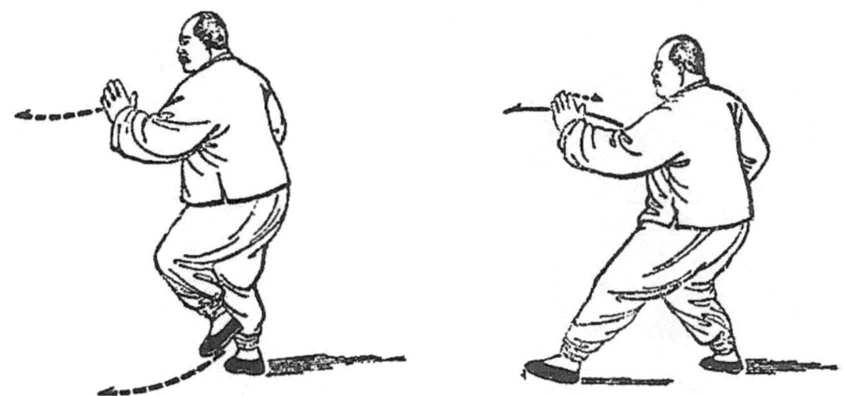

And then, turning the torso westward
while shifting the weight westward into a left bow stance,
cudgel the right fist upward and westward
while drawing the left hand northeastward
toward the right shoulder
as the right forearm glides westward past the left palm
until the right arm is nearly straight
with the left palm facing the right elbow and nearly touching it.
The gaze follows the left palm before shifting to the right fist

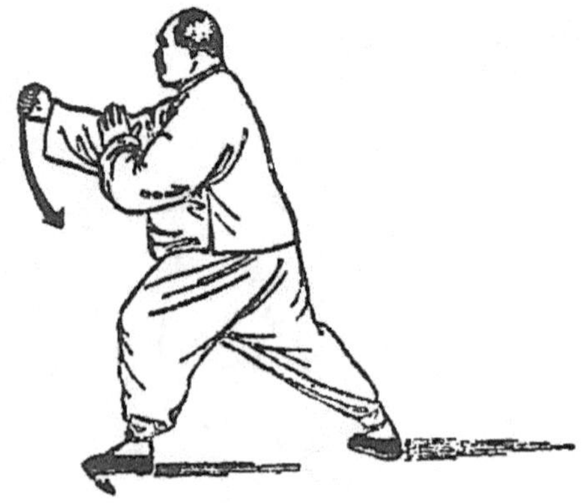

79.

攬雀尾式

Lǎn què wěi shì
Grasp Sparrow Tail Form.

Arrow Quiver Cover (Ward-Off).

Shifting the left foot on its heel southwestward
to turn the torso southwestward,
arc the right hand downward to the level of the abdomen
while opening it and turning its palm downward
and shifting the left elbow southeastward
to shift the left wrist downward to the level of its elbow
for its palm to face downward and westward.
And then, shifting all of the weight to the left leg
to lift the right knee westward,
circle the right hand downward and southeastward
and then upward
while shifting the left hand downward and eastward
 to turn the palms to face one another as if to hold a sphere.
The gaze is briefly toward the left forearm
before shifting toward the right arm
and then levelly southwestward.

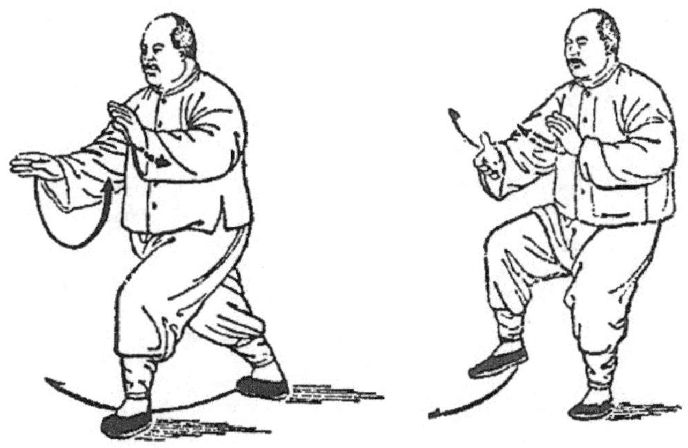

Then, stepping the right foot westward
to touch its heel to the ground *xū*,
shift the right hand westward and upward
while turning its palm southeastward
and shifting the left hand westward.
And then, shifting the weight westward into a right bow stance
while shifting the right hand further westward and upward
to west of the face for its palm to face the face,
shift the left hand with the right hand
while settling its wrist for its fingertips to point further upward.

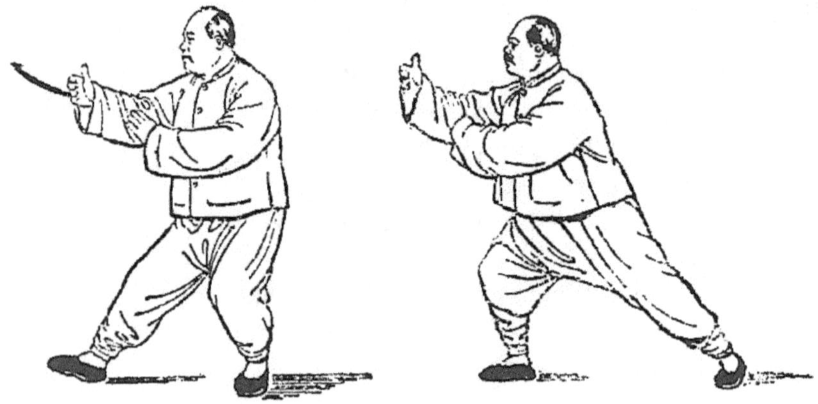

Stroke (Rollback).

Turning the right palm downward and westward
while turning the left palm toward the north,
begin to roll the hands downward and eastward.
Then, to continue rolling the hands downward and eastward,
bend the left knee to straighten the right leg
to shift the weight eastward onto the left leg.

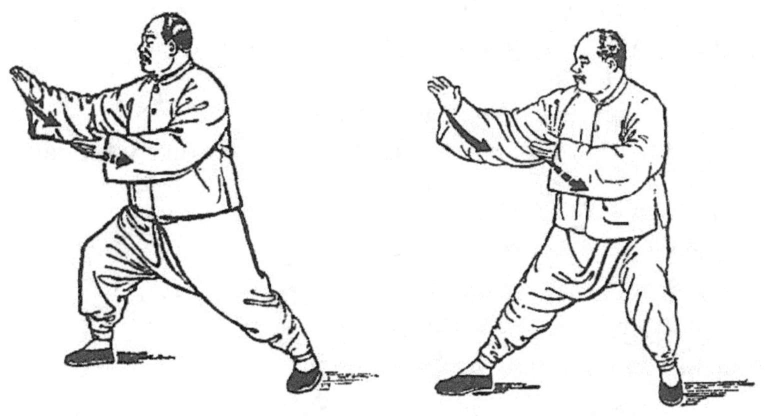

And then, keeping the elbows at least a fist's width from the torso,
roll the hands further downward and eastward
while turning the right palm southeastward.
The gaze attends to the left hand before following the right hand.

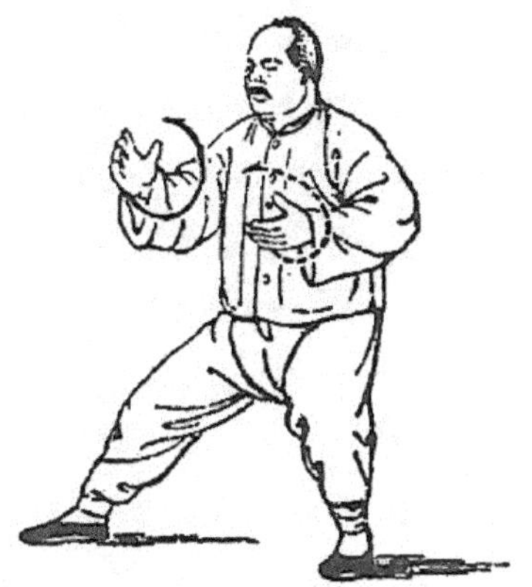

Press.

Beginning to shift the weight westward,
circle both hands downward and southeastward
and then upward and westward
to turn the left palm downward and westward
while turning the right palm eastward.
And then, completing the shift of the weight
westward again into a right bow stance
press the back of the right hand westward and upward
for its palm to face the face,
and push the left hand westward and upward
while settling its wrist to press the right forearm further westward.
The gaze is toward the right wrist.

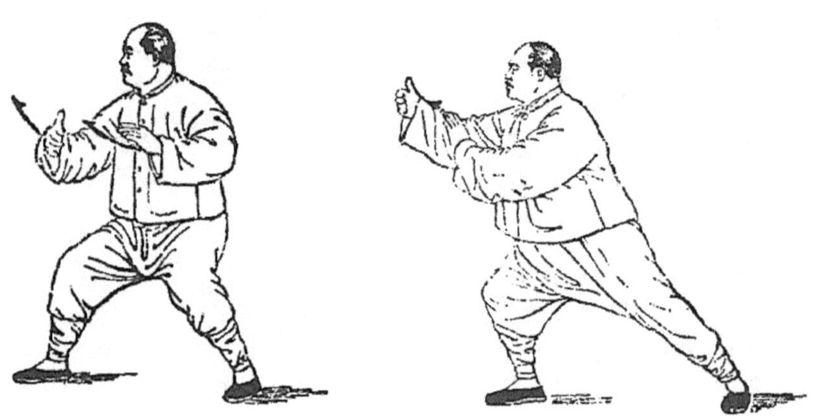

Push.

Turning the torso westward,
shift the right hand down to shoulder-level,
and pass the left hand over the right wrist
while turning both palms downward
to spread them shoulder-width apart.
Then, turning the palms to face one another
for their fingers to point upward and westward,
sink the elbows to draw the hands eastward toward the sternum
while bending the left knee to straighten the right leg
to shift the weight to the left leg.
The gaze is level and westward.

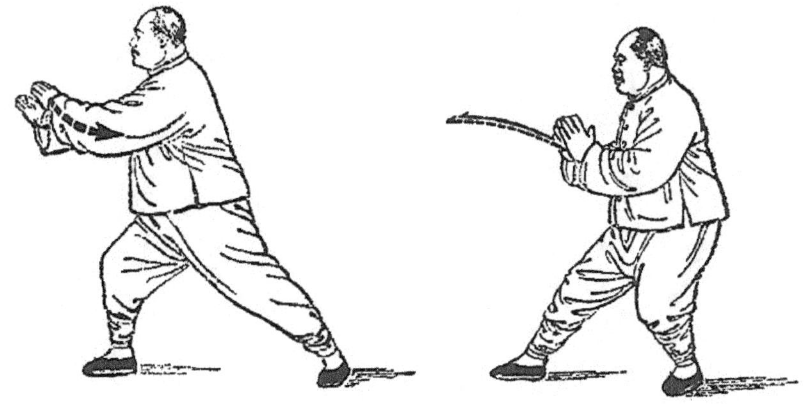

261

And then quickly straighten the wrists
to turn the palms downward
to push them upward and forward while settling their wrists
and shifting the weight westward again into a right bow stance.
The gaze remains level and forward.

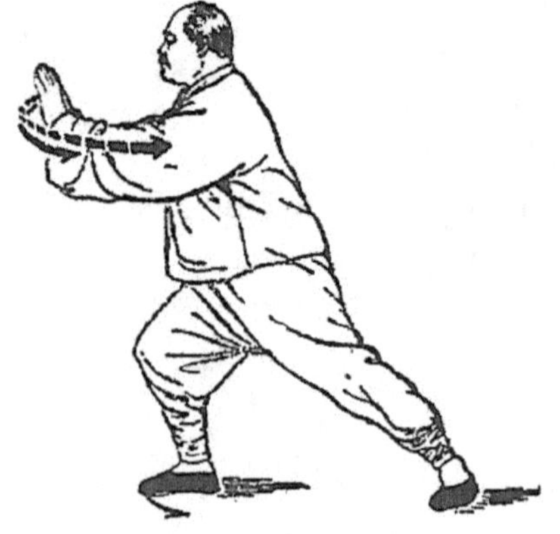

80.

單鞭式

Dān biān shì

Solitary Whip Form.

Bending the left knee and straightening the right leg
to shift the weight to the left leg, turn the torso southwestward,
and turn the right foot on its heel southwestward
while swinging the hands with the turn
and beginning to turn the palms downward.
And then, turning the torso southeastward
while swinging the arms with the turn
and continuing to turn the palms downward,
turn the left foot on its ball northwestward,
and turn the right foot on its ball also northwestward
while bending the right knee while straightening the left knee
to shift the weight to the right leg.
The gaze levelly shifts with the turn.

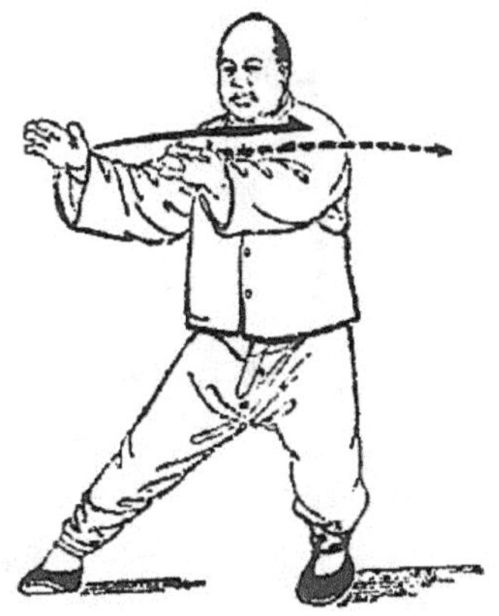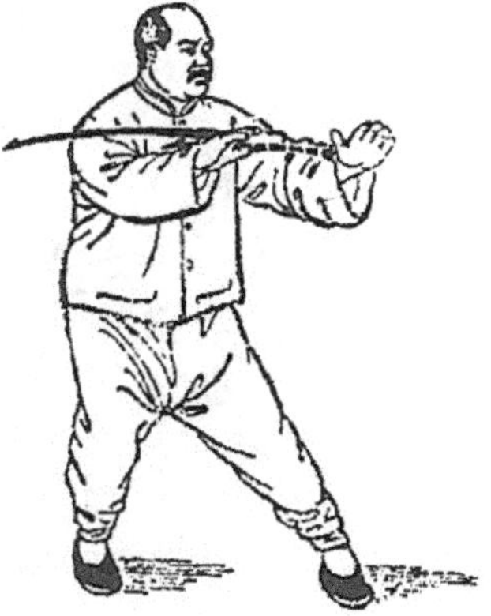

Then, keeping the weight on the right leg,
turn the torso again southwestward
while swinging the arms with the turn
and also shifting the gaze with the turn.
And then, again turning the torso southeastward
while shifting the left hand
upward and eastward to southeast of the chin
to turn its palm toward the chin,
lift the left knee eastward,
and *sōng* the right wrist while extending its hand westward
and gathering its fingers and thumb to each other
for the hand to hang downward
to form a hook shape with its wrist.
The gaze shifts levelly with the turn.

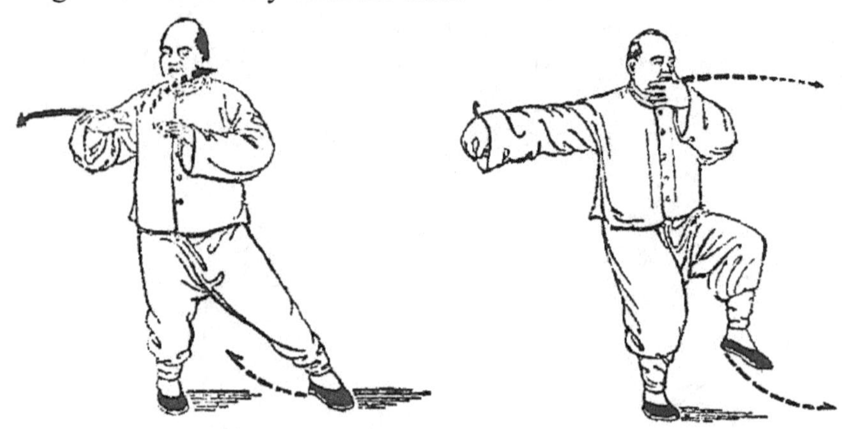

Then, shifting the right hand upward
until its fingertips are at shoulder-level,
step the left foot eastward into a left bow stance
while extending the left hand eastward
and turning its palm downward
before settling its wrist and turning its palm southeastward.
The gaze shifts levelly with the motion of the left hand.

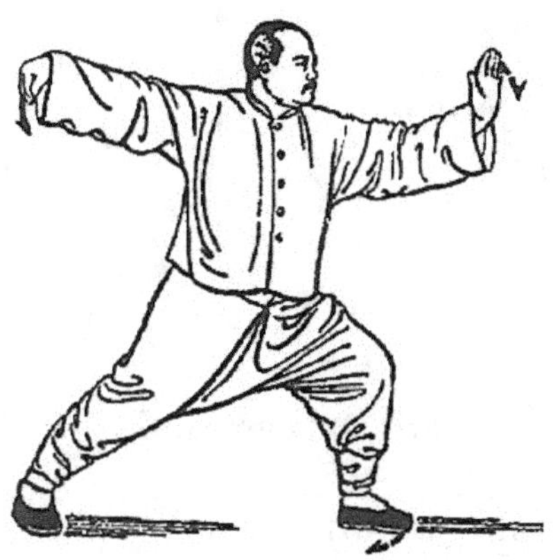

81.
扽手
Yǔn shǒu
Cloud Hands.

Right.

Lifting the left toes
to turn the left foot on its heel toward the south,
sōng the right hand while turning the left palm toward the south,
and begin to arc both hands downward.
Then, settling the left foot flat,
lift the right heel northeastward
to shift all the weight onto the left leg
while turning the torso to the south
and promptly arcing the right hand downward and eastward
while settling its wrist
for its palm to face downward and northeastward
from southwest of the *yāo*
and shifting the left hand down to southeast of the abdomen
while turning its palm downward for its fingers to point south.
The gaze shifts levelly to the southwest.

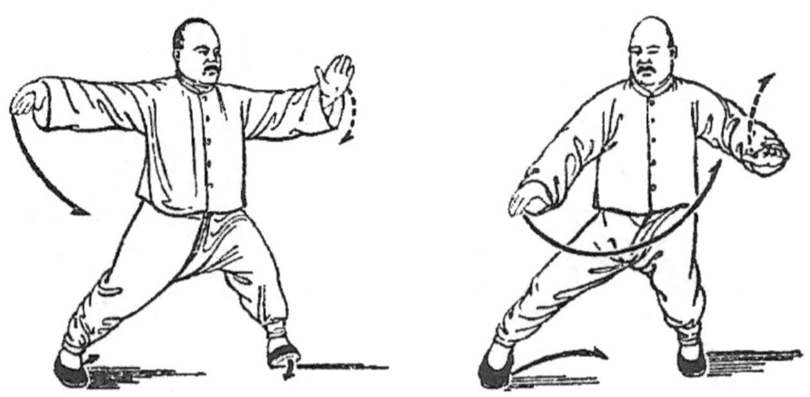

Then, lifting the right knee toward the south
while turning the torso southeastward,
shift the left hand up to shoulder-level for its palm to face south
with its fingers upward and eastward,
and continue the arc of the right hand downward and eastward
and then upward for its palm to face north with its fingers eastward
and its thumb at the level of the right elbow.
The gaze follows the right hand.
And then, turning the torso again to the south,
set the right foot on the ground flat to settle into the horse stance
while arcing the right hand upward and westward
for its palm to face the face from southwest of the face
and arcing the left hand downward and westward
for its palm to face the abdomen from south of the abdomen.
The gaze continues to follow the right hand.

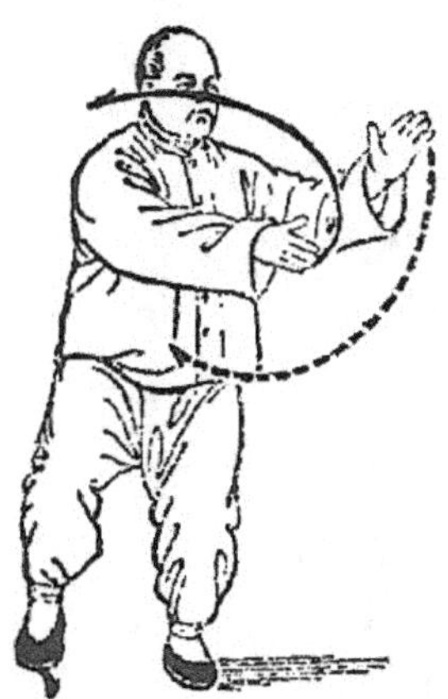 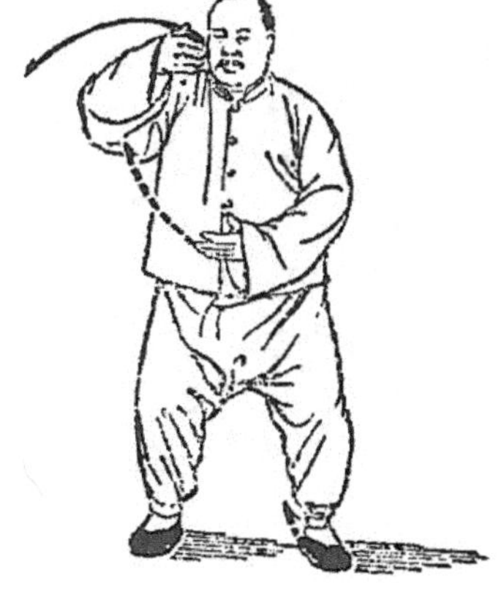

Left

Lifting the left knee to the south
while turning the torso southwestward,
arc the right hand westward for its palm to face south
with its fingers pointing upward and westward,
and arc the left hand westward and upward
while turning its palm downward and northwestward.
The gaze continues to follow the right hand.
And then, turning the torso again to the south,
step the left foot eastward into a wide horse stance,
and, arcing the left hand upward and eastward
for its palm to face the face from southeast of the face,
arc the right hand downward and eastward and upward
for its palm to face the abdomen from south of the abdomen.
The gaze shifts to the left palm.

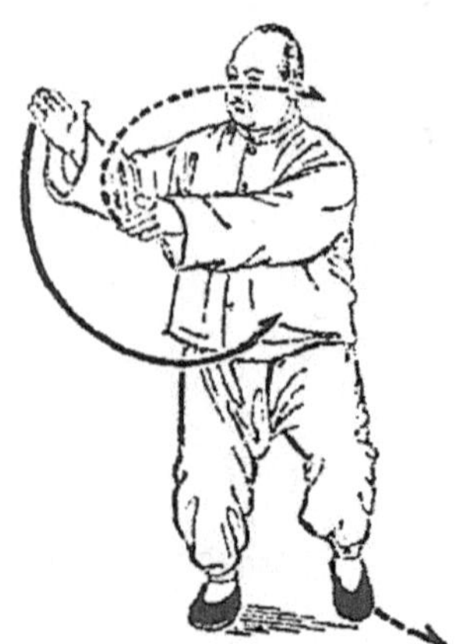 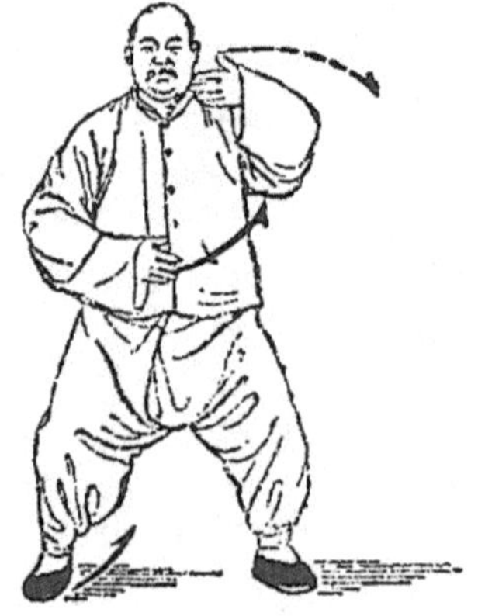

Right.

Lifting the right knee toward the south
while turning the torso southeastward,
arc the left hand eastward
while turning its palm toward the south
to point its fingers upward and eastward,
and arc the right hand eastward and upward
for its fingers to point eastward
with its thumb south of the left elbow.
The gaze continues to follow the left hand.
And then, turning the torso again to the south,
set the right foot on the ground flat to settle into the horse stance
while arcing the right hand upward and westward
for its palm to face the face from southwest of the face
and arcing the left hand downward and westward
for its palm to face the abdomen from south of the abdomen.
The gaze shifts to the right palm.

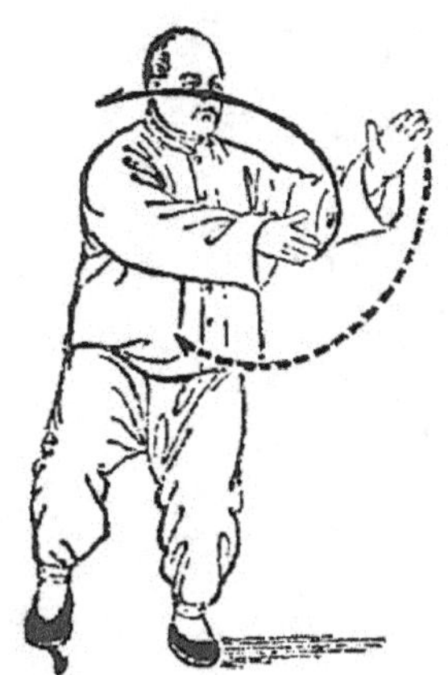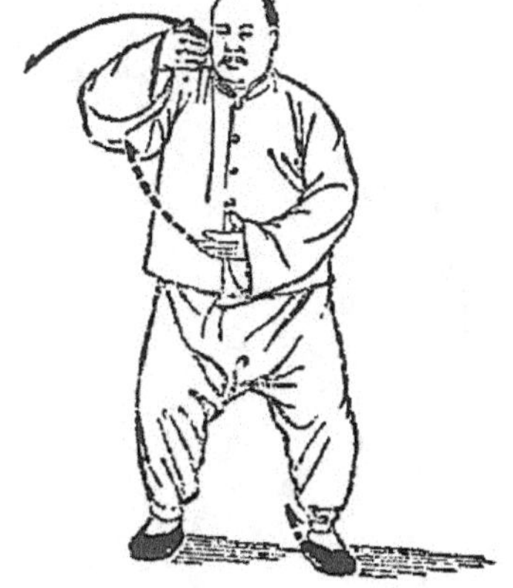

Left

Lifting the left knee to the south
while turning the torso southwestward,
arc the right hand westward for its palm to face south
with its fingers pointing upward and westward,
and arc the left hand westward and upward
while turning its palm downward and northwestward.
The gaze continues to follow the right hand.
And then, turning the torso again to the south,
step the left foot eastward into a wide horse stance,
and, arcing the left hand upward and eastward
for its palm to face the face from southeast of the face,
arc the right hand downward and eastward and upward
for its palm to face the abdomen from south of the abdomen.
The gaze shifts to the left palm.

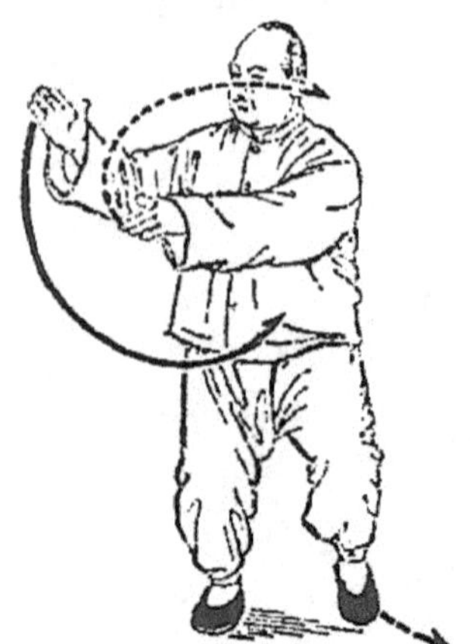 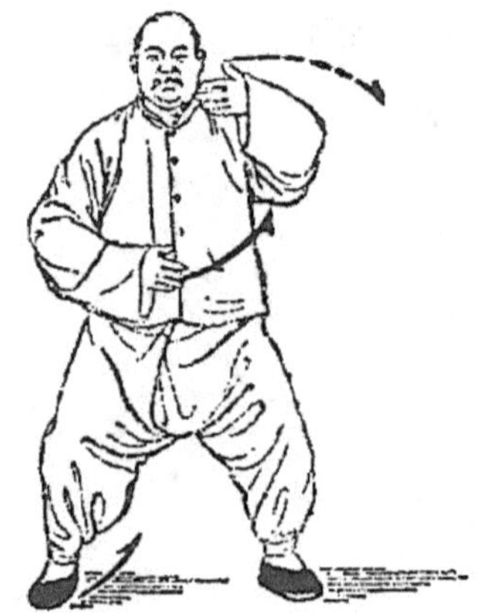

Right.

Lifting the right knee toward the south
while turning the torso southeastward,
arc the left hand eastward
while turning its palm toward the south
to point its fingers upward and eastward,
and arc the right hand eastward and upward
for its fingers to point eastward
with its thumb south of the left elbow.
The gaze continues to follow the left hand.
And then, turning the torso again to the south,
set the right foot on the ground flat to settle into the horse stance
while arcing the right hand upward and westward
for its palm to face the face from southwest of the face
and arcing the left hand downward and westward
for its palm to face the abdomen from south of the abdomen.
The gaze shifts to the right palm.

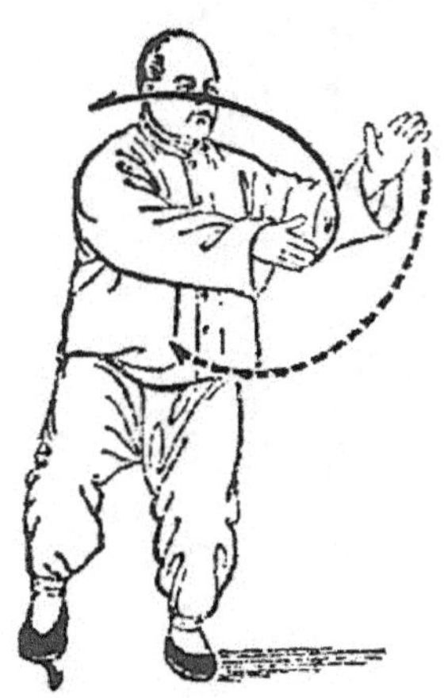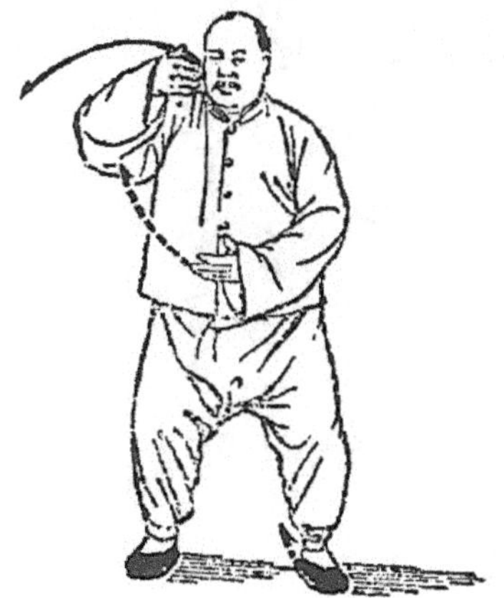

Left

Lifting the left knee to the south
while turning the torso southwestward,
arc the right hand westward for its palm to face south
with its fingers pointing upward and westward,
and arc the left hand westward and upward
while turning its palm downward and northwestward.
The gaze continues to follow the right hand.
And then, turning the torso again to the south,
step the left foot eastward into a wide horse stance,
and, arcing the left hand upward and eastward
for its palm to face the face from southeast of the face,
arc the right hand downward and eastward and upward
for its palm to face the abdomen from south of the abdomen.
The gaze shifts to the left palm.

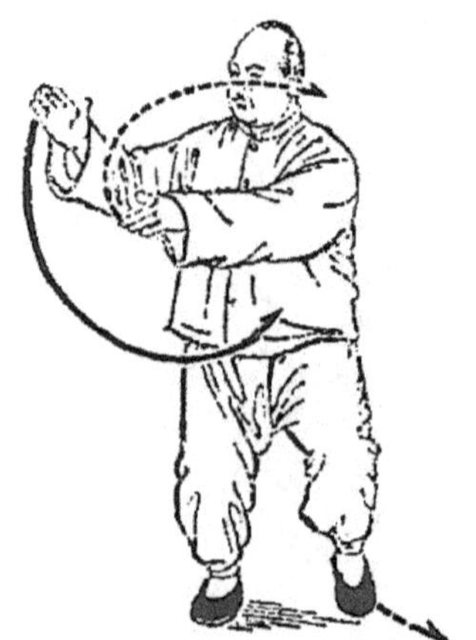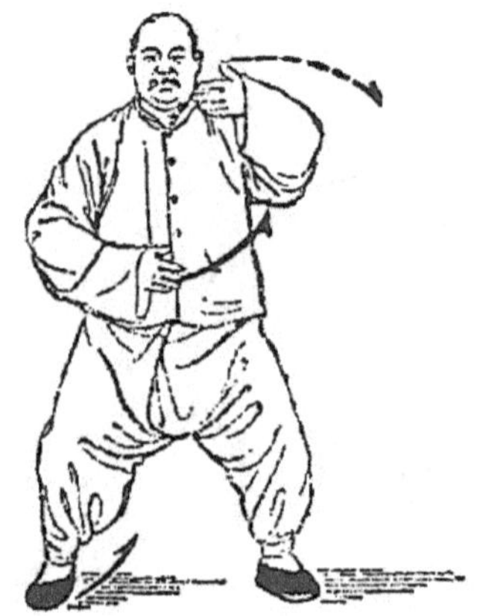

Right.

Lifting the right knee toward the south
while turning the torso southeastward,
arc the left hand eastward
while turning its palm toward the south
to point its fingers upward and eastward,
and arc the right hand eastward and upward
for its fingers to point eastward
with its thumb south of the left elbow.
The gaze continues to follow the left hand.
And then, turning the torso again to the south,
set the right foot on the ground flat to settle into the horse stance
while arcing the right hand upward and westward
for its palm to face the face from southwest of the face
and arcing the left hand downward and westward
for its palm to face the abdomen from south of the abdomen.
The gaze shifts to the right palm.

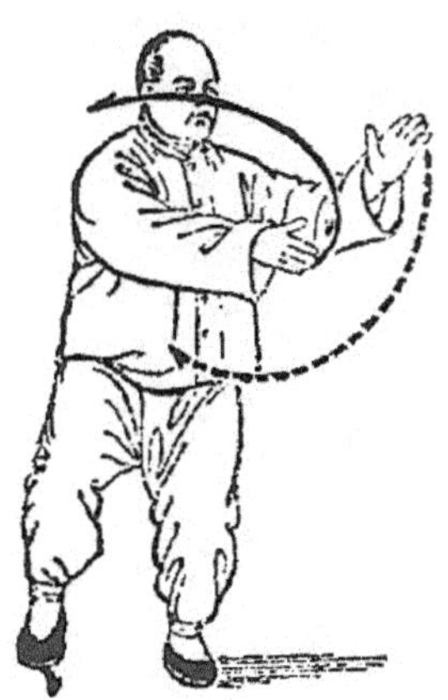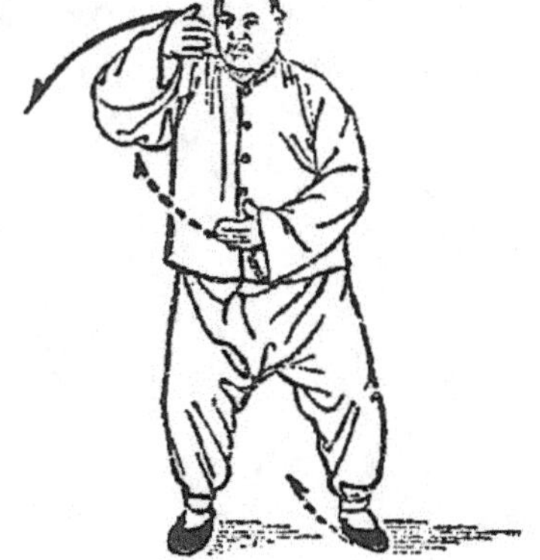

82.
單鞭
Dān biān
Solitary Whip.

Shifting the right foot on its ball northwestward
and shifting the weight to the right leg
to lift the left knee southeastward
while turning the torso southwestward,
sōng the right wrist while arcing it westward and downward
to the level of the sternum
and arcing the left hand westward and upward
while turning its palm downward and toward the north.
And then, turning the torso southeastward,
extend the right arm fully westward
while gathering its fingers and thumb to each other
for the hand to form a hook shape with its wrist
and arcing the left hand upward and eastward
to southeast of the chin while turning its palm toward the chin.
The gaze, after following the movement of the right hand,
shifts to the southeast over the left hand.

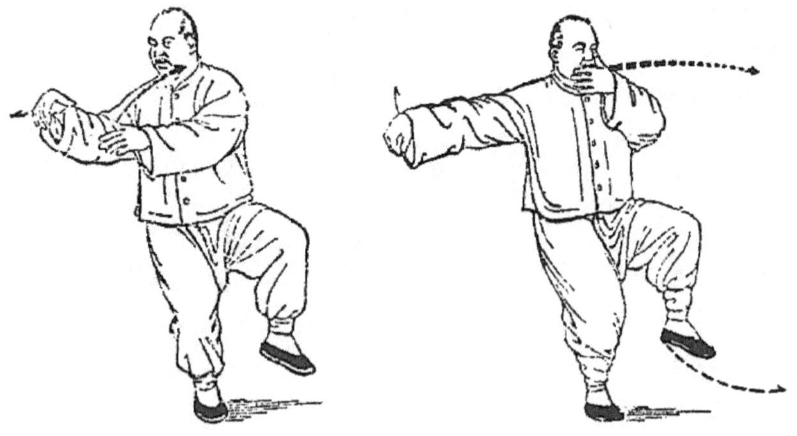

And then, shifting the right hand up to shoulder-level
while stepping the left foot eastward into a left bow stance,
extend the left hand eastward while turning its palm downward
before settling its wrist and turning its palm southeastward.
The gaze shifts levelly with the motion of the left hand.

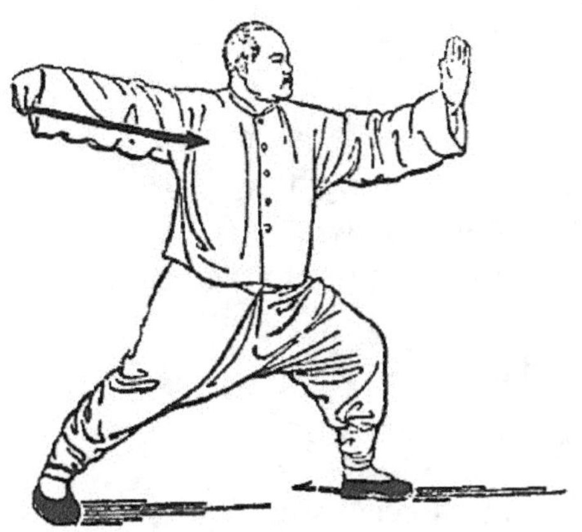

83.

高探馬代穿掌

Gāo tàn mǎ dài chuān zhǎng
High Search of Horse Generating Piercing Palm.

Bending the right leg while straightening the left leg
to shift the weight westward to the right leg,
raise the left toes from the ground,
and *sōng* the right hand while quickly arcing it eastward
to southwest of the sternum while straightening its wrist
and turning its palm downward and northeastward
while straightening the left wrist to turn its palm to the south.
The gaze is toward the left palm.
Then, arcing the right hand upward and eastward
and then to the north
for its palm to face downward from east of the chin,
lift the left knee eastward to turn the torso eastward
while drawing the left hand downward and westward
for the palms to face one another as if holding a sphere.

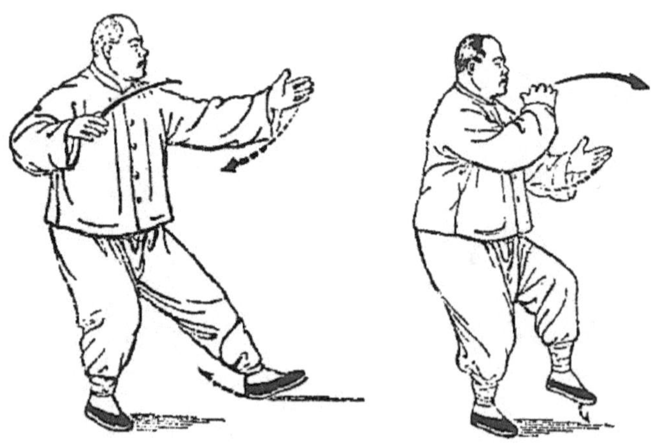

Then, setting the left foot on the ground
a half step east of the right heel,
extend the right hand eastward
for its palm to face downward and northeastward
from east of the face,
and draw the left hand downward and northwestward
to east of the left side of the abdomen
while turning its palm upward.
The gaze is toward the right hand extending.

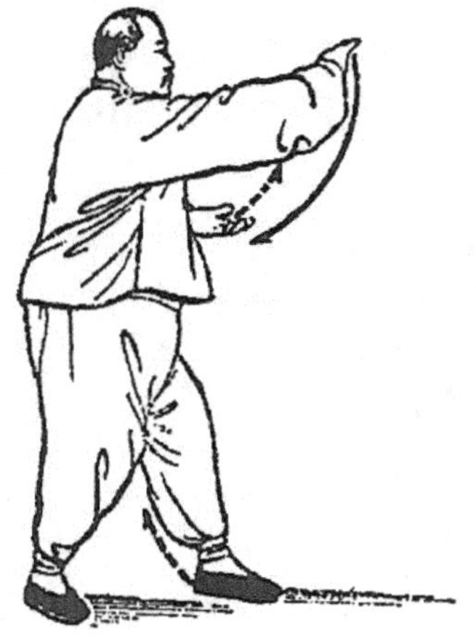

Left piercing palm.

Then, lifting the left knee eastward,
shift the left hand southeastward and upward
to east of the clavicle while turning its palm toward the clavicle,
and arc the right hand downward and northwestward
to east of the left forearm while turning its palm westward.
And then, stepping the left foot eastward into a left bow stance,
extend the left hand eastward for its palm to face upward,
and draw the right hand northwestward
to below the left elbow while turning its palm downward.
The gaze briefly shifts toward the withdrawal of the right hand
before returning levelly to the east.

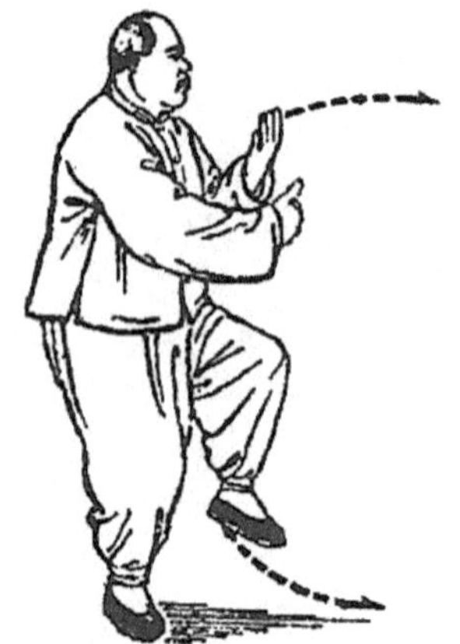
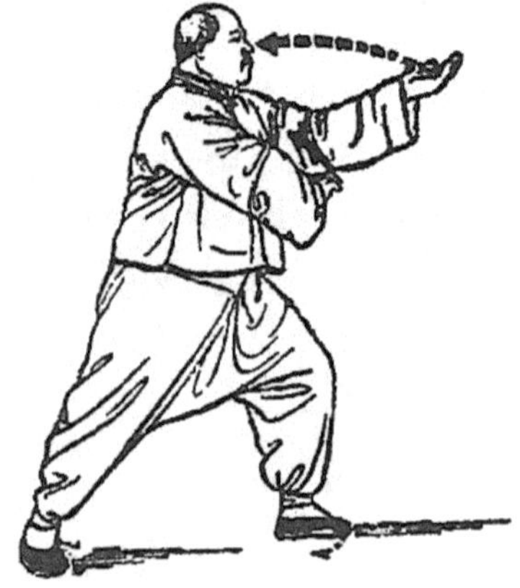

84.

十字單擺蓮

Shí zì dān bǎi lián
Ten *Zì* Solitary Swinging Lotus.

Turning the left foot on its heel southwestward
to turn the torso to the south,
shift the right foot on its heel southwestward
while shifting the right hand upward and southwestward
to southeast of the sternum while turning its palm toward the north
and drawing the left hand southwestward to southeast of the face
while turning its palm northwestward toward the face.
And then lift the right knee westward
to turn the torso southwestward while swinging the arms with turn
and shifting the left hand downward
while shifting the right hand upward
to cross the hands in front of the sternum
with the right hand on the outside.
The gaze shifts levelly with the turn.

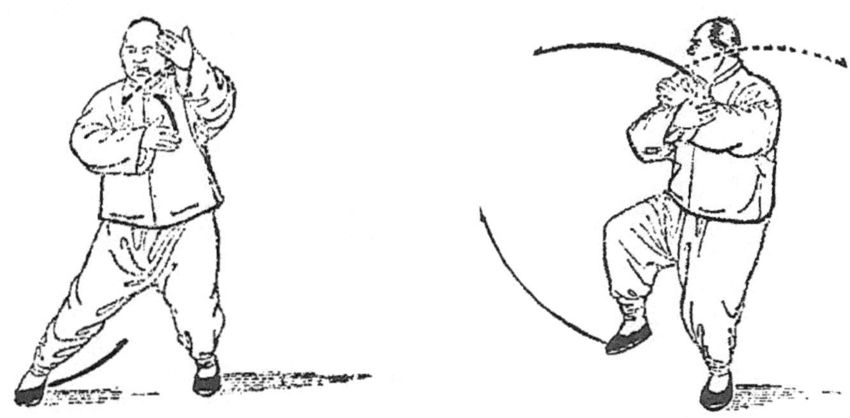

And then, continuing to lift the right knee,
straighten it to kick the right foot westward
for its toes to point upward at the level of the *yāo*,
and arc the left hand upward and southeastward
while arcing the right hand upward and northwestward
for the left palm to face south
with the right palm facing southwestward.
The gaze is toward the right hand.

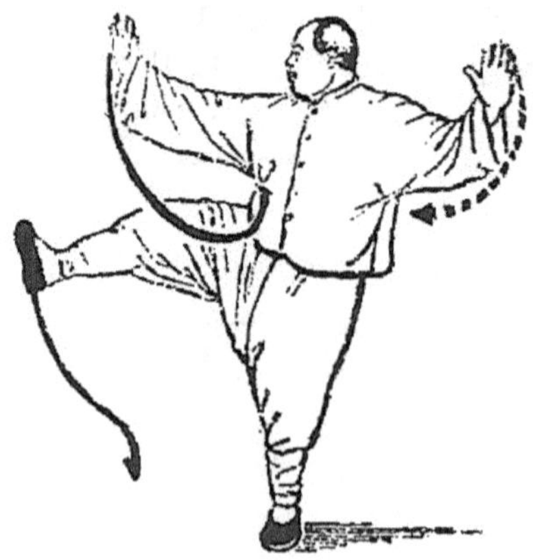

85.
進步指襠捶
Jìn bù zhǐ dāng chuí
Advance Step Directing Crotch Cudgel.

Settling onto the left leg while quickly lowering the right leg,
close the right hand into a fist
while arcing it downward and southeastward
and then upward to southwest of the center of the abdomen
while turning its heart downward and eastward
and quickly arcing the left hand downward and westward
to southeast of the sternum
while turning its palm downward and southwestward.
The gaze remains levelly toward the west.
And then, shifting the left foot on its ball northeastward
to turn the torso westward,
step the right foot northwestward into a right bow stance
with its toes pointing northwestward
while circling the right fist upward and westward
and then downward to northwest of the center of the abdomen
while turning its heart upward and toward the south
and arcing the left hand westward
while turning its palm downward and toward the north.
The gaze is toward the arcing of the left hand.

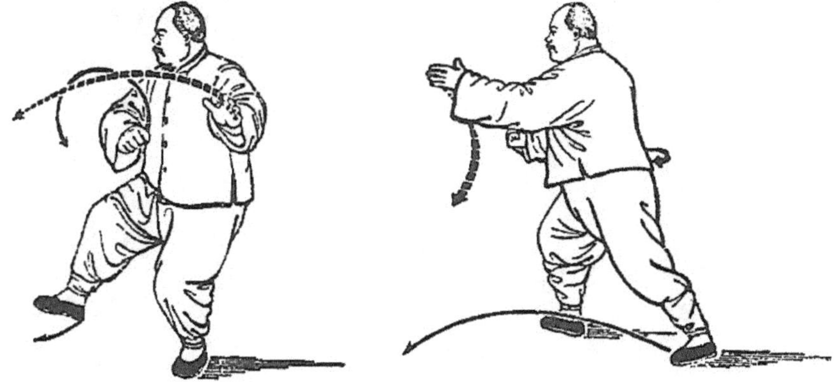

Then, stepping the left foot westward past the right ankle
to touch its heel to the ground *xū*, turn the torso northwestward,
and draw the right fist eastward to northeast of the *yāo*
while arcing the left hand downward
to the level of the *yāo* while turning its palm downward.
The gaze remains level and toward the west.
And then, shifting the weight westward into a left bow stance
while turning the torso westward,
quickly brush the left palm over the left knee
and downward to southeast of the knee
while leaning the torso westward
to cudgel the right fist westward
while turning its heart to the south.
The gaze includes the left palm brushing toward the south
before shifting toward the right fist cudgeling westward.

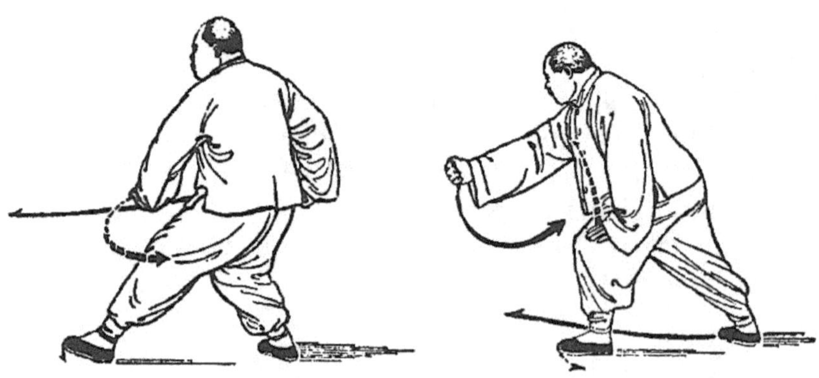

86.

上步攬雀尾

Shàng bù lǎn què wěi
Up Step Grasp Sparrow Tail

Turning the left foot on its heel southwestward,
return the torso to *xū líng dǐng jìn*
while lifting the right knee westward
to turn the torso southwestward
while arcing the left hand upward to southwest of the sternum
while turning its palm northwestward and downward
and opening the right hand while arcing it downward
and then eastward and then upward
while turning its palm toward the left palm as if to hold a sphere.
The gaze follows the convergence of the arms.

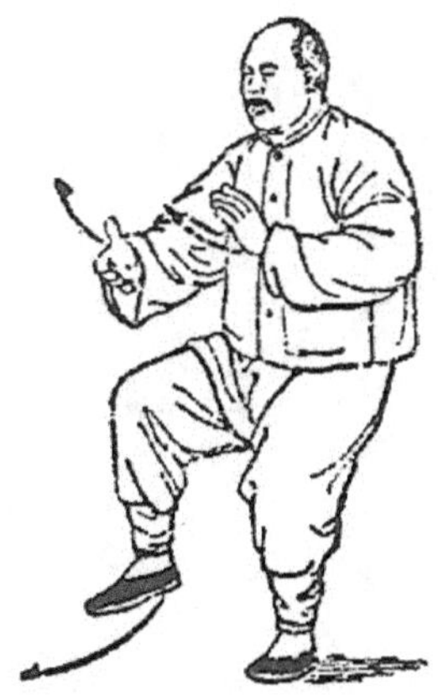

Yang Chengfu doesn't explain why, while this up step is a
component of each Grasp Sparrow Tail form he describes, he calls
but two of the Grasp Sparrow Tail repetitions in the sequence Up
Step Grasp Sparrow Tail.

Arrow Quiver Cover (Ward-Off).

Then, stepping the right foot westward
to touch its heel to the ground *xū*,
press the back of the right hand westward and upward
to west of the clavicle
while beginning to shift the left hand also westward.
And then, shifting the weight westward into a right bow stance
while shifting the right hand further westward and upward
to west of the face for its palm to face the face,
shift the left hand with the right hand
while settling its wrist for its fingertips to point further upward

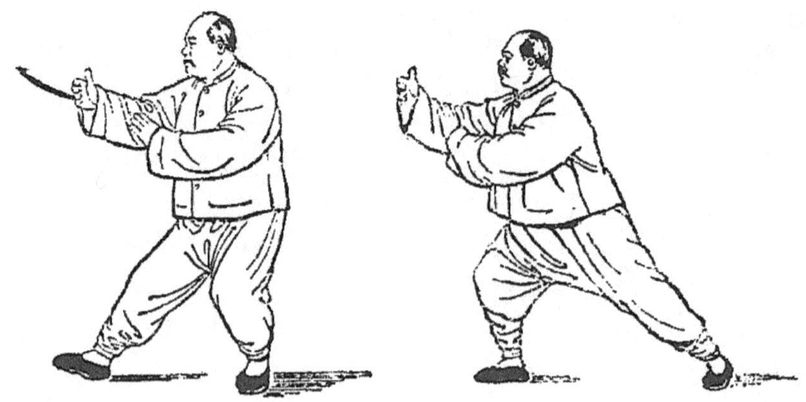

Stroke (Roll Back)

Turning the right palm downward and westward
while turning the left palm upward and toward the north,
begin to roll the hands downward and eastward.
Then, straightening the right leg and bending the left leg,
shift the weight to the left leg
to continue the downward and eastward roll of the hands.

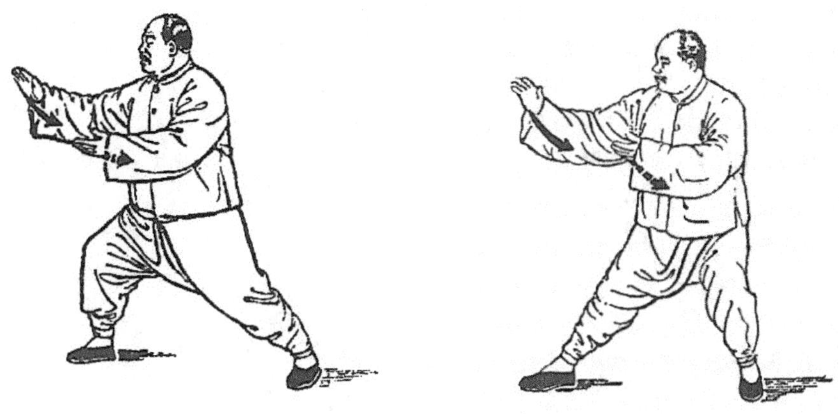

And then, keeping the elbows at least a fist's width from the torso,
continue rolling the hands downward and eastward
while turning the right palm southeastward
and turning the left palm toward the north.
The gaze attends to the left hand before following the right hand.

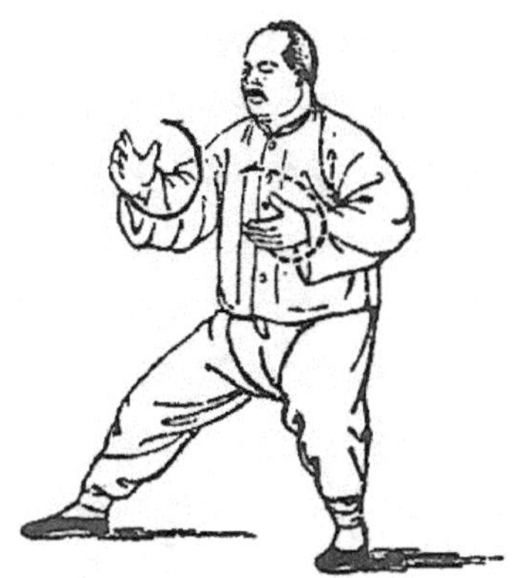

Press.

Beginning to shift the weight westward,
circle both hands downward and southeastward
and then upward and westward
to turn the left palm downward and westward
while turning the right palm eastward.
And then, completing the shift of the weight
westward again into a right bow stance
press the back of the right hand westward and upward
for its palm to face the face,
and push the left hand westward and upward
while settling its wrist to press the right forearm further westward.
The gaze is toward the right forearm.

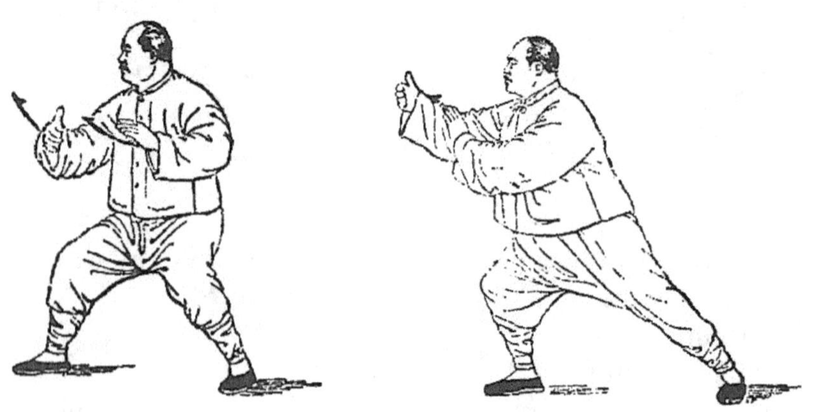

Push.

Turning the torso westward,
shift the right hand down to shoulder-level,
and pass the left hand over the right wrist
while turning both palms downward
to spread them shoulder-width apart.
Then, turning the palms to face one another
for their fingers to point upward and westward,
sink the elbows to draw the hands eastward toward the sternum
while bending the left knee to straighten the right leg
to shift the weight to the left leg.
The gaze is level and westward.

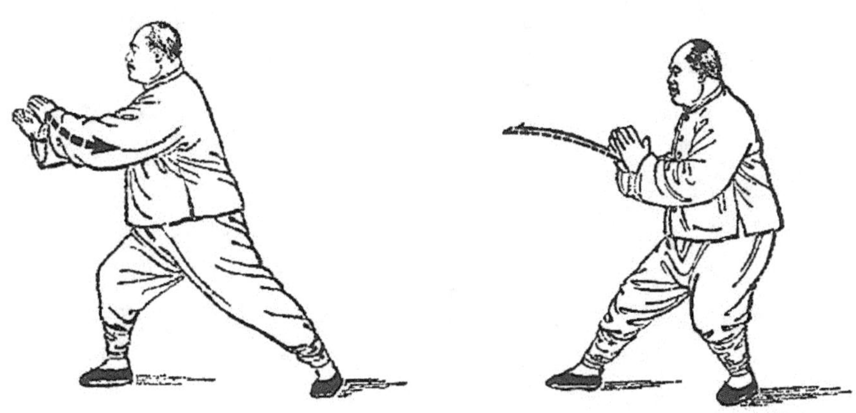

And then quickly straighten the wrists
to turn the palms downward
to push them upward and forward while settling their wrists
and shifting the weight westward again into a right bow stance.
The gaze remains level and forward.

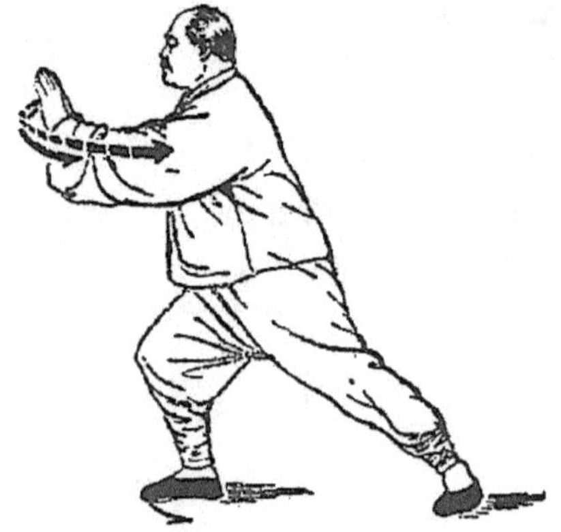

87.

單鞭下式

Dān biān xià shì
Solitary Whip Low Form.

Bending the left knee and straightening the right leg
to shift the weight to the left leg, turn the torso southwestward,
and turn the right foot on its heel southwestward
while swinging the hands with the turn
and beginning to turn the palms downward.
And then, turning the torso southeastward
while swinging the arms with the turn
and continuing to turn the palms downward,
turn the left foot on its ball northwestward,
and turn the right foot on its ball also northwestward
while bending the right knee while straightening the left knee
to shift the weight to the right leg.
The gaze levelly shifts with the turn.

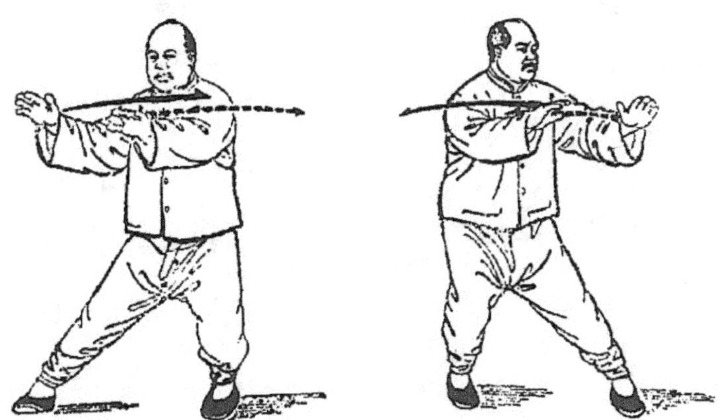

Then, keeping the weight on the right leg,
turn the torso again southwestward
while swinging the arms with the turn
and shifting the gaze with the turn.
And then, again turning the torso southeastward
while shifting the left hand
upward and eastward to southeast of the chin
to turn its palm toward the chin,
lift the left knee eastward,
and *sōng* the right wrist while extending its hand westward
and gathering its fingers and thumb to each other
for the hand to hang downward
to form a hook shape with its wrist.
The gaze shifts levelly with the turn.

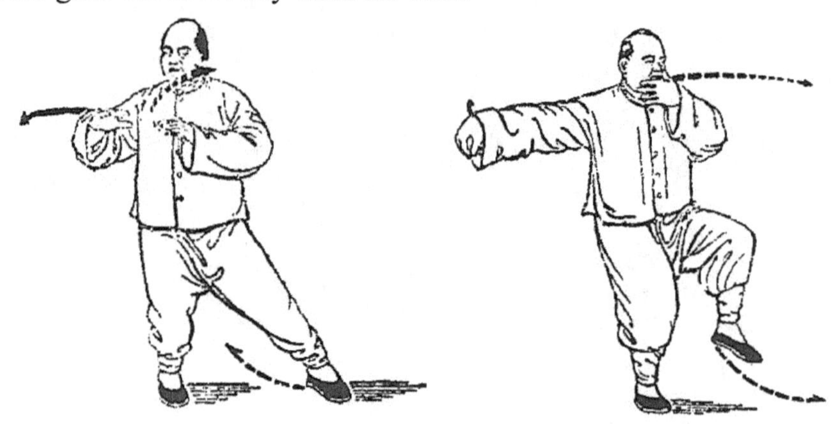

And then, stepping the left foot eastward
into a left bow stance, shift the right hand upward
until its fingertips are at shoulder-level,
and extend the left hand eastward
while turning its palm downward
before settling its wrist and turning its palm southeastward.
The gaze shifts levelly with the motion of the left hand.
Then, bending the right knee
and turning the right foot on its heel southwestward
while straightening the left leg
to shift the weight westward onto the right leg,
settle low onto the right foot,
and arc the left hand southwestward and downward
while turning its palm to the south.

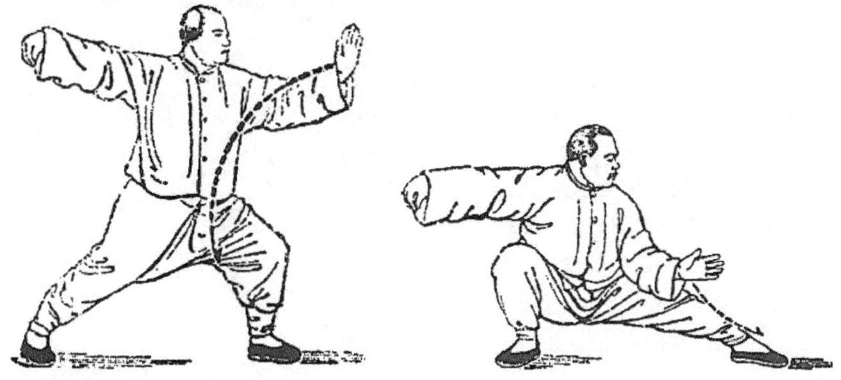

And then, bending the torso southeastward,
shift the left hand downward and eastward
to above and to the south of the left ankle.
The gaze follows the left hand.

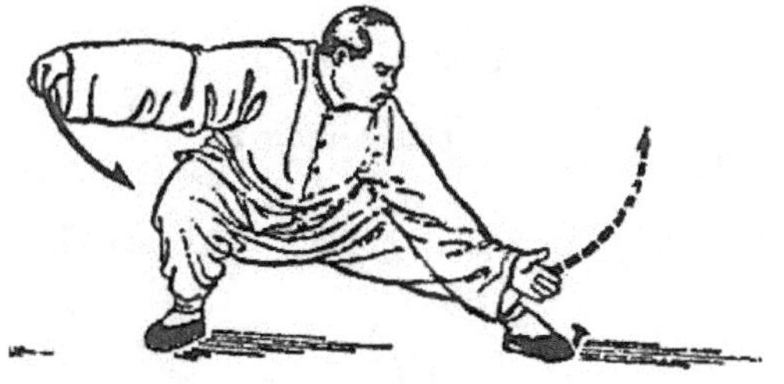

88.

上步七星

Shàng bù qī xīng
Up Step to Seven Stars.

Turning the left foot on its heel northeastward
and straightening the right leg while bending the left knee
to shift the weight to the left leg,
return the torso to *xū líng dǐng jìn* while turning it eastward
and lifting the right knee eastward
while arcing the right hand eastward to south of the abdomen
while closing it into a fist
and turning its heart downward and toward the north
while arcing the left hand eastward and upward
while closing it into a fist with its heart toward the south.
Then, stepping the right foot a half step eastward,
continue the arc of the right fist eastward and upward
to cross the hands east of the clavicle
with the right fist on the outside
with its heart downward and toward the north
and the heart of the left fist southwestward.
The gaze is forward and includes the fists warding off.

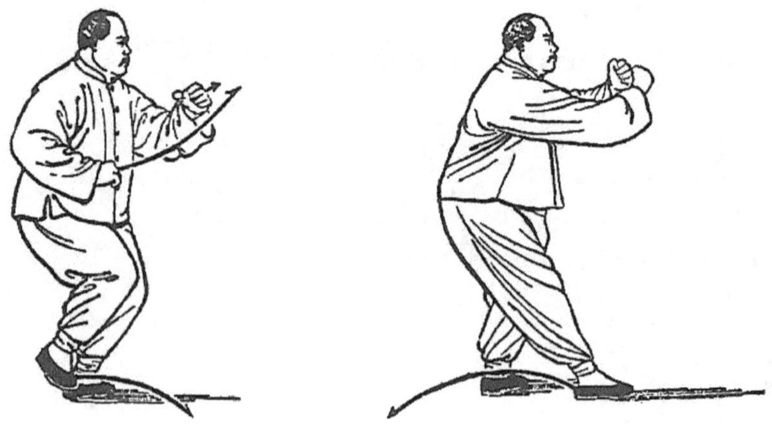

The seven stars are the constellation *Ursa Major*.

89.

退步跨虎式

Tuì bù kuà hǔ shì

Retreat Stepping Across Tiger Form.

Opening both hands and settling lower onto the left leg,
retreat the right foot southwestward past the left ankle
to touch it to the ground with its heel northwestward.
Then, straightening the left leg
while turning its foot on its heel eastward,
shift the weight to the right leg
while sweeping the right hand downward and southwestward
and then upward and northeastward
to above and to the east of the forehead
while turning its palm eastward
for its fingers to point upward and toward the north
and arcing the left hand downward and toward the north
for its palm to face downward
from above and to the north of the left knee.
The gaze is toward the right palm's
beginning to arc southwestward
and then shifts forward to include both palms
as the right palm moves upward before leveling forward.

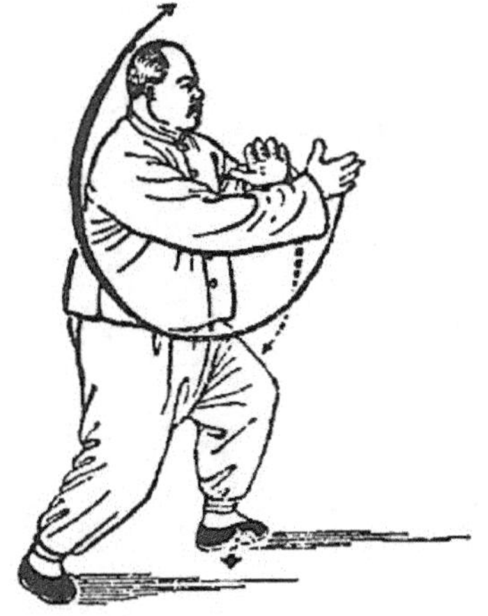 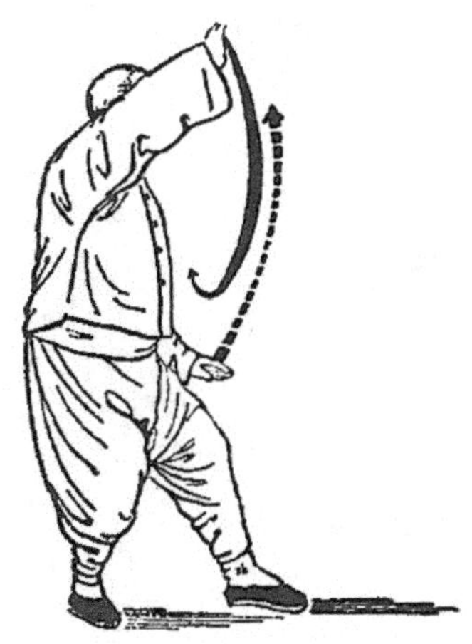

90.

轉身雙擺蓮

Zhuǎn shēn shuāng bǎi lián
Turning Body Doubly to swing Lotus.

Arcing the left hand upward to east of the forehead
while turning its palm southeastward
to point its fingers upward and southwestward,
arc the right hand downward
and then to the north to east of the abdomen
while turning its palm downward
and beginning to lift the left knee.
Then, promptly pivoting the right foot on its ball northeastward,
turn the torso southwestward
while swinging the arms with the turn
and beginning to swing the left leg toward the south
while arcing the left hand downward
to southwest of the sternum
while turning its palm downward and southwestward
and shifting the right hand upward to southwest of the clavicle
for its palm to face downward with its fingers southeastward.
The gaze levelly follows the turn.

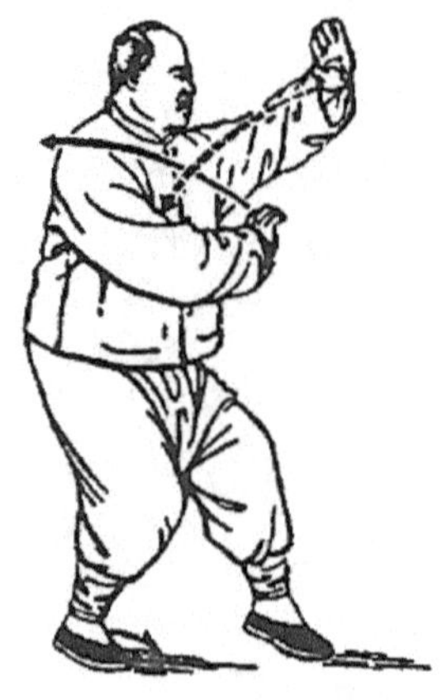
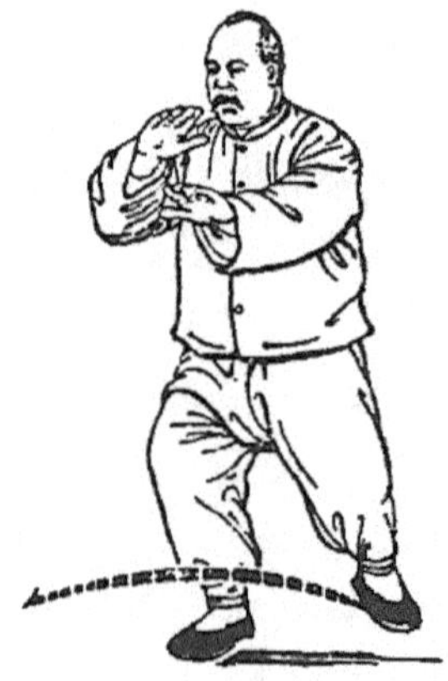

Then, continuing the pivot
to swing the left leg southwestward and then westward,
continue the turn of the torso westward and then northwestward
while swinging the arms with the turn.
And then, continuing the pivot to swing the left leg
northeastward to turn the torso eastward,
swing the right hand with the turn to extend it eastward
while turning its palm downward and eastward
and swinging the left hand with the eastward turn of the abdomen
while turning its palm downward and southeastward
and setting the left foot on the ground *shí*
pointing northeastward a half step northwest of the right foot
to bend the left knee
to settle the right foot flat but *xū* pointing eastward.
The gaze follows the hands swinging with the turn.

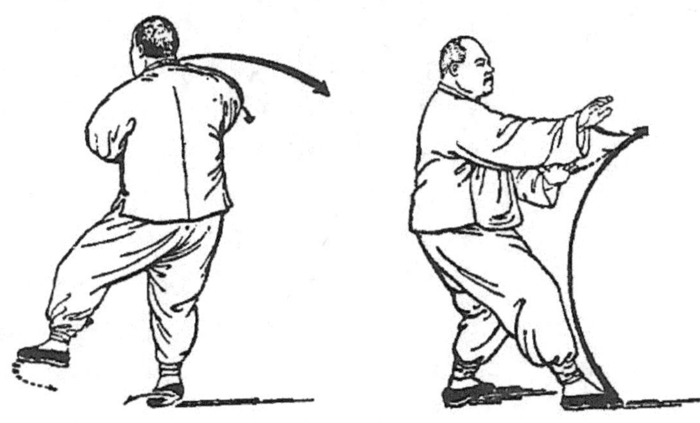

And then straighten the left leg to lift the right knee
to sweep its foot swiftly to the north and upward
and then toward the south to east of sternum
while shifting the left hand northeastward and upward
while shifting the right hand down to the level of the sternum
to turn its palm toward the north.
And then slap the left side of the right foot with the left hand
before slapping its right side with the right hand, and then,
settling the wrists while turning the palms downward and eastward,
begin to lower the right foot southeastward and downward.
The gaze is over the palms slapping the foot.

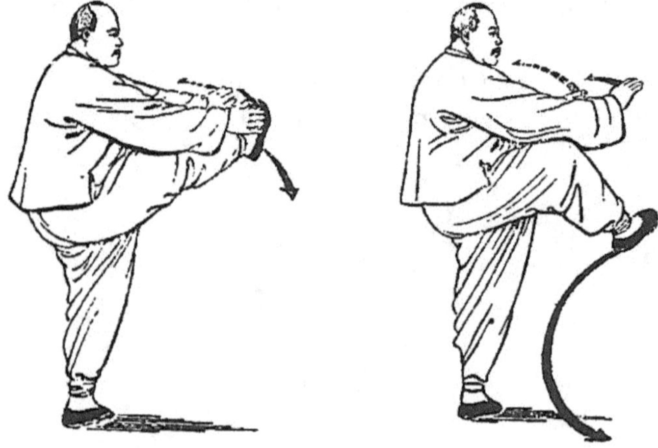

For none of the kicks in the sequence does Yang Chengfu direct
swiftness as he does for this sweep.

91.

彎弓射虎

Wān gōng shè hǔ
Bend Bow to Shoot Tiger.

Settling again onto the left leg, *sōng* the right knee
to swing the right foot westward and downward
before stepping it southeastward
while promptly shifting the right hand northwestward
to turn its palm toward the sternum
while arcing the left hand upward and northwestward
to turn its palm northeastward and downward.
The gaze follows the northwestward motion of the hands.
Then, shifting the right foot on its heel southeastward
to turn the torso southeastward,
arc the right hand downward and southwestward
to south of the right side of the *yāo*
while turning its palm northeastward
and arcing the left hand toward the south and downward
to southeast of the abdomen,
while turning its palm downward.

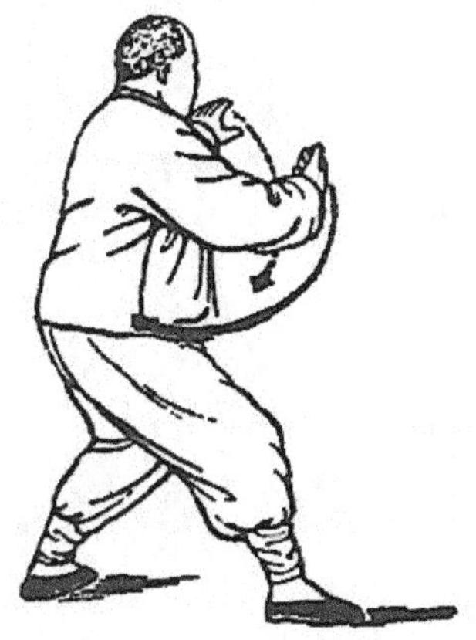
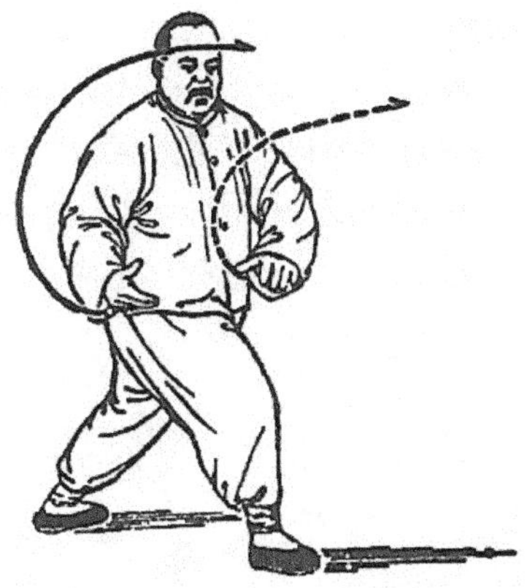

And then, turning the torso again eastward
while shifting the right foot on its heel again eastward,
shift the weight eastward into a right bow stance
while sweeping the right hand westward and upward
and then eastward past the right ear to southeast of the face
while closing it into a fist and turning its heart southeastward
and arcing the left hand southwestward and upward
and then northeastward to east of the left shoulder
while closing it into a fist and turning its heart toward the south.
The gaze follows the hands coiling upward and eastward.

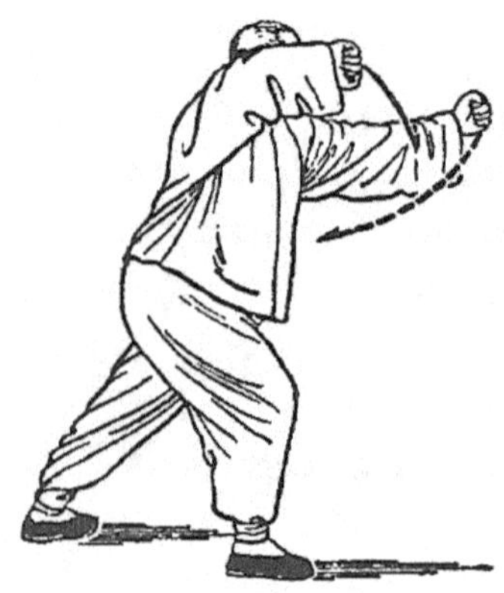

92.

進步搬攔捶

Jìn bù bān lán chuí
Advance Step Shift Block Cudgel.

Bending the left knee and straightening the right leg
to shift the weight northwestward onto the left leg,
turn the torso northeastward
while rolling the left fist downward and westward
and sinking the right elbow to shift its fist
eastward and downward to shoulder-level
while turning its heart downward and toward the north.
And then, continuing to sink the right elbow,
shift its fist downward and westward toward the sternum
while turning its heart westward and downward
and continuing the westward roll of the left fist.

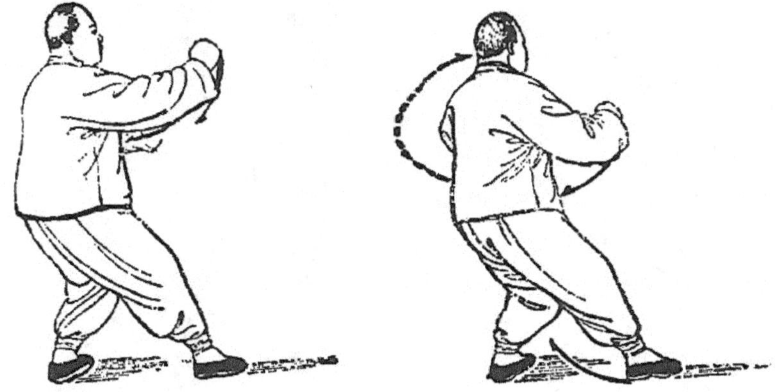

And then, straightening the left leg somewhat
to lift the right knee eastward,
coil the right fist downward and westward to northeast of the *yāo*
while arcing the left hand westward and upward and eastward
to northwest of the left ear
while opening it and turning its palm eastward.
The gaze shifts with the motion of the hands
before returning levelly southwestward.
Then, turning the torso eastward
and stepping the right foot southeastward
to set its heel on the ground *xū* to turn its toes southeastward,
arc the right fist upward and eastward,
and shift the left hand southeastward and downward
to cross the hands with the left palm facing south
and the heart of the right fist facing northwestward.

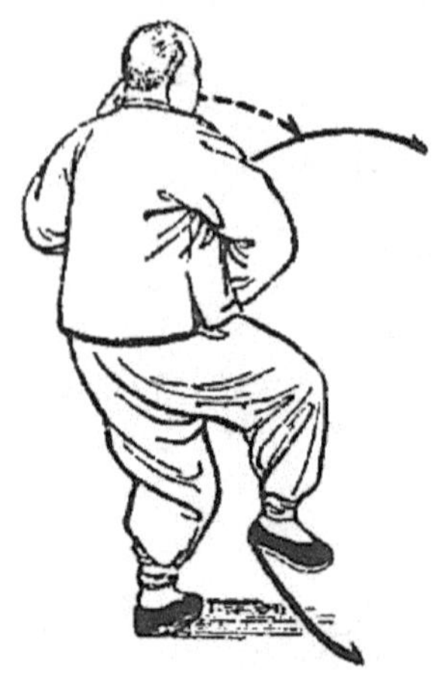 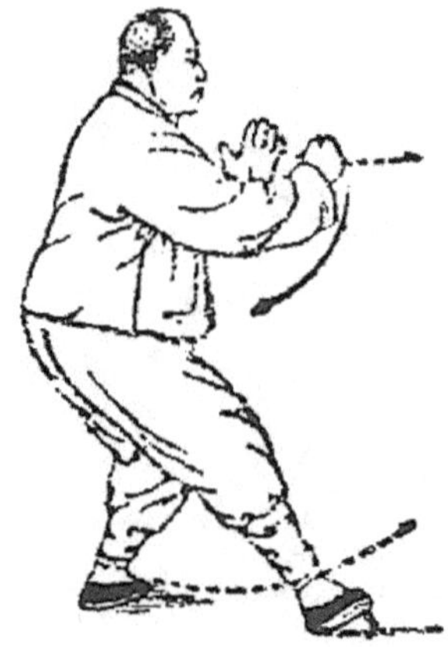

Then, settling the right foot flat and *shí*,
bend the right knee to shift the weight to the right leg
to lift the left knee eastward
while arcing the right fist downward and southwestward
to east of the right side of the abdomen
and beginning to extend the left hand eastward.
The gaze is toward the tips of the left fingers.
Then step the left foot eastward
to touch its heel to the ground *xū*
while continuing to extend the left hand eastward
and continuing the arc of the right fist westward.

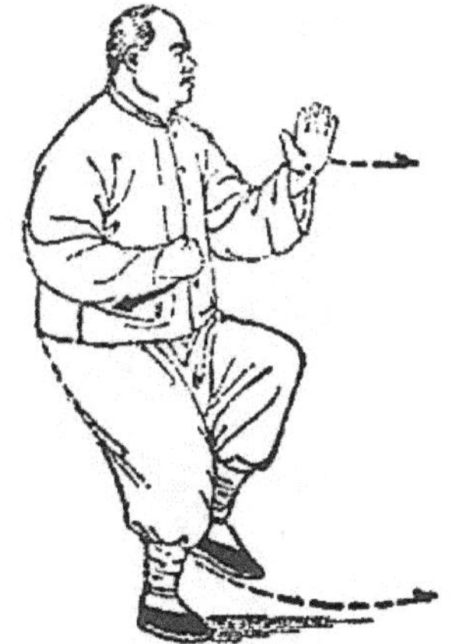
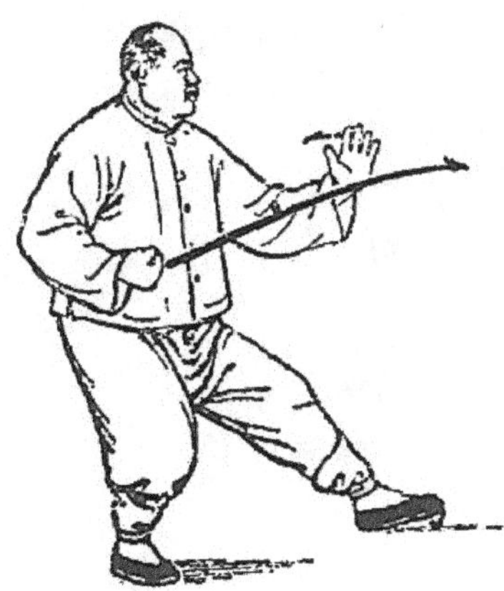

And then, turning the torso eastward
and shifting the weight eastward into a left bow stance,
cudgel the right fist upward and eastward
while drawing the left hand southwestward
toward the right shoulder
as the right forearm glides eastward past it
until the right arm is nearly straight
with the left palm facing the right forearm
with its thumb nearly touching the right elbow.
The gaze follows the left palm before shifting to the right fist.

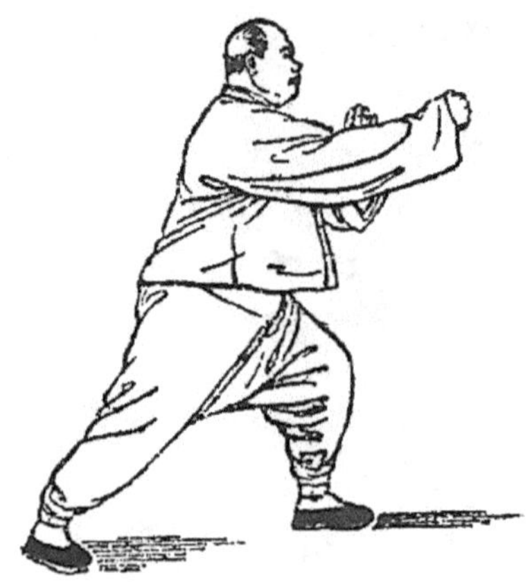

93.

如封似閉

Rú fēng shì bì
As Sealing Like Closing.

Thread the left hand beneath the right elbow
and to the southeast of it to turn the left palm southwestward
while opening the right hand
and turning its palm upward and northwestward.
Then, bending the right knee to shift the weight westward onto it,
sink the right elbow to draw its hand westward toward the clavicle
while shifting the left hand upward to cross the hands
for both palms to face the clavicle with the left hand on the outside
with its fingers pointing upward and toward the south
while the right fingers point upward and toward the north.
The gaze includes the palms.

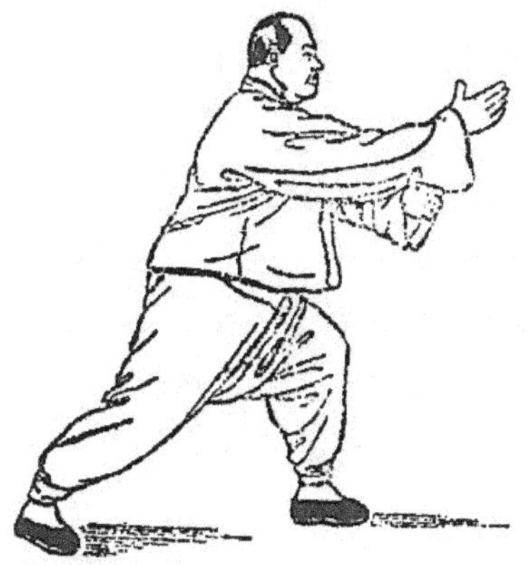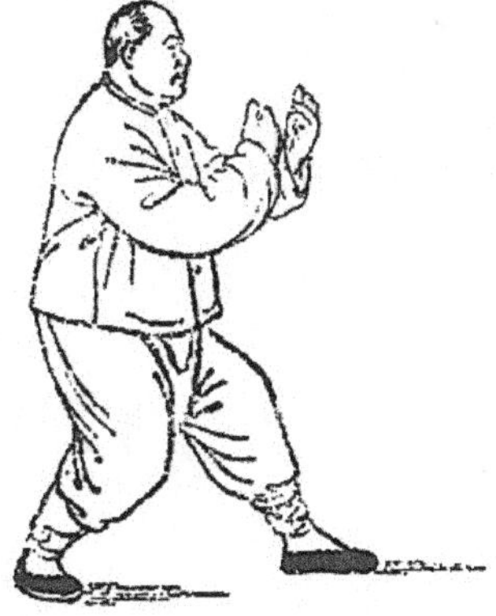

Then, shifting the left hand downward and northwestward
while shifting the right hand downward and southeastward,
turn the palms to face one another at the level of the sternum.
And then, shifting the weight eastward into a left bow stance,
push both hands upward and eastward to east of the clavicle
while settling their wrists and turning their palms eastward.
The gaze is levelly eastward.

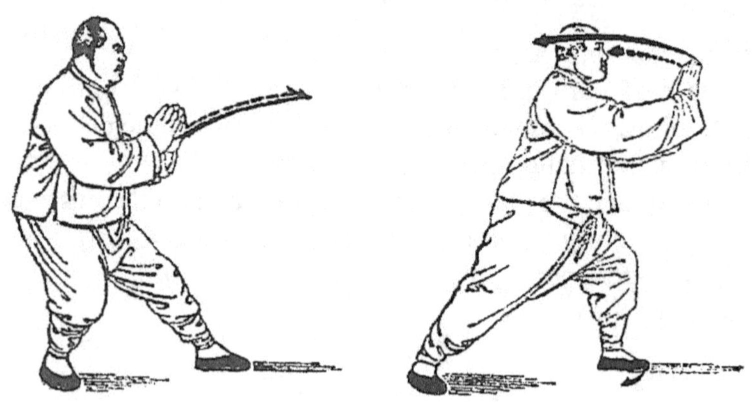

94.

十字手式變為合太極

Shí zì shǒu shì biàn wèi hé tài jí

Ten *Zì* Hands Form Changing to Actuating Closing *Tàijí*.

Keeping the weight on the left leg
while turning its foot on its heel to the south,
quickly turn the torso to the south
while swinging the hands with the turn
and turning the right foot on its heel southwestward
while spreading the elbows apart
for the right fingers to point upward and eastward
from southeast of the face
while the left fingers point upward and westward
from southwest of the face.
Then arc the hands upward and away from one another
and then downward to shoulder-level
for the right fingers to point upward and westward
while the left fingers point upward and eastward.

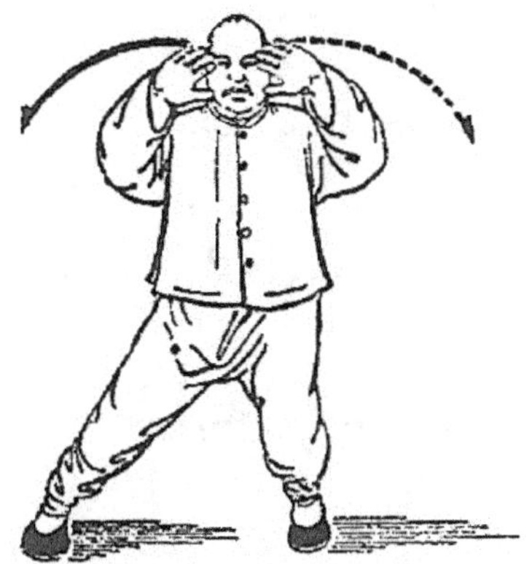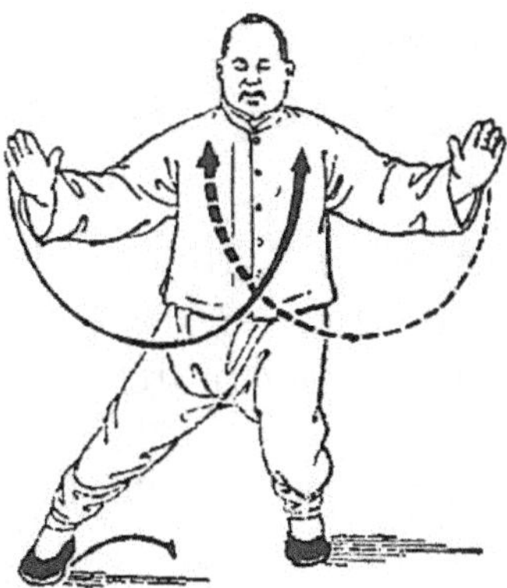

And then, stepping the right foot toward the left foot
into the horse stance,
arc the hands downward and toward one another and then upward
to cross them in front of the clavicle
with the palms facing inward with the right hand on the outside.
The gaze is over the intersection of the wrists.
And then, turning the palms toward the south
while beginning to spread them eastward and westward,
begin to extend them toward the south
while straightening the legs.

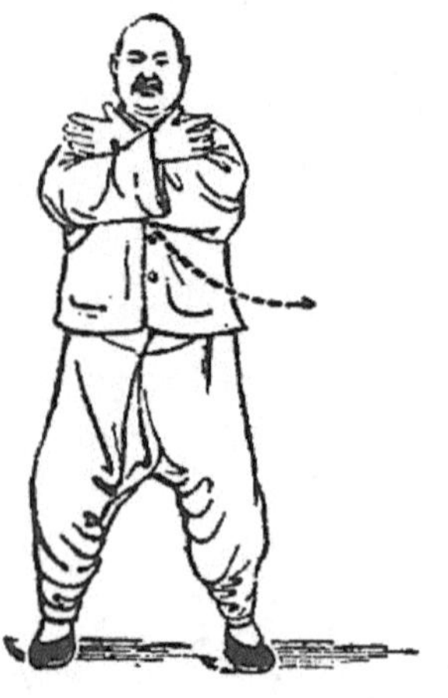 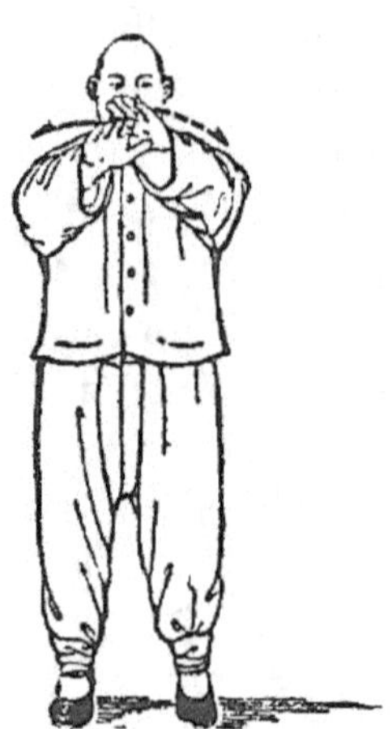

The reason the arrows and the positions of the feet in the first of
these two drawings would put the left hand and both feet in
positions different from their positions in the second of these two
drawings is that these drawings of the cross hands form are copies
of those illustrating the 16th and 53rd segments.

Then, turning the palms downward and toward the south,
continue the spread of the hands to the width of the shoulders
while extending the hands to the south
until the arms are approximately horizontal
with the fingers pointing upward and toward the south.
And then, sinking the elbows while settling the wrists
to keep the fingers pointing toward the south
lower the hands until they're below
and to the southwest and southeast of the *yāo*.

.

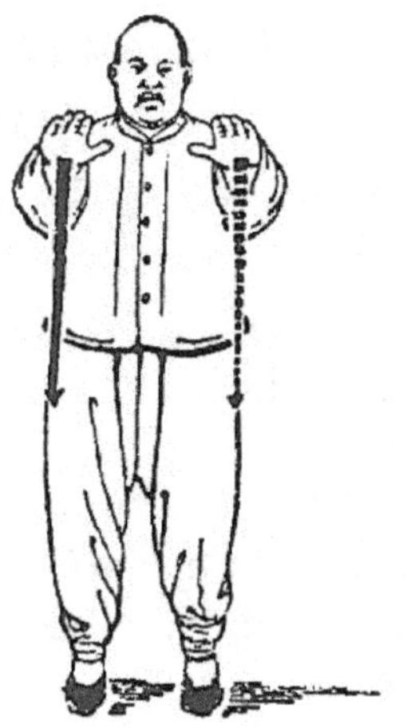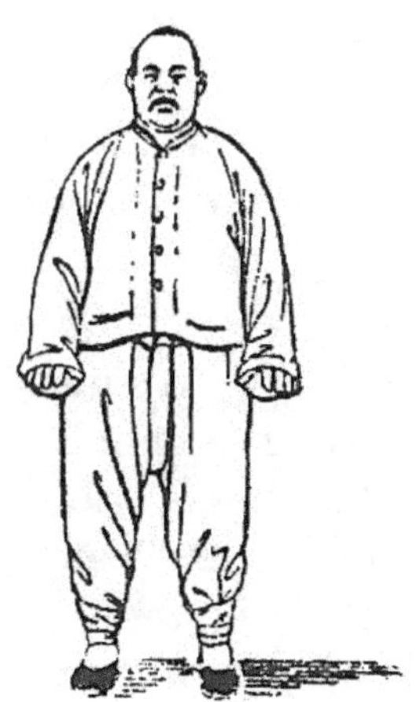

And then *sōng* the arms and wrists to return to the *wújí* stance. The gaze is levelly toward the south.

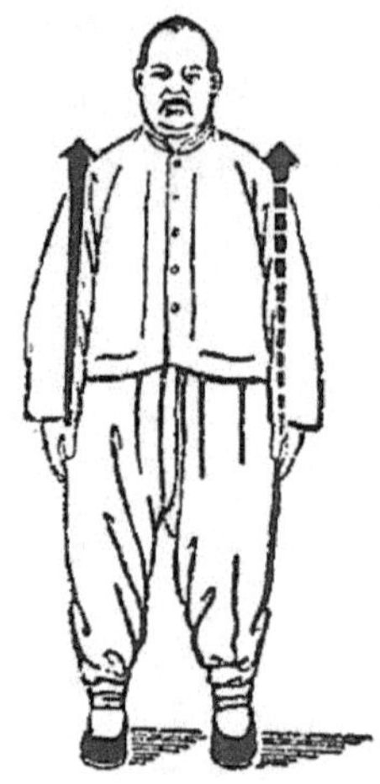

  This is Louis Swaim's translation of Yang Chengfu's comment on the closing form in his 1934 book:

  "Students must not overlook the fact that Closing Taiji means the uniting of Yin and Yang (*liang yi*), the four images (*si xiang*), the eight trigrams (*ba gua*), and the sixty-four hexigrams (*liu shi si gua*), then again returning to Taiji. Also, it means collecting the mind and consciousness, the *qi* and the breath, to become whole and return to the *dantian*. Concentrate the spirit and still anxieties (*ning shen jing*). Knowing when to stop with certainty (*zhi shi you ding*), you must not become scattered and lost, thus you will avoid making a fool of yourself before adepts."

  Note that, while describing the return to the *wújí* state, these injunctions close with an injunction assigning primacy to ego disparity and that the second use of the term "Taiji" here is as though it means "*wújí*". And also pertinent is that neither Yang Chengfu nor Fu Zhongwen repeats for this closing segment the illustration of the *wújí* stance with which they illustrate the opening of the sequence. But you, the reader, may estimate the significance of all that for yourself.

Principal Abiding Writings

The translations in this section are of Yang Chengfu's presentations in his 1931 book.

My presentation of each of the five begins with what Benjamin Pang Jeng Lo and his collaborators call each in their book *The Essence of T'ai Chi Ch'uan: the Literary Tradition*, and their Wade-Giles spelling of the name of the author to whom they attribute it, if they attribute it to anyone. But next, in *zì* and *pīnyīn* and English, is what Yang Chengfu calls each in his 1931 book. And next, also in *zì* and *pīnyīn* and English, is the abiding text.

The original texts are columns of *zì* with no punctuation, no grammatical inflection or equivalent of the English verb "to be", no articles and few conjunctions, and no line breaks. But in my translations, to facilitate both comprehensibility in English and verifiability, I've divided the texts into line segments and added punctuation and, for grammatical purposes, some words. And, also to accord with English grammar, I've somewhat changed the syntax.

But you easily can ignore the punctuation. And I've neither omitted words nor placed the translation of any word in a line segment other than that of its *zì*. So you can use any Chinese-English dictionary or electronic translation application including Chinese and English to verify how literal the translation is.

My motive, both for presenting my translations and not others' here and for making mine easy to verify, is that I found in others' translations much interpretation and extrapolation for martial arts purposes. So I've tried to avoid any bias either for or against martial arts or any epistemology or religion. But some bias is inherent in the writings.

Many passages in them are plainly paraphrases of the *Dào Dé Jīng*. And, because "zen" is a Japanese pronunciation of "*chán*", pertinent to the questions of whether Bodhidharma originated *Tàijíquán* and whether Zhang Sanfeng was a Buddhist monk or a Daoist monk is that Yang Chengfu calls the *Tàijíquán Jīng* Lu Chan Master's Original Text. And relevance of that is in that *Lù Chán* isn't Yang Luchan's name but a title he earned that literally means "Zen revealer".

So, if any of this translation is misrepresentation, it isn't by any intentional means of mine. And, also for literal accordance with Yang Chengfu's presentations, any ambiguity in these translations is also in the original. And I've presented the five writings in the order of their dispersal in Yang Chengfu's 1931 book:

T'ai Chi Ch'uan Ching, beginning on the next page;

Song of the Thirteen Postures, beginning on page 320;

Song of Hand-Pushing, page 323;

Expositions of Insights into the Practice of the Thirteen Postures, beginning on page 324;

and *T'ai Chi Ch'uan Lun*, beginning on page 332.

[And, rather than departing from the literal to clarify relationships the context doesn't make clear, I placed any clarification I thought necessary in brackets after the translation of the line segment to which it refers.]

T'ai Chi Ch'uan Ching
Chang San-feng

露禪師原文

Lù chán shī yuán wén
Revealing Zen Master's Original Text

一舉動周
Yī jǔ dòng zhōu
One motion moves all.

身俱要輕靈
Shēn jù yào qīng líng
The entire body desires lightness and alertness

尤須貫串
Yóu xū guàn chuàn
and especially must string together.

氣宜皷盪
Qì yí gǔ dàng
Qì should drum vibrantly.

.

神宜內歛
Shén yí nèi hān
Spirit should converge within.

毋使有缺陷處

Wú shǐ yǒu quē xiàn chù

Have no making having lacking or trapping places.

毋使有凸凹處

Wú shǐ yǒu tū āo chù

Have no making having protruding or receding places.

毋使有斷續處

Wú shǐ yǒu duàn xù chù

Have no making having severing or unremitting places.

.

練拳宜求圓滿

Liàn quán yí qiú yuan mǎn

Practicing the *quán* should seek circularity fully.

不可參差不齊

Bù kě cēn cī bù qí

Not being able to join differences isn't similar to [it].

[Chinese usage implies "it" at the end of this sentence.]

宜緩慢而不使間斷

Yí huǎn màn ér bù shǐ jiàn duàn

[It] should be gradual and slow while not making parts sever.

[Chinese usage often omits pronouns when they're inferable.]

其根在脚發於腿

Qí gēn zài jiǎo fā yú tuǐ

It roots in the feet and issues from the legs.

[The only reasonable antecedent of "*qi*" here and of the pronoun
the previous two lines imply is the practicing the *quán* of *Tàijíquán*
to which the line segment preceding these three segments refers.]

主宰于腰

Zhǔ zǎi yú yāo

Main control is from the *yāo*.

形于手指

Xíng yú shǒu zhǐ

Shaping is from the hands and fingers.

由脚而腿而腰

Yóu jiǎo ér tuǐ ér yāo

Leaving the feet, while in the legs and while in the *yāo*,

總須完整一氣

Zǒng xū wán zhěng yī qì

all must be completely and wholly one *qì*.

向前退後

Xiàng qián tuì hòu

Advancing forward and retreating rearward

乃能得機得勢

Nǎi néng dé jī dé shì

is then ability to attain the opportunity to attain potential.

有不得機

Yǒu bù dé jī

Having not attained opportunity,

得勢處身

Dé shì chǔ shēn

attaining potential places the body

便散亂
biàn sàn luàn
in easily scattered disorder.

其病必於腰腿求之
Qí bìng bì yú yāo tuǐ qiú zhī
Its disfunction must be sought in the *yāo* and its legs.

上下前後左右
Shàng xià qián hòu zuǒ yòu
Upward and downward, forward and backward, left and right,

皆然
jiē rán
all are so.
.
凡此皆是意不在外面
Fán cǐ jiē shì yì bù zài wài miàn
Where this is all, that's *yì* and isn't on the outer side.

有上即有下
Yǒu shàng jí yǒu xià
Having upward reaches having downward.

有前則有後
Yǒu qián zé yǒu hòu
Having forward then has backward,

有左則有右
Yǒu zuǒ zé yǒu yòu
Having left then has right.

如意要向上
Rú yì yào xiàng shàng
Yì demanding desiring upward

即寓下意
Jí yù xià yì
reaches implying downward *yì*,

若將物掀起
Ruò jiāng wù xiān qǐ
like initiating lifting immobile things

而加以挫之力
Ér jiā yǐ cuò zhī lì
while adding by oppressing their *lì*.

斯其根自斷
Sī qí gēn zì duàn
So their root severs itself.
[The antecedent of "their" here is immobile things or opponents.]

乃攘之速而無疑
Nǎi rǎng zhī sù ér wú yí
Then is resisting their quickness while having no doubt.

虛實宜分清楚
Xū shí yí fēn qīng chǔ
Xū and *shí* should be distributed clearly and distinctly.

一處有一處虛實處
Yī chù yǒu yī chù xū shí chù
One place having one place, a *xū* and *shí* place,

處總此一虛實
Chù zǒng cǐ yī xū shí
the place gathers this one *xū* and *shí*.

周身節節貫
Zhōu shēn jié jié guàn
External body parts and parts internal

串毋令絲毫間斷耳
Chuàn wú lìng sī háo jiàn duàn ěr
string to have no letting a thread or hair sever between sides.
[A hair is a Chinese unit of measurement equal to about a
hundredth of an inch.]

長拳者如長江大海
Chǎng quán zhě rú cháng jiāng dà hǎi
Long *quán* is one's being like a long river and a great sea
[*Tàijíquán* practitioners have called *Tàijíquán* long *quán*.]

滔滔不絕也
Tāo tāo bù jué yě
flowing and flowing and not exhausting also.

十三勢者
Shí sān shì zhě
The thirteen potentialities are one's
[*Tàijíquán* practitioners also have called *Tàijíquán* the thirteen
potentialities as in the Thirteen Potentialities Song.]

掤捋擠按採挒肘靠北
Bīng lǚ jǐ àn cǎi liè zhǒu kào běi
bīng, *lǚ*, *jǐ*, *àn*, plucking, splitting, elbowing, and leaning north

八卦也
Bā guà yě
and are the *bāguà* also.

進步退步
Jìn bù tuì bù
Advancing steps, retreating steps,

左顧右盼
Zuǒ gù yòu pàn
considering the left, anticipating the right,

中定
Zhōng dìng
and fixing the center:

此五行也
Cǐ wǔ háng yě
These are the five conducts also.
[The five conducts are traditional categories of Chinese occupations.]

掤捋擠按即乾坤坎離
Bīng lǚ jǐ àn jí qián kūn kǎn lí
Bīng, lǚ, jǐ, and *àn,* reaching *qián, kūn , kǎn,* and *lí,*
[*Qián, kūn , kǎn,* and *lí* are four of the *bāguà*.]

四正方也
Sì zhèng fāng yě
are the four main directions also.
[The four main directions are north, south, east, and west.]

採挒肘靠
Căi liè zhǒu kào
Plucking, splitting, elbowing, and leaning,

即巽震兌艮
Jí xùn zhèn duì gěn
reaching *xùn, zhèn, duì,* and *gěn,*
[*Xùn, zhèn, duì,* and *gěn* are the other four of the *bāguà.*]

四斜角也
Sì xié jiǎo yě
are the four oblique corners also.
[The four oblique corners are northeast, etc.]

進退顧盼定
Jìn tuì gù pàn dìng
Avancing, retreating, considering, expecting, and firming

即金木水火土也
Jí jīn mù shuǐ huǒ tǔ yě
reach metal, wood, water, fire, and earth also.
[These, traditionally, are the five elements and are basic *Yì Jīng* interpretations of five of the *bāguà.* So that, in the context of the other references to the *bāguà* above, suggests that the assertion above that leaning north is also one of the *bāguà* may be a reference to the traditional orientation from the north of the method of augury the Zhōu Dynasty used to extrapolate from *bāguà* into the *Yì Jīng.* And many presentations of the *Tàijíquán Jīng* omit all of this presentation of it beginning with the reference to long *quán.* And Yang Chengfu doesn't comment on this portion of it. So it may be an addendum by him or another contributor.]

原注云此係
Yuán zhù yún cǐ xì
An original note says this connects to

武當山張三峯老師
Wǔ dāng shān zhāng sān fēng lǎo shī
Wudang Mountain old teacher Zhang Sanfeng's

遺論欲天下豪傑
Yí lùn yù tiān xià háo jié
leaving a treatise desiring sky's below's outstanding heroes'

延年益壽
Yán nián yì shòu
extensive years of beneficially living,

不徒作技藝之末也
Bù tú zuò jì yì zhī mò yě
not merely making skill, but art in the end also.

[This closing, referring to Zhang Sanfeng from the third person point of view, may be a kind of signature by Zhang Sanfeng or a note by Wang Zongyue or Yang Luchan or another person passing this *jīng* on.]

Song of the Thirteen Postures

十三勢歌

Shí sān shì gē
Thirteen Potentialities Song

十三勢來莫輕視
Shí sān shì lái mò qīng shì
The thirteen potentialities come to no one's light regard.

命意源頭在腰際
Mìng yì yuan tóu zài yāo jì
Yì commanding, root and head meet in the *yāo*.

變轉虛實須留意
Biàn zhuǎn xū shí xū liú yì
Shifting and turning, *xū* and *shí* must remain in *yì*.

氣遍身軀不少滯
Qì biàn shēn qū bù shǎo zhì
Qì, throughout the person's body, isn't small or stagnant.

靜中觸動動猶靜
Jìng zhōng chù dòng dòng yóu jìng
Still, the center touches the movement, and the movement, yet still,

因敵變化示神奇
Yīn dí biàn huà shì shén qí
causes opponents to shift and change, revealing spirit and wonder.

勢勢存心揆用意
Shì shì cún xīn kuí yòng yì
Potential potentially retains considering the mind using *yì*

得來不覺費功夫
Dé lái bu jué fèi gōng fū
to attain coming not to sense cost of men's achievement.
["Men's achievement" is a literal translation of "*gōng fū*" or what
English-speaking people often transliterate "kung fu".]

刻刻留心在腰間
Kè kè liú xīn zài yāo jiān
Moment to moment remaining in the mind and the *yāo*,

腹內鬆淨氣騰然
Fù nèi sōng jìng qì téng rán
the abdomen *sōng* within, the *qì* soars purely so.

尾閭中正神貫頂
Wěi lǘ zhōng zhèng shén guàn dǐng
The *wěilǘ* central and straight, the spirit penetrating the head-top,

滿身輕利頂頭懸
Mǎn shēn qīng lì ding tóu xuán
the body completes lightly beneficial head-top head suspension.

仔細留心向推求
Zǐ xì liú xīn xiàng tuī qiú
Minutely and finely keeping the mind toward advancing, seeking,

屈伸開合聽自由
Qū shēn kāi hé tīng zì yóu
bending, extending, opening, and closing, listen by the self.

入門引路須口授
Rù mén yǐn lù xū kǒu shòu
Entering the gate and guiding the path must be oral teaching.

321

功夫無息法自休
Gōng fū wú xī fǎ zì xiū
Men's achievement having no ceasing, the method rests in the self.

若言體用何為準
Ruò yán tǐ yòng hé wèi zhǔn
As words, bodies use what actuating standard?

意氣君來骨肉臣
Yì qì jūn lái gǔ ròu chén
Yì and *qì* come to rule bones and administer flesh.

想推用意終何在
Xiǎng tuī yòng yì zhōng hé zài
The desire is to push how to use *yì* to end in

益壽延年不老春
Yì shòu yán nián bù lǎo chūn
beneficially living and prolonging years, a spring not aging.

歌兮歌兮百四十
Gē xī gē xī bǎi sì shí
Sing, oh sing, oh hundred forty

字字眞切義無遺
Zì zì zhēn qiè yì wú yí
zì, *zì* genuine, corresponding rightly, and having no omission,

若不向此推求去
Ruò bù xiàng cǐ tuī qiú qù
as not guiding this advancing seeks leaving

枉費工夫貽嘆息
Wǎng fèi gōng fū yí tàn xí
vainly expending men's work, bequeathing breathing sighs.

Song of Hand-Pushing

[Yang Chengfu ascribes to this short poem no title or author.]

掤捋擠按須認眞
Bīng lǔ jǐ àn xū rèn zhēn
Bīng, *lǔ*, *jǐ*, and *àn* must be accurately recognized.

上下相隨人難進
Shàng xià xiāng suí rén nán jìn
Above and below mutually following, humans' entry is difficult,

任他巨力來打我
Rèn tā jù lì lái dǎ wǒ
letting their huge *lì* coming to hit me

牽動四両撥千斤
Qiān dòng sì liǎng bō qiān jīn
lead to moving four *liǎng* to deflect a thousand *jīn*.
[A *liǎng* is about an ounce. A *jīn* is about a pound.]

引進落空合即出
Yǐn jìn luò kōng hé jí chū
To guide entering falling into air, approach closely, and issue,

粘連黏隨不丟頂
Zhān lián nián suí bù diū dǐng
adhere, connect, stick, and follow, not deflecting the head-top.

Expositions of Insights
into the
Practice of the Thirteen Postures
Wu Yu-hsiang

王宗岳原序

Wáng zōng yuè yuán xù
Wang Zongyue's Original Order

以心行氣務令沈着
Yǐ xīn xíng qì wù lìng chén zhuó
By mind conduct *qì* to engage commanding sinking and touching.

乃能收歛入骨
Nǎi néng shōu hān rù gǔ
Then can be receiving and gathering into the bones.

以氣運身務令順遂
Yǐ qì yùn shēn wù lìng shun suì
By *qì* conduct the body's affairs to make smooth fulfilment.

乃能便利從心
Nǎi néng biàn lì cóng xīn
Then can pass beneficially following the mind.

精神能提得起
Jīng shén néng tí dé qǐ
Fine spirit can lift to attain rising.

則無遲重之虞
Zé wú chí zhòng zhī yú
Then is having no slow heavy apprehension.

所謂頂頭懸也
Suǒ wèi ding tóu xuán yě
Wherein is called head-top head suspension also,

意氣須換得靈
Yì qì xū huàn dé líng
yì and *qì* must exchange to attain alertness.

乃有圓活之趣
Nǎi yǒu yuán huó zhī qù
Then is having lively interest and circularity.

所謂變動虛實也
Suǒ wèi biàn dòng xū shí yě
Wherein is called moving and transforming *xū* and *shí* also,

發勁須沉着鬆靜
Fā jìn xū chén zhuó sōng jìng
issuing *jìn* must sink and touch completely *sōng*

須專主一方
Xū zhuān zhǔ yī fāng
and must concentrate mainly in one direction.

立身須中正安舒
Lì shēn xū zhōng zhèng ān shū
Standing, the body must be centered, straight, quiet, and placid

撐支八面
Chēng zhī bā miàn
to support bearing the eight sides.
[The eight sides are the main directions and the oblique corners.]

行氣如九曲珠
Xíng qì rú jiǔ qū zhū
Conduct *qì* like a nine bend bead,
[Nine-bend beads were for developing girls' stitching dexterity.]

無往不利
Wú wǎng bù lì
having no wending not beneficial.

氣遍身軀之謂運勁
Qì biàn shēn qū zhī wèi yùn jìn
Qì everywhere in a person's body is called transporting *jìn*.

運勁如百鍊鋼
Yùn jìn rú bǎi liàn gang
Transporting *jìn* as a hundred chains of steel,

何堅不摧
Wú jiān bù cuī
how is firmness not destroyed?

形如搏兔之鶻
Xíng rú bó tù zhī hú
The form is like a falcon seizing a rabbit,
[Yang Chengfu, in his commentary on this notion in his 1931
book, says the intention of this analogy isn't cruelty.]

神如捕鼠之貓
Shén rú bǔ shǔ zhī māo
The spirit is like a cat capturing a mouse.
[But he also says in that commentary on these similes that the cat
captures fiercely.]

靜如山岳動若江河
Jìng rú shān yuè dòng ruò jiāng hé
Stillness is like a mountain peak, movement like a flowing river.

蓄勁如張弓
Xù jìn rú kāi gōng
Storing *jìn* is like drawing a bow.

發勁如放箭
Fā jìn rú fàng jiàn
Issuing *jìn* is like releasing an arrow.

曲中求直
Qū zhōng qiú zhí
Bending, the center seeks the straight.

蓄而後發
Xù ér hòu fā
Store while afterward issuing.

力由脊發
Lì yóu jí fā
Force is by the spine issuing.

步隨身換
Bù suí shēn huàn
Stepping follows the body's changes.

放即是收
Shōu jí shì fàng
Discharging and reaching: That's receiving.

斷而復連
Duàn ér fù lián
Sever while again connecting.

往復須有摺疊
Wǎng fù xū yǒu zhé dié
Wending and repeating must have folding and piling.

進退須有轉換
Jìn tuì xū yǒu zhuǎn huàn
Advancing and retreating must have turning and changing.

極柔軟而後極堅剛
Jí róu ruǎn ér hòu jí jiān gāng
Soft pliant polarity, while afterward is firm hard polarity,

能呼吸然後
Néng hū xī rán hòu
enables exhaling and inhaling correctly

能靈活
Néng líng huó
and enables alertness afterward.

氣以直養而無害
Qì yǐ zhí yǎng ér wú hài
Qì, by directly rising, is while having no harm.

勁以曲蓄而有餘
Jìn yǐ qū xù ér yǒu yú
Jìn, by bending and storing, is while having surplus.

心為令氣為旗
Xīn wèi lìng qì wèi qí
Mind acts as the commander. *Qì* acts as the flag.

腰為纛
Yāo wèi dào
The *yāo* acts as the banner.

先求開展
Xiān qiú kāi zhǎn
First seek open expansion.

後求緊湊
Hòu qiú jǐn còu
Afterward seek compact gathering.

乃可臻於縝密也
Nǎi kě zhēn yú zhěn mì yě
Then can be reaching into comprehensive concentration also.

又曰
Yòu yuē
Also spoken:

先在心後在身
Xiān zài xīn hòu zài shēn
Initially in the mind, afterward in the body,

腹鬆靜氣斂入骨
Fù sōng jìng qì hān rù gǔ
the abdomen *sōng* and still, *qì* gathers and enters the bones.

刻刻在心切記
Kè kè zài xīn qiè jì
Engrave. Engrave in the mind, and cut the mark:

一動無有不動
Yī dòng wú yǒu bù dòng
Once moving, have no having not moving;

一靜無有不靜
Yī jìng wú yǒu bù jìng
once still, have no having not being still.

牽動往來氣貼背
Qiān dòng wǎng lái qì tiē bèi
Lead movement's wending to come to the *qì*'s adhering to the back

歛入脊骨
Hān rù jǐ gǔ
to gather to enter the spine and bones.

內固精神外示安逸
Nèi gù jīng shén wài shì ān yì
Inside, firmly refine the spirit. Outside, show quiet ease.

邁步如貓行
Mài bù rú māo xíng
Walking and stepping like cats' conduct

運勁如抽絲
Yùn jìn rú chōu sī
and transporting *jìn* like drawing silk,

全身意在精
Quán shēn yì zài jīng
the whole body and *yì* are in refinement.

神不在氣在氣則
Shén bù zài qì zài qì zé
Spirit not in the *qì*, the *qì* is then stagnant.

有氣者無力
Yǒu qì zhě wú lì
Having *qì*, one has no *lì*.

無氣者純剛
Wú qì zhě chún gāng
Having no *qì*, one is purely hard.

氣如車輪腰似車軸
Qì rú chē lún yāo shì chē zhóu
Qì is like a cart's wheels. The *yāo* is like a cart's axles.

又曰
Yòu yuē
Also spoken:

彼不動己不動
Bǐ bù dòng jǐ bù dòng
Others not moving already, don't move.

彼微動己先動
Bǐ wēi dòng jǐ xiān dòng
Others minimally moving already, move first.

勁似鬆非鬆
Jìn shì sōng fēi sōng
Jìn seeming *sōng* but contrary to *sōng*

將展未展
Jiāng zhǎn wèi zhǎn
will extend having no extension.

勁斷意不斷
Jìn duàn yì bù duàn
Severing *jìn* doesn't sever *yì*.

T'ai Chi Ch'uan Lun

Wang Tsung-yueh

王宗岳太極論

Wáng zōng yuè tài jí lùn

Wang Zongyue's *Tàijí Lùn*

太極者無極

Tài jí zhě wú jí

Tàijí and one's *wújí*,

而生陰陽之母也

Ér shēng yīn yáng zhī mǔ yě

while being life and *yīn* and *yáng*, are their mother also.

動之則分靜之則合

Dòng zhī zé fēn jìng zhī zé hé

Their movement then fragments. Their stillness then unites.

無過不及隨

Wú guò bu jí suí

Have no passing not reaching following.

曲就伸

Qū jiù shēn

Bend already extending.

人剛我柔為之走
Rén gāng wǒ róu wéi zhī zǒu
Humans being rigid, our pliancy actuates their yielding.

我順人背為之黏
Wǒ shùn rén bèi wéi zhī nián
We go along with humans and afterward actuate their cohesion.

動急則急應
Dòng jí zé jí yīng
Movement being urgent, then urgently follow.

.

動緩則緩隨
Dòng huǎn zé huǎn suí
Movement being gradual, then gradually follow.

雖變化萬端
Suī biàn huà wàn duān
Though changes transform ten thousand ends,

而理為一貫
Ér lǐ wéi yī guàn
while managing, actuate one throughout.

由着而漸悟懂勁
Yóu zhe ér jiàn wù dǒng jìn
By touching while gradually comprehending, understand *jìn*.

由懂勁而階及神明
Yóu dǒng jìn ér jiē jí shén míng
By understanding *jìn* while stepping, reach spiritual light.

然非用力之久不能豁
Rán fēi yòng lì zhī jiǔ bù néng huō
So, contrarily, using *lì* is its long not being able to open.
[The antecedent of this possessive pronoun is spiritual light.]

然貫通焉
Rán guàn tōng yān
So string and connect wherein is

虛靈頂勁氣沉丹田
Xū líng dǐng jìn qì chén dān tián
xū líng dǐng jìn and *qì* sinking to the *dāntián*.

不偏不倚
Bù piān bù yǐ
Don't lean. Don't incline.

忽隱忽現
Hū yǐn hū xiàn
Suddenly conceal. Suddenly reveal.

左重則左虛
Zuǒ zhòng zé zuǒ xū
The left is heavy. Then the left is *xū*.

右重則右杳
Yòu zhòng zé yòu yǎo
The right is heavy. Then the right disappears.

仰之則彌高
Yǎng zhī zé mí gāo
Its looking up is then fully high.

俯之則彌深
Fǔ zhī zé mí shēn
Its looking down is then fully deep.

進之則彌長
Jìn zhī zé mí zhǎng
Its advancing is then fully distant.
.

退之則愈促
Tuì zhī zé yù cù
Its retreating is then more urgent.
[The antecedent of the possessive pronoun in those four line
segments may be the entire *Tàijíquán* approach.]

一羽不能加蠅虫不能落
Yī yǔ bù néng jiā yíng chóng bù néng luò
One feather isn't able to be added. Insects aren't able to land.

人不知我我獨知人
Rén bù zhī wǒ wǒ dú zhī rén
Humans not knowing us, we alone know humans.

英雄所向無敵
Yīng xióng suǒ xiàng wú dí
Brave men's wherein is toward having no enmity.

蓋皆由此而及也
Gài jiē yóu cǐ ér jí yě
By covering all this while reaching also,

斯技旁門甚多
Sī jì pang mén shén duō
other gates to such skill are quite many.

雖勢有區
Suī shì yǒu qū
Though potentialities have divisions,

別概不外乎
Bié gài bù wài hū
the separateness generally isn't outside mostly

壯欺弱
Zhuàng qī ruò
the strong bullying the weak,

335

慢讓快耳
Ěr màn ràng kuài
the slow side yielding to the fast,

有力讓無力
Yǒu lì ràng wú lì
having *lì* yield having no *lì*,

手慢讓手快
Shǒu màn ràng shǒu kuài
and slow hands yield to fast hands.

此皆先天自
Cǐ jiē xiān tiān zì
This is all prior to the sky's self.
[*Tàijí* after *wújí* is prior to returning to *wújí*.]

然之能非關學力而有也
Rán zhī néng fēi guān xué lì ér yǒu yě
So its ability contrarily severs study while having *lì* also.

察四両能撥千斤
Chá sì liǎng néng bō qiān jīn
Observe four ounces able to deflect a thousand pounds,

之力顯非力盛
Zhī lì xiǎn fēi lì shèng
Its *lì* displays contrariety to abundant *lì*'.

觀耄耋能禦衆
Guān mào dié néng yù zhòng
Observe old age able to resist a throng,

之形快何能為
Zhī xíng kuài hé néng wéi
what its fast form can actuate.

立如平準活似車輪
Lì rú píng zhǔn huó shì chē lún
Stand like a balance level. Be lively like a cart's wheel.

偏沉則隨
Piān chén zé suí
Lean and sink, and then follow.

雙重則滯
Shuāng chóng zé zhì
Double weighting, then being sluggish,

每見數年純功
Měi jiàn shù nián chún gōng
each year sees repeating simple work

不能運化
bù néng yùn huà
not able to transport or transform

者率皆自為
Zhě lǜ jiē zì wéi
one's leading all self action.

人制雙重
rén Zhì shuāng chóng
Humans' making double weighting,

之病未悟耳
Zhī bìng wèi wù ěr
its disease is having no comprehending sides.

預避此病
Yù bì cǐ bìng
Preparing to avoid this disease

須知陰陽
Xū zhī yīn yáng
must be knowing *yīn* and *yáng*.

粘即是走
Zhān jí shì zǒu
Adhering's reaching: That's leaving.

走即是粘
Zǒu jí shì zhān
Leaving's reaching: That's adhering.

陰不離陽陽不離陰
Yīn bù lí yáng yáng bù lí yīn
Yīn doesn't depart from *yáng*. *Yáng* doesn't depart from *yīn*.

陰陽相濟
Yīn yáng xiāng jì
Yīn and *yáng* mutually aid.

方為懂勁
Fāng wéi dǒng jìn
Squarely actuate understanding *jìn*.

懂勁
Dǒng jìn
Understanding *jìn*

後愈練愈精
hòu yù liàn yù jīng
is after more progress and more refinement.

默識揣摩漸
Mò shí chuǎi mó jiàn
Silently estimating knowledge rubs gradually

至從心所欲
Zhì cóng xīn suǒ yù
engaging arriving wherein is the mind's desire.

本是捨己從人
Běn shì shě jǐ cóng rén
Rooting: That's abandoning the self to follow humans.

多誤捨近求遠
Duō wù shě jìn qiú yuǎn
Many erroneously abandon the near to seek the distant,

所謂差之釐毫
Suǒ wèi chà zhī lí háo
wherein is called a thousandth of a hair's discrepancy,

謬逾千里
Miù yú qiān lǐ
an error exceeding a thousand miles.

學者不可不詳辨
Xué zhě bù kě bù xiáng biàn
Learning one's not being able not to discern detail:

焉是為論
Yān shì wèi lùn
That's how to actuate the *lùn*.

Basic Chinese Terms

Àn - 按 ：Push.

Bāguà - 八卦 ：Eight augury trigrams of three *yīn*s or *yáng*s.

Bīng or peng - 掤 ：Arrow quiver cover or ward-off.

Dāntián - 丹田 ：Elixir field, the center of the *yāo*.

Jǐ - 擠 ：Press.

Jìn - 勁 ：Strength.

Jīng - 經 ：Literally abiding, idiomatically abiding writing.

Lì - 力 ：Force.

Lǚ - 捋 ：Rollback or stroke.

Lùn - 論 ：Treatise.

Qì - 氣 ：Breath.

Shēn - 身 ：Body.

Shén - 神 ：Spirit.

Shí - 實 : Full or solid.

Sōng - 鬆 : Loose or flowing, not tense.

Tàijíquán - 太極拳 : Extreme polarity fist.

Wěilú - 尾閭 : Literally a tail gate, idiomatically the coccyx.

Wújí - 無極 : Having no polarity.

Xīn - 心 : Mind.

Xū - 虛 : Empty or void.

Xū líng dǐng jìn - 虛靈頂勁 : Empty alert head-top strength.

Yáng - 陽 : Illumination, brightness before shade.

Yāo - 腰 : The pelvic region.

Yì - 意 : Intention.

Yīn - 陰 : Shade, darkness before illumination.

Zì - 字 : Pictographs the Chinese use for writing.

Pīnyīn
phonetics
(approximate English equivalents)

Pīnyīn	Equivalent	*Pīnyīn*	Equivalent	*Pīnyīn*	Equivalent
.. *a*	f**a**r	*iong*	*y* + *u* + *ng*	*uang*	*ua* + *ng*
ai	k**i**te	*iu*	**yo**ke	*üe*	*ü* + *e*
an	f**a**n	*j*	**g**enial	*ueng*	**wa**s + *ng*
ang	**o**n + *ng*	*k*	**k**ey	*ui*	**way**
ao	h**ow**	*l*	**l**aw	*un*	p**u**t + pu**n**
b	**b**ee	*m*	**m**ind	*ün*	*ü* + pu**n**
c	i**ts**	*n*	**n**ow	*uo*	**wa**ll
ch	**ch**oose	*ng*	si**ng**	*w*	**w**alk
d	**d**ay	.. *o*	**o**ff	*x*	**sh**eer
e	y**es**	*ong*	p**u**t + *ng*	*y*	**y**es
ei	w**ay**	*ou*	**ow**n	*z*	be**ds**
en	w**en**d	*p*	**p**ut	*zh*	**j**oy
eng	s**u**ng	*q*	**ch**eer	**Tone marks**	
f	**f**an	*r* ..	mira**ge**	(The diacritical	
g	**g**ive	.. *r*	fa**r**	marks over vowels,	
h	**h**ave	*s*	**s**ing	indicating pitch)	
.. *i*	s**ee**m or s**i**t	*sh*	**sh**ine	H**ī**gh	
ia	**ya**rd	*t*	**t**ime		
ian	**ya**n**k**	*u*	p**u**t	R**í**sing	
iang	**ya**rd + *ng*	*ü*	*u* + *i*		
iao	**y**on + b**ow**	*ua*	**wa**nd	Falling b**ě**fore rising	
ie	**ye**t	*uai*	**wi**se		
in	**in**	*uan*	**wan**gle	F**à**lling	
ing	s**ing**	*üan*	*ü* + *an*		

342

Books
by
Billy Lee Harman

Dust
a novel
2005

Ashes
some memories
2015

Angels
summaries of scripture
2020

Dao De Jing
a literal translation
2021

Tai Ji Quan
(fundamentally)
2021

Annie
(how children are)
2021

Space and Light
2023